John Strauss

(N) Vitals

RR    30-50 @birth
16-20 @6 yrs

HR    70-170 @birth
120-140 infant
80-140   1a
80-120   2a
70-115  >3a

# Handbook of
# Pediatric Emergencies

**Edited by**
**Gregory A. Baldwin, M.D., F.R.C.P. (C.)**
Clinical Research Fellow, Division of Emergency Medicine,
Department of Medicine, The Children's Hospital,
Harvard Medical School, Boston

Illustrations by **Jane Rowlands**
Charts and graphs by **Beth Crescent**

**Little, Brown and Company**
**Boston/Toronto/London**

Library of Congress Catalog Card No. 89-83471

ISBN 0-316-07919-7

Printed in the United States of America

FG

**To Karen**

# Contents

# Contributing Authors

**Gregory A. Baldwin, M.D., F.R.C.P. (C.)**
Clinical Research Fellow, Division of Emergency Medicine, Department of Medicine, The Children's Hospital, Harvard Medical School, Boston

**Richard D. Beauchamp, M.D., F.R.C.S. (C.)**
Clinical Associate Professor, Department of Orthopaedics, University of British Columbia Faculty of Medicine; Active Staff, Department of Orthopaedics, British Columbia's Children's Hospital, Vancouver

**Derek Blackstock, M.D., F.R.C.P. (C.)**
Clinical Assistant Professor, University of British Columbia Faculty of Medicine; Staff Anaesthetist, British Columbia's Children's Hospital, Vancouver

**Geoffrey K. Blair, M.D., F.R.C.S. (C.)**
Clinical Assistant Professor, Department of Surgery, University of British Columbia Faculty of Medicine; Attending Paediatric Surgeon, Department of Surgery, British Columbia's Children's Hospital, Vancouver

**James E. Carter, M.B., Ch.B., F.R.C.P. (C.)**
Associate Professor, Department of Paediatrics, University of British Columbia Faculty of Medicine; Consultant, Division of Paediatric Nephrology, British Columbia's Children's Hospital, Vancouver

**David D. Cochrane, M.D., F.R.C.S. (C.)**
Assistant Professor, Department of Surgery (Neurosurgery), University of British Columbia Faculty of Medicine; Attending Surgeon, British Columbia's Children's Hospital, Vancouver

**Gerald U. Coleman, M.D., F.R.C.S. (C.)**
Clinical Associate Professor, Division of Urology, Department of Surgery, University of British Columbia Faculty of Medicine; Head, Department of Urology, British Columbia's Children's Hospital, Vancouver

**Robert M. Couch, M.D., F.R.C.P. (C.)**
Assistant Professor, Department of Paediatrics, University of British Columbia Faculty of Medicine; Endocrinologist, Department of Paediatrics, British Columbia's Children's Hospital, Vancouver

**John M. Dean, M.B.B.S., F.R.C.P. (C.)**
Clinical Associate Professor, Department of Paediatrics, University of British Columbia Faculty of Medicine; Allergy Department, British Columbia's Children's Hospital, Vancouver

**Gary D. Derkson, D.M.D.**
Associate Professor of Paediatric Dentistry, University of British Columbia Faculty of Dentistry; Head, Department of Dentistry, British Columbia's Children's Hospital, Vancouver

**Kevin Farrell, M.B., F.R.C.P. (C.)**
Associate Professor, Department of Paediatrics, University of British Columbia Faculty of Medicine; Director, Seizure Clinic, British Columbia's Children's Hospital, Vancouver

**Loretta Fiorillo, M.D., F.R.C.P. (C.)**
Resident, Division of Dermatology, University of British Columbia Faculty of Medicine, Vancouver

**Graham C. Fraser, M.B., F.R.C.S. (Edin., Eng., C.), F.A.C.S.**
Clinical Associate Professor, Department of Surgery, University of British Columbia Faculty of Medicine; Head, General Paediatric Surgery, British Columbia's Children's Hospital, Vancouver

**Anne C. Halstead, M.D., F.R.C.P. (C.)**
Clinical Assistant Professor, Department of Pathology, University of British Columbia Faculty of Medicine; Medical Biochemist, Pathophysiology, Department of Pathology, British Columbia's Children's Hospital, Vancouver

**Eric Hassall, M.D., F.R.C.P. (C.)**
Associate Professor, Department of Paediatrics, University of British Columbia Faculty of Medicine; Head, Division of Gastroenterology, British Columbia's Children's Hospital, Vancouver

**Jean Hlady, M.D., F.R.C.P. (C.)**
Clinical Assistant Professor, University of British Columbia Faculty of Medicine; Department of Paediatrics, British Columbia's Children's Hospital, Vancouver

**David S. Lirenman, M.D., F.R.C.P. (C.)**
Professor, Department of Paediatrics, University of British Columbia Faculty of Medicine; Medical Director, Renal Unit, Head, Division of Paediatric Nephrology, British Columbia's Children's Hospital, Vancouver

**Gillian Lockitch, M.D., F.R.C.P. (C.)**
Assistant Professor, Department of Pathology, University of British Columbia Faculty of Medicine; Program Head, Pathophysiology, Department of Pathology, British Columbia's Children's Hospital, Vancouver

**Christine A. Loock, M.D., F.R.C.P. (C.)**
Clinical Assistant Professor, University of British Columbia Faculty of Medicine; Attending Paediatrician, Youth Clinic and Emergency Services, British Columbia's Children's Hospital, Vancouver

**Andrew J. Macnab, M.D., M.R.C.S., F.R.C.P. (C.)**
Clinical Associate Professor, Department of Paediatrics, University of British Columbia Faculty of Medicine; Consulting Paediatrician, Intensive Care Unit, British Columbia's Children's Hospital, Vancouver

**John J. Macready, B.Sc., B.Sc.Phm.**
Clinical Instructor of Pharmacy, University of British Columbia Faculty of Pharmacy; Clinical Pharmacist,

Intensive Care Unit, British Columbia's Children's
Hospital, Vancouver

**Andrew Q. McCormick, M.D., C.M.**
Clinical Associate Professor, Department of
Ophthalmology, Associate, Department of Paediatrics,
University of British Columbia Faculty of Medicine;
Attending Ophthalmologist, Department of Surgery,
British Columbia's Children's Hospital, Vancouver

**Albert R. McDougal, B.Sc.Phm.**
Clinical Instructor of Pharmacy, University of British
Columbia Faculty of Pharmacy; Clinical Pharmacist,
Pharmacy Department, British Columbia's Children's
Hospital, Vancouver

**Ross E. Petty, M.D., Ph.D., F.R.C.P. (C.)**
Department of Paediatrics, University of British Columbia
Faculty of Medicine; Head, Division of Rheumatology,
British Columbia's Children's Hospital, Vancouver

**Shirley A. Reimer, M.D., F.R.C.S. (C.)**
Lecturer, Department of Obstetrics and Gynecology,
University of British Columbia Faculty of Medicine;
Attending Gynecologist, Sunny Hill Hospital, Vancouver

**Keith H. Riding, M.D., F.R.C.S. (C.)**
Clinical Associate Professor, University of British
Columbia Faculty of Medicine; Head, Department of
Otolaryngology, British Columbia's Children's Hospital,
Vancouver

**Paul C. Rogers, M.B., M.R.C.P. (U.K.), F.R.C.P. (C.)**
Associate Professor, Department of Paediatrics, University
of British Columbia Faculty of Medicine; Acting Head,
Oncology/Hematology, British Columbia's Children's
Hospital, Vancouver

**George G. S. Sandor, M.B., Ch.B., F.R.C.P. (C.)**
Associate Professor, Department of Paediatrics, University
of British Columbia Faculty of Medicine; Head, Division of
Cardiology, British Columbia's Children's Hospital,
Vancouver

**David W. Scheifele, M.D., F.R.C.P. (C.)**
Professor, Department of Paediatrics, University of British
Columbia Faculty of Medicine; Head, Division of Infectious
Diseases, British Columbia's Children's Hospital,
Vancouver

**Leslie A. Scott, M.D., F.R.C.S. (C.)**
Assistant Professor of Surgery, Queen's University Faculty
of Medicine; Paediatric Surgeon, Department of General
Surgery, Hotel Dieu Hospital, Kingston, Ontario

**Michael Seear, M.B., F.R.C.P. (C.)**
Clinical Assistant Professor, University of British
Columbia Faculty of Medicine; Attending Physician,
Intensive Care Unit, British Columbia's Children's
Hospital, Vancouver

**David Smith, M.D., F.R.C.P. (C.)**
Clinical Associate Professor, Department of Paediatrics, University of British Columbia Faculty of Medicine; Head, Emergency Department, British Columbia's Children's Hospital, Vancouver

**Derryck H. Smith, M.D., F.R.C.P. (C.)**
Clinical Assistant Professor, University of British Columbia Faculty of Medicine; Head, Department of Psychiatry, British Columbia's Children's Hospital, Vancouver

**Alfonso J. Solimano, M.D., F.R.C.P. (C.)**
Clinical Assistant Professor, Department of Paediatrics, University of British Columbia Faculty of Medicine; Staff Neonatologist, British Columbia's Children's Hospital, Vancouver

**David P. Speert, M.D., F.R.C.P. (C.)**
Associate Professor, Department of Paediatrics, University of British Columbia Faculty of Medicine; Attending Physician, Division of Infectious Diseases, Department of Paediatrics, British Columbia's Children's Hospital, Vancouver

**Wah Jun Tze, M.D., F.R.C.P. (C.)**
Professor, Department of Paediatrics, University of British Columbia Faculty of Medicine; Director, Metabolic Investigation Unit, British Columbia's Children's Hospital, Vancouver

**Louis D. Wadsworth, M.B., Ch.B., F.R.C.P. (C.), F.R.C.Path. (C.)**
Clinical Professor, Department of Pathology, University of British Columbia Faculty of Medicine; Program Head, Hematopathology/Immunohematology, British Columbia's Children's Hospital, Vancouver

**Karen Wardill, M.B., Ch.B., M.H.Sc.**
Attending Physician, Downtown Community Health Clinic, Medical Officer of Health, Public Health Department, City of Vancouver

**David F. Wensley, M.B.B.S., F.R.C.P. (C.)**
Clinical Assistant Professor, Department of Paediatrics, University of British Columbia Faculty of Medicine; Assistant Director, Intensive Care Unit, British Columbia's Children's Hospital, Vancouver

**Robert White, M.D., F.R.C.P. (C.)**
Clinical Assistant Professor, Department of Paediatrics, University of British Columbia Faculty of Medicine; Attending Physician, Emergency Department, British Columbia's Children's Hospital, Vancouver

**Gerald Wittenberg, D.M.D.**
Head, Division of Oral and Maxillofacial Surgery, British Columbia's Children's Hospital, Vancouver

# Preface

Few aspects of medicine are as demanding of one's time and energy as the care of acutely ill and injured children. The purpose of this book is to save time for physicians by providing a pocket-sized practical guide to the diagnosis and treatment of pediatric emergencies. Although designed for students and emergency and pediatric house staff, I believe that emergency physicians, pediatricians, and family physicians will also find it useful.

Over 40 chapters are included, each containing a brief review of diagnosis, treatment, and patient disposition, with a list of key points to reinforce important information. I have tried to create a functional format, with chapters and sections organized by presenting sign or symptom rather than by diagnosis. Supplementing the text are illustrations showing over 20 procedures and an informative formulary of emergency medications for neonates and children.

For conciseness, discussion of pathophysiology and controversial aspects of diagnosis and therapy have been minimized. In most cases, therapeutic regimens are based on data from the literature, but when this was lacking, tried and true protocols currently used by the various departments of medicine and surgery at Children's Hospital in Vancouver have been substituted. The reader is advised that differing therapies are often acceptable—the danger of strictly adhering to protocols in all emergency treatment situations cannot be overstated. Those wishing more information on a particular subject are encouraged to consult the bibliographies at the end of the chapters or any authoritative text in the field.

Production of this volume was a truly cooperative effort, and could not have been accomplished without the intellectual, emotional, and moral support of the following persons: Dr. Gary Fleisher, one of the great leaders in the field, for his review of material that pertains to the American readership; Dr. Volker Ebelt, for his painstaking review from the standpoint of the generalist pediatrician; Dr. David Scheifele, for his review of areas pertaining to infectious disease; Dr. David Steward, for his review of the resuscitation section; Dr. Charles Snelling, for his review of the chapters on burns and smoke inhalation and on frostbite; Gillian Willis, M.P.S., for her review of the toxicology chapter; Susan Pioli, Senior Editor, and Jon Sarner, Production Editor, at Little, Brown and Company, for their enthusiasm and patience in guiding this project; and the patients, parents, and medical, nursing, and other staff of B.C.'s Children's Hospital, who provided the inspiration.

G.A.B.

# Resuscitation

# Respiratory Failure

## Derek Blackstock

Respiratory failure occurs when there is inadequate delivery of oxygen to or removal of carbon dioxide from the pulmonary circulation. Ensuring adequate ventilation is the first priority in the management of the ill child.

**I. Diagnosis.** Respiratory failure may be due to upper or lower airway obstruction, restrictive lung disease, or inefficient gas transfer (Table 1-1). Common causes are infections (croup, epiglottitis, pneumonia), asthma, chest trauma, and depression of the respiratory center secondary to head injury, meningitis, or toxic ingestion. An awareness of the factors that can interact to cause respiratory failure is vital to early diagnosis and treatment (Fig. 1-1).

The **definitive diagnosis** is made by arterial blood gas analysis (see Table 1-2). Alternative but less accurate diagnostic methods are capillary and transcutaneous blood gas measurements. Pulse oximetry and end-tidal carbon dioxide monitoring are excellent for continuous monitoring of respiratory status. The **clinical manifestations** of respiratory failure in the child include: (1) **respiratory dysfunction** with cyanosis, chest retraction, grunting, tachypnea, and apnea; (2) **cerebral dysfunction** causing agitation, restlessness, headache, convulsions, and coma; and (3) **cardiovascular dysfunction** including dysrhythmia and cardiac arrest.

**II. Assessment and management** (Fig. 1-2)

  **A. Initial assessment.** If the patient is conscious and responding appropriately with adequate respiratory and cardiac function, these signs usually indicate sufficient oxygenation. Initial assessment is the same in all cases:

   **1.** Look for respiratory effort.

   **2.** Listen for air entry at the chest or over the trachea.

   **3.** Feel for air exchange at the mouth, nose, or artificial airway.

  Further evaluation of the airway is essential to detect subtle degrees of obstruction. Following the initial respiratory assessment, determine cardiovascular function—auscultate the heartbeat and assess capillary filling, pulses, and blood pressure.

  **B. Opening the airway**

   **1. Head tilt and jaw lift** (Fig. 1-3). Extend the cervical spine and atlantoaxial joint and lift the bony portion of the chin forward, placing the child in the "sniffing position." This is often sufficient to improve respiration in the unconscious child. Avoid hyperextension because airway obstruction may result. When cervical injury is suspected, have an assistant stabilize the head in the neutral position with cranial traction while performing the jaw thrust.

   **2. Jaw thrust** (Fig. 1-4). Because children have a relatively large tongue, the jaw lift may force the tongue against the posterior pharyngeal wall, caus-

**Table 1-1. Causes of respiratory failure**

| Type | Cause |
| --- | --- |
| Obstructive | |
| Upper | Croup |
| | Epiglottitis |
| | Trauma |
| | Foreign body |
| | Congenital anomalies |
| | Laryngospasm |
| Lower | Foreign body |
| | Pneumonia |
| | Asthma |
| | Secretions |
| | Congenital anomalies |
| Restrictive | Pneumonia |
| | Pneumothorax |
| | Pulmonary edema |
| | Polio, botulism |
| | Congenital anomalies |
| Inefficient gas transfer | Pulmonary edema |
| | Depression of respiratory center: |
| |   Cerebral injury, infection |
| |   Toxic ingestion |
| |   Asphyxia |

Source: Modified from R. Pagtakhan and V. Chernick. Respiratory failure in the pediatric patient. *Pediatr. Rev.* 3: 250, 1982.

ing obstruction. This can usually be rectified by lifting the jaw at the posterior angles of the mandible with the index fingers. Alternatively, the mandible can be grasped with the thumb hooked behind the incisors in the mouth and then pulled anteriorly. This position can be maintained by "locking" the lower incisors over the upper incisors. A number of positions may need to be tried until a clear airway is achieved. The jaw thrust maneuver may close the lips; an oral airway is then required. Grasp either of the lips to keep them apart if an oral airway is not tolerated.

    **3. Choking.** A foreign body in the pharynx may be removed under direct vision using Magill forceps. Blind probing is not recommended. For specific management of the choking child see Chap. 3.

**C. Oxygen.** Ideally, 100% inspired oxygen should be given to all children with respiratory failure. A partial rebreathing mask with a reservoir will deliver 60–80% oxygen. A face mask (35–65%), nasal prongs (25–45%), or oxygen hood (30–60%) may also be used as appropriate. Oxygen should always be humidified.

**D. Bag and mask ventilation.** If there is no respiratory effort, immediately suction the oropharynx with a large

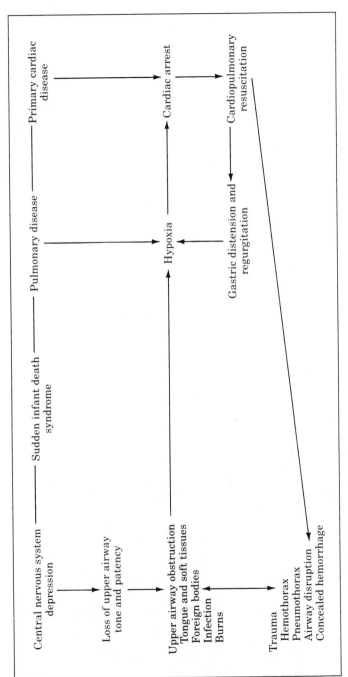

**Fig. 1-1. Factors that interact to cause hypoxia.**

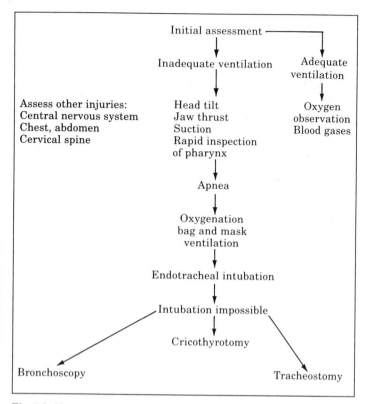

**Fig. 1-2. Airway management.**

rigid suction catheter. Apply a suitably sized mask (see Table 1-3), ensure that there is a good seal, and ventilate while maintaining the jaw lift or jaw thrust position. (See Table 3-2 for appropriate ventilation rates for age.) A partial rebreathing bag should be used to ensure maximal oxygen delivery. If bag-mask ventilation is ineffective, insert an oral airway and reattempt to ventilate the patient (for size of oral airway see Table 1-3). Failure to ventilate after oral airway insertion may be due to foreign body obstruction; when this is suspected use the laryngoscope to inspect the upper airway (see **III.A.**).

**E. Endotracheal intubation.** Each clinical situation will determine the urgency of intubation. The child in cardiac arrest and the patient who cannot be ventilated with a bag and mask require immediate intubation, which is usually performed without premedication. When elective or semielective intubation is planned, the skills of an anesthetist or the most experienced person available should be sought (see **III.A.**).

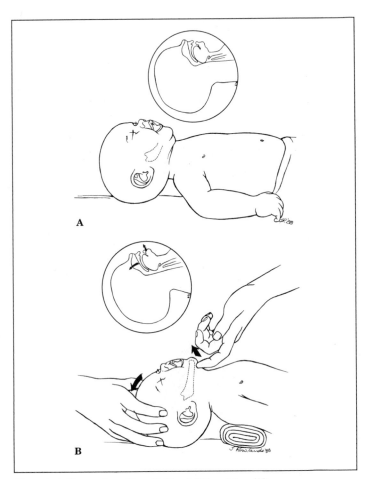

**Fig. 1-3. A. Neutral position. B. Head tilt and jaw lift.**

**F. Cricothyroidotomy** (Fig. 1-5). If the airway is completely occluded, as in patients with laryngeal trauma, inaccessible foreign body, or congenital malformation, cricothyroidotomy can be lifesaving. **It is a hazardous procedure that is rarely indicated and is especially difficult in infants and young children.** When possible it should be performed by a surgeon.

To perform a surgical cricothyroidotomy, locate the cricothyroid notch between the cricoid and thyroid cartilages, incise the superficial tissue horizontally with a scalpel blade, and dissect in the midline until the cricothyroid membrane is seen. Dissect through the membrane to form an opening large enough to insert an en-

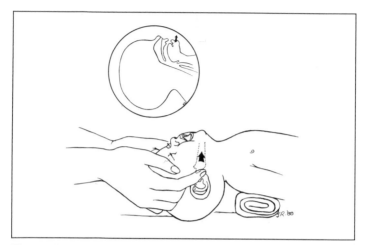

**Fig. 1-4. Jaw thrust.**

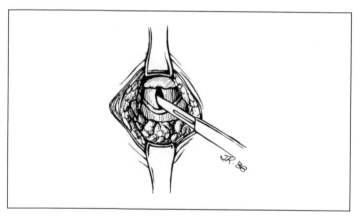

**Fig. 1-5. Incision for surgical cricothyroidotomy.**

dotracheal or tracheostomy tube. For a description of needle cricothyroidotomy, see Chap. 32.

**G. Ventilation.** After stabilization, children should be transferred to an intensive care unit for monitoring or mechanical ventilation. Decisions regarding ventilation should be guided by the clinical assessment and blood gas analyses.

**H. Determination and treatment of the cause.**
   **1.** When the child is stable, take a complete history. Inquire about recent infection, cough, wheeze, stridor, drooling, toxic ingestion (narcotics, barbiturates), asthma, and trauma. In the infant with unexplained

**Table 1-2. Diagnosis of respiratory failure**

| Parameter | Manifestations |
| --- | --- |
| Clinical finding | |
|   Cerebral | Uncontrolled restlessness; anxious expression; lack of response to physical stimuli |
|   Cardiac | Severe tachycardia; severe bradycardia; peripheral collapse |
|   Ventilatory | Decreased breath sounds despite vigorous effort; weakening respiratory effort |
|   General physical | Loss of ability to cry; limpness |
| Laboratory—arterial blood gas ($FIO_2 = 1.0$) | |
|   $PaO_2$ | <40–50 mm Hg (newborn) |
| | <50–60 mm Hg (older child) |
|   $PaCO_2$ | >60–65 mm Hg (newborn) |
| | >55–60 mm Hg (older child) |
| | Rapidly rising (> 5 mm Hg/hr) |

Note: Both clinical and laboratory findings must be considered and either or both may dictate the diagnosis of respiratory failure and the need for a mechanical aid to breathing.
Modified from R. Pagtakhan and V. Chernick. Respiratory failure in the pediatric patient. *Pediatr. Rev.* 3:250, 1982.

    apnea or respiratory failure, ask about prematurity and related lung disease.

  **2.** Thoroughly examine the child (Table 1-2). Note the respiratory status including color, respiratory effort, wheeze, and stridor. Examine the cardiovascular system including heart rate and rhythm, blood pressure, and central venous pressure, if available, and determine if hepatomegaly is present. Perform a complete central nervous system examination including mental status, and test for neck stiffness. For specific diagnosis and management of disorders causing respiratory failure, see appropriate subsequent chapters.

**III. Procedure**

  **A. Endotracheal intubation**

    **1. Indications**

      **a.** To establish an airway when simple maneuvers such as positioning or bag-mask ventilation are ineffective

      **b.** To protect the lungs from soiling by gastric contents, blood, or pus

      **c.** To assist in pulmonary toilet

      **d.** To treat cardiorespiratory arrest

    **2. Equipment**

      **a. Laryngoscope blades.** Test the light source before the procedure

        **(1)** Straight (for infants and young children)

          **(a)** Oxford

**Table 1-3. Intubation equipment by age**

| Age | Weight (kg) | Tube size (mm) | Length (cm) Oral | Length (cm) Nasal | Suction catheter (F) | Oral airway F/cm | Scope blade | Mask size* |
|---|---|---|---|---|---|---|---|---|
| Premature | <2.5 | 2.5 | 10 | 12 | 6 | 000/3.5 | W, M | 0 |
| Premature | 2.5 | 2.5–3.5 | 11 | 13.5 | 6 | 000/3.5 | W, M | 0 |
| Newborn | 3.5 | 3–3.5 | 12 | 14 | 8 | 00/5 | O, W, M | 0 |
| 12 mo | 10 | 4.0 | 13 | 15 | 8 | 0/6 | O, M, W | 1 |
| 2 yr | 12 | 4.5 | 14 | 16 | 8 | 0/6 | MA, W | 1 |
| 4 yr | 16 | 5.0 | 15 | 17 | 10 | 0/6 | MA, W | 2 |
| 6 yr | 20 | 5.5 | 17 | 19 | 10 | 2/7 | MA, W | 2 |
| 8 yr | 25 | 6.0 | 19 | 21 | 10 | 3/8 | MA, W | 2 |
| 10 yr | 30 | 6.5 | 20 | 22 | 10 | 4/9 | MA, W | 3 |
| 12 yr | 40 | 6.5–7.0 | 21 | 22 | 10 | 4/9 | MA, W | 3 |
| 14 yr | 45 | 7.5 | 22 | 23 | 10 | 5/10 | MA, W | 3 |
| 16 yr | 50 | 7.5–8.0 | 23 | 24 | 10 | 5/10 | MA, W | 3 |

Key: W = Wisconsin, O = Oxford, M = Miller, MA = Macintosh
*Mask sizes vary with different manufacturers; these are average sizes. Larger or smaller sizes may be tried

          **(b)** Wisconsin
          **(c)** Seward
     **(2)** Curved (for older children).
          **(a)** Macintosh

**b. Endotracheal tubes** (Portex)
     **(1)** Always have three tubes available, including one larger and one smaller than the calculated size
     **(2)** Uncuffed tubes should be used in children less than 8 years old
     **(3)** Size
          **(a)** May be calculated by the formula:

$$\frac{\text{Age} + 16}{4}$$

= internal diameter in millimeters

          **(b)** Tube diameter is approximately equal to that of the child's little finger
          **(c)** Table 1-3 is a guide to endotracheal equipment for each age

**c. Other equipment**
     **(1)** High-volume suction
     **(2)** Airway (Guedel)
     **(3)** Magill forceps
     **(4)** Flexible laryngoscope (optional)
     **(5)** Rigid bronchoscope (optional)

**3. Premedication**
   **a. Preoxygenation** by bag-mask ventilation is indicated in all cases. Insufflation of oxygen through the side port of the laryngoscope will help to prevent hypoxia during intubation in the awake child.
   **b.** In cardiorespiratory arrest and in resuscitation of the newborn, premedication is not indicated. If possible, all other children should be given **atropine** 0.01–0.02 mg/kg (minimum dose 0.1 mg) to prevent severe bradycardia during laryngoscopy.
   **c.** Intubation while the patient is awake is the procedure of choice in young infants or children with an abnormal airway. **Do not sedate or paralyze the patient with an abnormal airway; if intubation is unsuccessful, bag-mask ventilation may be impossible.**
   **d.** Older infants and children may require the use of **sedatives** or **hypnotics** and **muscle relaxants.** These agents should be given only after airway patency has been established with bag-mask or mouth-to-mouth ventilation. They should be used by qualified personnel skilled in airway management; in most cases this means an anesthetist. For sedation and relaxation, give Pentothal 4–6 mg/kg IV push, and succinylcholine 1–2 mg/kg IV push, each administered over 15–30 seconds after atropine administration (see sec. **III.A.3.b** above). Pentothal may cause hypotension and

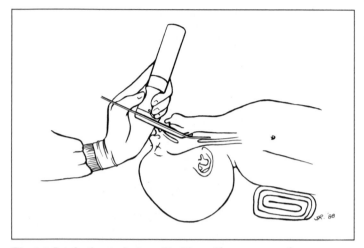

**Fig. 1-6. Intubation technique. Position of laryngoscope for endotracheal intubation.**

myocardial depression in children who are hypovolemic. Succinylcholine should be avoided when hyperkalemia is suspected; in this case pancuronium 0.08–0.10 mg/kg IV is a suitable alternative.

**e. Lidocaine** 1 mg/kg IV should be given 3 minutes prior to intubation in children with suspected brain injury (e.g., trauma, meningitis, coma, space-occupying lesion). This helps to blunt the rise in intracranial pressure associated with the procedure.

**4. Anatomy and positioning.** The infant has a relatively larger tongue, thicker epiglottis, and larger head in proportion to body size compared to an adult or older child. This difference may cause difficulty in exposing the vocal cords during direct laryngoscopy. An assistant should be available to stabilize the head, assist in positioning, and provide cricoid pressure if necessary. A malleable stylet may be helpful in maneuvering the tube; it should be kept 1–2 cm from the distal end of the tube. In the infant and younger child the narrowest portion of the airway is the cricoid ring.

**5. Method** (Fig. 1-6)

**a.** Place the child on a cardiac monitor, and if available, attach a pulse oximeter.

**b.** Preoxygenate the child and give atropine and other premedications. Oral intubation is the initial procedure of choice in most cases. Nasotracheal intubation is contraindicated in children with large adenoids, nasopharyngeal tumor, or basilar skull fracture.

c. Hold the laryngoscope in the left hand and open the mouth by pulling down on the chin with the right hand. Insert the blade in the right side of the mouth, and advance it while lifting and sweeping the tongue to the left.

(1) Use a straight laryngoscope blade in the **infant.** The tip of the blade is inserted under the epiglottis and then lifted anteriorly while being withdrawn until the vocal cords come into view.

(2) In **older children** a curved laryngoscope blade is preferred. The head should be placed on a small pillow or towel. This puts the child in the "sniffing" position and provides an optimal view of the larynx and vocal cords. Lifting the occiput slightly or having an assistant apply gentle pressure on the cricoid cartilage may further help to bring the larynx into view. An attempt at intubation should not interrupt ventilation. If it takes longer than 30 seconds or is associated with severe bradycardia (heart rate <80 in an infant, <60 in a child) or hypoxia, resume bagmask or mouth-to-mouth ventilation.

d. When the larynx is visible, advance the tube down the right side of the mouth and through the vocal cords. The tip of the endotracheal tube should lie in the midtrachea; most endotracheal tubes are marked with a black line, which should lie at the level of the vocal cords. A leak around the tube at an airway pressure of 20 cm of water is desirable to prevent subglottic pressure damage.

e. Following intubation of the trachea, perform auscultation over both axillae to confirm bilateral air entry. The continued well-being of the patient is an important sign. Deterioration following intubation usually indicates esophageal intubation.

f. The tube should be securely fastened in place with adhesive tape on skin that has been prepared with tincture of benzoin. Sedate and restrain the child as necessary to prevent self-extubation. Sedation can usually be achieved with diazepam 0.1 mg/kg IV q2h prn, and morphine 0.025–0.10 mg/kg IV q4h prn.

g. Obtain a chest x ray and blood gas measurements to assess tube location and ventilation. In general, the arterial oxygen tension should be maintained above 80 mm Hg and the carbon dioxide tension kept between 30 and 40 mm Hg. These levels can be achieved by ventilation with a bag-valve-mask device or by using a modification of the Jackson-Rees T-piece system. For the inexperienced, a bag-valve-mask device is probably safer.

**B. Rapid-sequence intubation procedure**

**1. Indications.** When awake intubation is inappropriate or impossible (e.g., when an infant is vigorous, or when a child has elevated intracranial pressure or is unable to open the mouth owing to seizures or altered level of consciousness), a rapid-sequence technique will prevent aspiration of gastric contents in the child with a full stomach. Aspiration can occur when an uncuffed tube is used.

**2. Contraindications.** The child who cannot be ventilated by bag and mask should not be given a muscle relaxant.

**3. Method**

**a.** Correct hypovolemia and achieve oxygenation prior to administering drugs.

**b.** Following oxygenation, a sleep-inducing dose of Pentothal 4–6 mg/kg is given over 15–30 seconds IV, and atropine 0.01–0.02 mg/kg (minimum dose 0.1 mg), followed by succinylcholine 1–2 mg/kg. Ketamine 2–4 mg/kg IV may be substituted for Pentothal if the child is hypovolemic and intravascular volume cannot be fully restored. In brain-injured children, lidocaine 1 mg/kg should be given 3 minutes prior to intubation to blunt the associated rise in intracranial pressure.

**c.** Have an assistant apply pressure to the cricoid using the thumb and finger of one hand while the cervical spine is supported posteriorly by counterpressure with the other hand. Maintain pressure on the cricoid until the child is successfully intubated.

**IV. Disposition.** Admit all patients with respiratory failure to an intensive care unit.

**V. Key points**

**A.** Respiratory insufficiency is the most common cause of cardiac arrest in children.

**B.** Recognize patients at high risk for respiratory arrest and use a systematic approach to diagnosis and treatment.

**C.** Preoxygenate patients prior to intubation.

**D.** Do not use muscle relaxants or sedatives in the child with an abnormal airway.

**E.** Attempts at intubation should not interrupt ventilation for more than 30 seconds.

**Bibliography**

Badgwell, J. M., McLeod, M. E., and Friedberg, J. Continuing medical education article: Airway obstruction in infants and children. *Can. J. Anaesth.* 34:90, 1987.

Donegan, J. C. P. R. 1986. *Can. Anaesth. Soc. J.* 33:S43, 1986.

Marsden, A. K., and McGowan, A. Resuscitation in the accident and emergency department. *Br. Med. J.* 292:1316, 1986.

Simons, R. S., and Howells, T. H. The airway at risk. *Br. Med. J.* 292:1722, 1986.

Standards for C.P.R. and E.C.C., Part V: Pediatric advanced life support. *J.A.M.A.* 255:2961, 1986.

Zideman, D. Resuscitation of infants and children. *Br. Med. J.* 292:1584, 1986.

# Emergency Vascular Access

Gregory A. Baldwin

The optimal site and method of emergency vascular access are dependent on the nature of the illness, the age of the child, and the experience of the physician. In most instances, emergency administration of fluids and medications is best done by infusing the agent directly into the venous system. In the intubated child atropine, epinephrine, and lidocaine can be administered via the endotracheal tube if there is difficulty in establishing vascular access. In the child with shock or cardiac arrest, follow a protocol for establishing access, beginning with a peripheral vein in a familiar location (Fig. 2-1).

I. **Scalp vein access.** In the young infant and newborn, scalp veins are generally prominent and easy to cannulate with a 25- or 27-gauge butterfly needle. Frontal veins that course over the forehead are preferred, followed by superficial temporal, posterior auricular, and occipital veins (Fig. 2-2). (Arteries resemble veins but may be differentiated by the presence of pulsations.) When there is no alternative, scalp veins *can* be used to resuscitate seriously ill or shocked infants. However, they are too small and fragile to be relied on for long-term use in infants and should be replaced by more suitable peripheral or central venous access as soon as possible.

II. **Peripheral vein access.** In the upper extremity, the veins in the hand and the cephalic, median basilic, and median antecubital veins are acceptable peripheral locations. A particularly reliable site in the infant and child is the fifth interdigital vein, which lies between the fourth and fifth metacarpals (Fig. 2-2). In the lower limb, good sites include the saphenous vein, the medial marginal vein, and the dorsal arch of the foot (Fig.2-2).

III. **Central vein access.** Central venous lines are useful for the treatment of shock; they allow high flow of fluids and may be used for hemodynamic monitoring. Two sites are appropriate for central venous access in the infant and child: the external jugular and femoral veins. Avoid subclavian and internal jugular venous line insertion in the emergency room—they are difficult procedures fraught with complications.

   A. **External jugular vein** (Fig. 2-3). Although the external jugular vein is not a true central vein, it allows for a rapid infusion rate and can be used for central pressure monitoring. Cannulation can be achieved using the direct catheter-over-needle method in the infant or child, or by using the Seldinger technique in the child over 1 year of age.

   B. **Femoral vein.** Access may be gained using the Seldinger technique. This is a useful method in a child who is severely volume depleted.

IV. **Greater saphenous vein cutdown.** This is the preferred method of emergency intravenous access if percutaneous at-

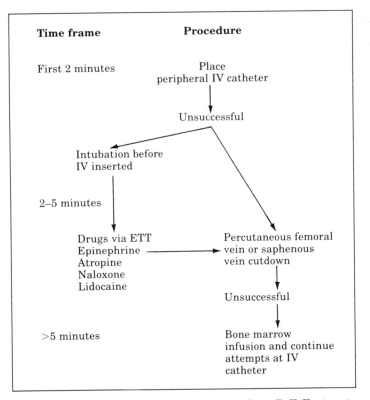

| Time frame | Procedure |

Fig. 2-1. Emergency vascular access algorithm. (From R. K. Kanter et al. Pediatric emergency intravenous access. *Am. J. Dis. Child.* 140[February]:133, 1986. Copyright 1986, American Medical Association.)

tempts fail. In life-threatening situations, an attempt at venous cutdown should proceed if percutaneous access has not been obtained within 2 minutes.

Saphenous vein cutdown can be performed at two sites. One site is at the ankle, anterior to the medial malleolus. This is the first choice in the young infant or neonate undergoing cardiopulmonary resuscitation because it is conveniently distant from resuscitative efforts at the airway and chest. The other cutdown site is in the groin, near the junction of the saphenous and femoral veins. Because this vein is big and easy to cannulate, it is preferred in the older child.

**V. Intraosseous infusion.** The child who is in shock or cardiac arrest needs immediate intravenous access. Percutaneous procedures are often unsuccessful, and a cutdown can be time-consuming. Fluids and resuscitative medications may be given by means of intraosseous infusion, achieving

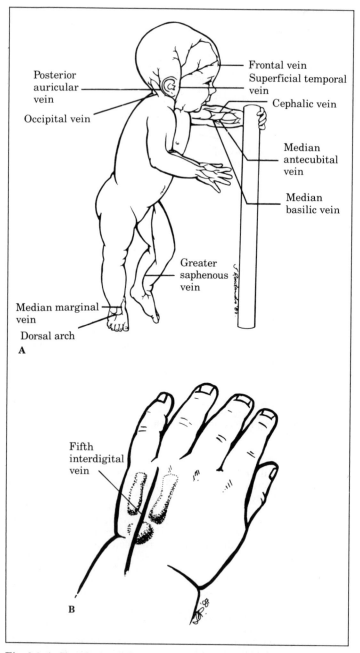

**Fig. 2-2. A.** Sites for peripheral intravenous access. **B.** Sites for peripheral intravenous access.

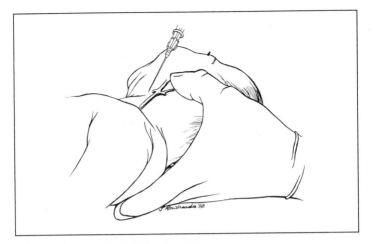

**Fig. 2-3. External jugular line insertion.**

a flow rate that probably equals that of a peripheral intra-venous line. The best location is the tibia, although the fe-mur and iliac crest can also be used. Intraosseous infusion should be attempted if peripheral intravenous access or cut-down venous access has not been obtained within 5 min-utes.

### A. Scalp vein cannulation
#### 1. Equipment
**a.** 25- or 27-gauge butterfly needle

**b.** 3–5 ml sterile normal saline, 2-ml syringe

**c.** Razor

**d.** Antiseptic solution (70% alcohol, 0.5% tincture of chlorhexidine)

**e.** Rubber band tourniquet

#### 2. Method
**a.** Shave the selected site clean of hair.

**b.** Cleanse with antiseptic.

**c.** If desired, apply a rubber band around the scalp to facilitate venous filling.

**d.** Firmly attach a syringe of saline to the butterfly needle and infuse saline through it.

**e.** With the needle at about a 30-degree angle, punc-ture the skin directly over the vein.

**f.** Advance the needle into the vein, and test the patency of the site by gently infusing normal sa-line.

**g.** Tape the needle in place.

#### 3. Complications
**a.** Arterial or venous laceration.

**b.** Infection of thrombosed scalp veins may cause persistent bacteremia. These veins communicate with the intracranial venous sinuses, and infection of the scalp vein may lead to intracranial infection.

**c.** Beware of calcium, bicarbonate, and epinephrine infusions, which if extravasated may burn the scalp.

## B. Peripheral vein cannulation

### 1. Equipment

**a.** Intravenous catheter-over-needle set

**b.** Tourniquet

**c.** 18- to 20-gauge needle for skin puncture

**d.** Antiseptic solution (70% alcohol or 0.5% tincture of chlorhexidine)

### 2. Method

**a.** Restrain the extremity and prepare with antiseptic solution.

**b.** Apply a tourniquet—an assistant squeezing the limb above the site will stabilize it and distend the veins.

**c.** Use an 18- or 20-gauge needle to puncture the skin 1 cm distal to the site of entry to the vein.

**d.** Perform a two-stage venipuncture, as in scalp vein cannulation.

**e.** When blood returns to the cannula, advance the cannula by 1–2 mm and thread the plastic catheter into the vein.

**f.** Remove the cannula and tape the catheter into place.

### 3. Complications

**a.** Arterial or venous laceration

**b.** Infection

**c.** Catheter fragment in the circulation

## C. Central vein cannulation

### 1. External jugular vein (Fig. 2-3)

#### a. Catheter-over-needle method

##### (1) Equipment

**(a)** Catheter-over-needle set

**(b)** Tincture of chlorhexidine or povidone-iodine antiseptic solution

**(c)** 1% plain lidocaine in 3-ml syringe

**(d)** 16-gauge straight needle, gloves, sterile drape

**(e)** Op-site dressing, Steri-strips, suture

**(2)** Place the child in 15- to 30-degree Trendelenburg position. In the young infant, place a small, rolled towel under the shoulders and back, hyperextending the neck over it.

**(3)** Encourage filling of the vein by making the child cry. Prepare the skin with a tincture of chlorhexidine. Achieve local anesthesia at the entry site with lidocaine, and make a small entry site with a 16-gauge needle point.

**(4)** Advance the cannula toward the vein with each cry. When blood returns to the hub, wait until the next cry and then advance the catheter into the distended vein.

     **(5)** As the catheter is advanced, it may tend to "catch" as it passes beneath the clavicle. This can be rectified by placing traction on the shoulder in a caudal and posterior direction.

     **(6)** Quickly remove the needle and place a gloved thumb over the catheter opening to prevent an air embolus. Attach an infusion set.

     **(7)** Secure the catheter in place with steri-strips and Op-site.

  **b. Seldinger method** (Fig. 2-4)

    **(1) Equipment**

      **(a)** Cook catheter (4 or 5 F): metal needle, guide wire, infusion catheter

      **(b)** Sterile drape, gloves, suture

      **(c)** T-connector, 3-way stopcock

      **(d)** Tincture of chlorhexidine or povidone-iodine antiseptic solution

      **(e)** Sterile gauze pads, 3–5 ml sterile normal saline, 5-ml syringe

      **(f)** Infusion fluid

    **(2)** Attach a 3-ml syringe containing normal saline to the metal needle, and use the method with aseptic technique, sec. **C.1.a.(2)–(4),** to advance the needle into the vein.

    **(3)** When there is venous blood return, advance the metal needle 1–2 mm and check again for blood return.

    **(4)** With the needle steadied using one hand, cover the open hub with the thumb until ready to advance the guidewire.

    **(5)** Grasp the soft end of the wire with the free hand and slowly advance it into the vein, several centimeters past the needle tip. If it does not advance easily, remove the wire and reestablish the needle until there is good blood flow, then replace the wire.

    **(6)** Hold the wire against the skin and carefully remove the metal needle.

    **(7)** Advance the proximal end of the infusion catheter over the wire, twisting at the entry site and advancing while holding the wire distally.

    **(8)** Withdraw the wire when the cannula is in place. There should be free flow of blood. Attach an infusion set and suture the catheter in place.

    **(9)** Complications

      **(a)** Arterial or venous laceration.

      **(b)** Infection

      **(c)** Catheter fragment in the circulation

      **(d)** Airway obstruction due to hematoma

      **(e)** AV fistula

      **(f)** Air embolism

**2. Femoral vein.** Use the same equipment and tech-

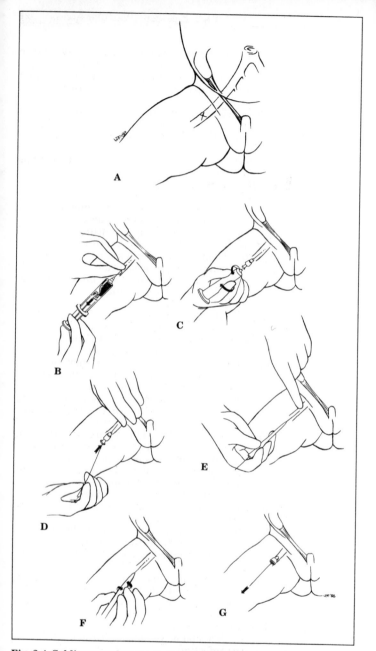

Fig. 2-4. Seldinger technique. A. Landmarks for femoral vein catheterization. B. Advance metal catheter into vein. Check for venous blood return. C, D. Detach syringe and advance guidewire into vein past catheter tip. E. Hold wire and remove metal catheter. F. Advance proximal end of infusion catheter over guidewire and into vein. G. Remove guidewire and attach infusion set.

nique as described for Seldinger cannulation (sec. **C.1.b.**).

   **a.** Restrain the lower extremities and trunk of the child. Externally rotate the hips to make palpation of the femoral pulse easier.

   **b.** Palpate the femoral artery 2 cm below the inguinal ligament, halfway between the symphysis pubis and the anterior superior iliac spine.

   **c.** Cleanse and puncture the skin and direct the catheter cephalad along the line of the artery and 0.5 cm medial to it, at an angle of 30 degrees to the horizontal while gently withdrawing on the syringe.

   **d. Complications**

   **(1)** Arterial or venous laceration

   **(2)** Avascular necrosis of the femoral head

   **(3)** Infection, including osteomyelitis of hip

   **(4)** Bowel perforation

**D. Intraosseous infusion** (Fig. 2-5)

   **1. Equipment**

   **a.** 13- and 18-gauge short Jamsheedie bone marrow needles or intraosseus needles

   **b.** Short 20-gauge LP needle for neonates

   **c.** Providone-iodine antiseptic solution

   **d.** 70% alcohol, sterile gauze

   **e.** 1% lidocaine

   **f.** Infusion set

   **2. Method**

   **a.** Using aseptic technique prepare the site. In the tibia, this is on the flat part of the bone 1–2 cm below and 1–2 cm medial to the tibial tuberosity. In the femur, the location is on the lower third of the bone in the midline, 3 cm above the external condyle. The site can be anesthetized with 1% lidocaine in the non-arrest situation.

   **b.** After penetration of skin, the needle is directed 10–15 degrees from the vertical—cephalad in the femur, caudad in the tibia—and pressure is applied while rotating to and fro. As the needle passes through the bony cortex a "trap door" effect is felt with sudden release of resistance. If a 13-gauge needle is used, bone marrow may be aspirated to confirm proper placement.

   **c.** The needle should stand without support. Flush with heparinized saline and attach an infusion set.

   **3. Complications**

   **a.** Osteomyelitis

   **b.** Subcutaneous abscesses

   **c.** Damage to epiphysis

   **d.** Fat embolism

**E. Greater saphenous vein cutdown** (Fig. 2-6)

   **1. Equipment**

   **a.** Nos. 11, 15 scalpel blades

   **b.** Curved hemostat

   **c.** Catheter-over-needle set

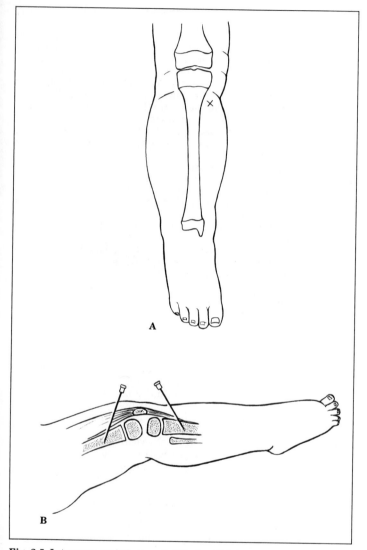

Fig. 2-5. Intraosseous infusion. A. Site for tibial access. B. Needle positions: femoral and tibial infusion.

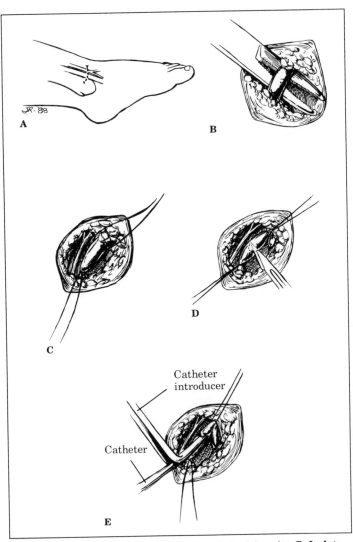

Fig. 2-6. Greater saphenous vein cutdown. A. Incision site. B. Isolate vein. C. Pass proximal and distal sutures beneath vein and tie the latter. D. Incise vein while applying tension on distal suture. E. Lift proximal flap of vein with BD introducer and advance IV catheter.

      **d.** 22-gauge needle

      **e.** BD catheter introducer

      **f.** Two 3–0 silk suture ties

      **g.** Silk 3–0 suture

      **h.** 0.5% chlorhexidine or povidone-iodine antiseptic solution

      **i.** Sterile gloves

      **j.** Sterile dressing

      **k.** 1% lidocaine

      **l.** Normal saline, 3-ml syringe

**2. Method**

      **a.** Cleanse the area with antiseptic.

      **b.** Drape area. Infiltrate with 1% lidocaine if the procedure is elective.

      **c.** Make a 2-cm incision proximal and anterior to the medial malleolus.

      **d.** Use a hemostat to spread the subcutaneous tissue along the course of the vein.

      **e.** Isolate the vein, pass one tie underneath proximally and one distally, tying the latter. Clamp the distal suture.

      **f.** Apply tension on the distal suture and incise the vein with a #11 scalpel blade.

      **g.** Bend a 22-gauge needle into a hook with the hemostat. Use the hook or a BD introducer to lift proximal flap of vein, exposing the lumen.

      **h.** Fill the IV catheter with IV solution; insert and advance into the lumen.

      **i.** Gently tie a proximal suture around the vein and catheter (if too tight, it will occlude catheter).

      **j.** Close skin with interrupted sutures, and apply sterile dressing.

**3. Complications**

      **a.** Infection

      **b.** Nerve laceration

      **c.** Catheter embolization

      **d.** Arterial catheterization

      **e.** Hemorrhage

**VI. Key points**

  **A.** Emergency vascular access in children is often difficult; use a protocol in cases of shock or cardiac arrest to prevent delay.

  **B.** Begin with a peripheral vein in a familiar location.

## Bibliography

American College of Surgeons. *Student Manual—Advanced Trauma Life Support Course.* American College of Surgeons, 1984.

American Heart Association. *Textbook of Advanced Cardiac Life Support.* Dallas: American Heart Association, 1986.

Fleisher, G., and Ludwig, S. *Textbook of Pediatric Emergency Medicine.* Baltimore: Williams and Wilkins, 1985.

Hodge, D. Intraosseous infusions: A review. *Pediatr. Emer. Care* 1:215, 1985.

Hughes, W. T., and Buescher, E. S. *Pediatric Procedures*. Philadelphia: Saunders, 1980.

Kanter, R. K., Zimmerman, J. J., Strauss, R. H., et al. Pediatric emergency intravenous access. *Am. J. Dis. Child* 140:132, 1986.

# Life Support

David F. Wensley

I. **Cardiorespiratory arrest.** In children, severe bradycardia or cardiac arrest usually follows respiratory arrest due to pulmonary or neurologic disease. Most victims are infants under 1 year of age. The outcome is dismal, with mortality in excess of 75% in arrests that occur outside of hospital.

   A. **Diagnosis and assessment.** In many cases, therapy is delayed because the event is unwitnessed or the collapse is not immediately recognized. **Sudden** respiratory arrest is most likely to occur in the following situations: (1) Severe stress in a young infant, who may become apneic; (2) infective upper airway obstruction, such as severe croup or epiglottitis; and (3) sudden onset of coma or seizures following neurologic insult. In contrast, the child with primary pulmonary pathology or cardiac failure usually presents with respiratory distress that slowly progresses to respiratory failure. When children present with severe respiratory distress or imminent respiratory failure, prepare a bag and mask and appropriately sized equipment for endotracheal intubation (see Chap. 1). Obtain assistance from people who are skilled in pediatric airway management.

   B. **Initiation of resuscitation.** If there is cardiorespiratory arrest:

      1. The first person on the scene must establish the diagnosis: look, listen, and feel for respiration and feel the pulses. Place the child on a firm, flat surface (arrest board), give four rapid mouth-to-mouth breaths, call for help, and initiate cardiopulmonary resuscitation (CPR).

      2. Whenever possible, use a team approach to resuscitation. The most experienced person should identify himself as the leader and stand at the child's head. The leader's responsibilities are airway management, ordering of medications, and delegation of tasks to other members, including vascular access, obtaining blood specimens, and recording information. In the ideal situation each team member knows his task and performs it automatically.

      3. One team member should be dispatched to take a history from parents, ambulance attendants, or witnesses. He or she should ask about respiratory and/or infectious symptoms, trauma, drug ingestion, past medical history, and congenital malformations.

      4. Equipment must be provided, including intubation equipment, a defibrillator/monitor, intravenous and intraosseous catheters, cutdown sets, and resuscitation drugs (for list of equipment needed in patients with multiple trauma see Chap. 32). Equipment should be located in a single secure location such as a crash-cart and should be periodically checked to

**Table 3-1. Causes of cardiorespiratory arrest**

| Type | Examples |
| --- | --- |
| Respiratory failure | See Table 1-1 |
| CNS | Meningitis, encephalitis, trauma, hypoxic-ischemic injury |
| Trauma | Multiple trauma, child abuse |
| Environmental | Hypothermia, anaphylaxis |
| Toxic | Cyclic antidepressants, narcotics, sedatives |
| Cardiac | Congenital heart disease, primary dysrhythmia, myocarditis |
| Metabolic | Hypoglycemia, hypocalcemia, hyperkalemia |

ensure that the contents are complete and in working order.

**C. Resuscitation protocol**

1. **Airway** (see also Chap. 1). Establishing an airway is the most important intervention and frequently is all that is necessary for resuscitation. In all cases attempt to open the airway and determine if the child is breathing. Detailed management of the pediatric airway is discussed in Chapter 1.

2. **Breathing** (see also Chap. 1)
   a. Look, listen, and feel for effective ventilation.
   b. For ventilation either a bag and endotracheal tube (preferred method) or a bag and mask is the best method (see Chap. 1). In all cases the oxygen supply should be connected to the bag with a reservoir to ensure the maximum concentration of inspired oxygen.
   c. For the unskilled, either mouth-to-mouth or mouth-to-mouth-and-nose ventilation is the most effective method. Inspired oxygen can be increased by placing a tube to an oxygen supply inside the corner of the mouth with the flow set at 6–8 liters/minute.
   d. If there is no response to ventilation, the patient's position may be faulty, or the airway may be obstructed by a foreign body.
   e. The rate of ventilation decreases with increasing age (Table 3-2). Smaller tidal volumes are required to ventilate a young child.
   f. When performing bag-mask or mouth-to-mouth ventilation, care should be taken to achieve slow symmetric chest expansion without stomach inflation.

3. **Circulation.** Place the child on a cardiac monitor and rapidly assess the carotid or femoral pulse. If a pulse is palpable, proceed to a more complete assessment of cardiac output including blood pressure, cap-

**Table 3-2. CPR guidelines in children**

| Age | Compression rate | Compression depth | Ventilation rate |
|-----|------------------|-------------------|------------------|
| Newborn | 120/min | 2 cm | 60/min |
| Infant | 100/min | 2 cm | 30–40/min |
| < 8 yr | 80/min | 2–3 cm | 20–30/min |
| > 8 yr | 60 | 3–4 cm | 16/min |
| Adult | 60 | 4–5 cm | 12/min |

illary filling, and extremity temperature. If the child is pulseless or if output is inadequate, perform cardiac massage by compressing the lower half to one-third of the sternum. Allow the sternum to return to a neutral position at the end of each compression, and allow equal periods of time for compression and relaxation.

   a. In the **newborn,** the operator's hand encircles the chest and the thumbs depress the sternum about 2 cm (Fig. 3-1).

   b. Hold the **young infant** in the palm of one hand and use the index finger of the other hand to depress the sternum about 2 cm at a point one and one-half finger breadths below the internipple line (Fig. 3-1).

   c. In the **child under age 8,** the heel of the hand is placed on the lower sternum; the depth of compression gradually increases as the child reaches adult proportions (Table 3-2).

   d. In **children over age 8** the method is similar to that used in adults.

   Effectiveness of cardiac massage is assessed by palpating the femoral, carotid, or umbilical pulse (in a newborn). Previous standards for CPR recommended pausing with every fifth compression for ventilation. Recent evidence suggests that it is the increase in intrathoracic pressure rather than direct cardiac compression that produces forward flow of blood through the great vessels, and simultaneous ventilation and compression may be more effective.

4. **Intravenous access.** The initial attempt at vascular access should be made at a peripheral vein in a familiar location. If the attempt at peripheral access is unsuccessful, an early attempt should be made at cutdown or intraosseous infusion (see Chap. 2). Until vascular access is obtained, epinephrine, atropine, and lidocaine may be given through the endotracheal tube.

5. **Treat the cause.** Treatment of the underlying cause of cardiorespiratory arrest is especially important in

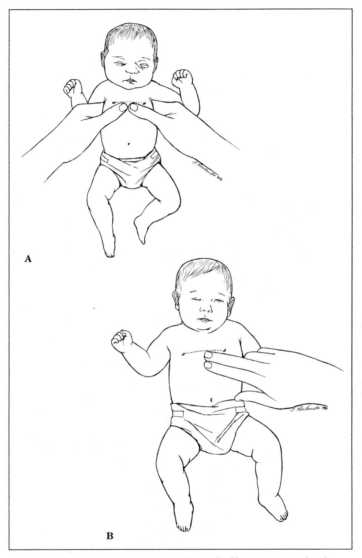

**Fig. 3-1. A. Chest compression in neonate. B. Chest compression in older infant.**

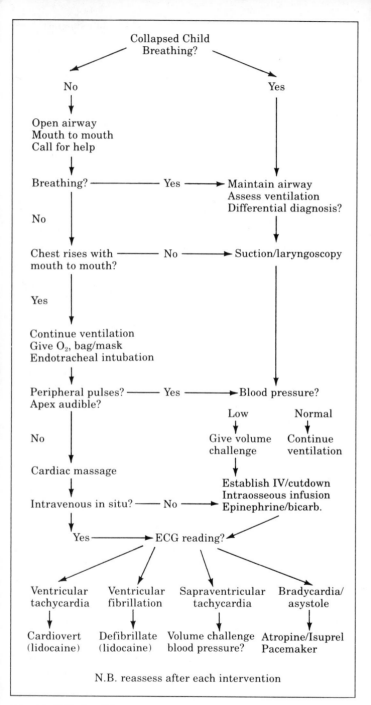

Fig. 3-2. CPR algorithm.

cases of hypothermia, shock, dysrhythmia, increased intracranial pressure, or cardiac pump failure (see appropriate chapters).

6. **Medications—first line** (Table 3-3). The initial aims of drug therapy in the child with cardiorespiratory arrest are to correct hypoxemia, accelerate the heart rate, and correct acidosis or hypotension. When different intravenous drugs are used, take care to flush the line after giving each medication. Calcium and bicarbonate will precipitate if mixed, and a strong alkaline solution will inactivate epinephrine, dopamine, and isoproterenol.

   a. **Oxygen.** Administer maximum inspired oxygen in all cases.

   b. **Epinephrine.** Epinephrine is used to increase the heart rate and support the blood pressure. It can be given by endotracheal tube (dilute to 2 ml with normal saline), intravenously, or by means of an intraosseous infusion every 5 minutes during cardiac arrest. It is less effective at a low pH, but if vascular access has not been established, do not wait to correct the acidosis; give epinephrine immediately through the endotracheal tube.

   c. **Bicarbonate.** Bicarbonate is indicated only when there is prolonged cardiac arrest or documented metabolic acidosis associated with organ dysfunction (dysrhythmia, myocardial dysfunction, hypotension). The dose is 0.5 mEq/kg in the infant and 1.0 mEq/kg in the older child, given once at the beginning of the resuscitation attempt. This dose is followed by 0.5 mEq/kg q10min as indicated by blood measurements (see Chap. 23, Acid-Base Disturbances). Excessive use may result in metabolic alkalosis with severe consequences.

   d. **Intravenous fluid (see Chap. 4).** Push aliquots of 10 ml/kg of colloid (plasma, 5% albumin, or blood) or crystalloid (normal saline, Ringer's lactate) should be given in patients with hypovolemia.

   e. **Glucose** (see Chap. 13, Hypoglycemia). Hypoglycemia secondary to stress is frequent in children with cardiorespiratory arrest. In infants, hypoglycemia may be the cause of cardiorespiratory arrest. If suspected, give 2.5 ml/kg of 10% D/W in newborns or 1 ml/kg of 25% D/W in children, followed by an infusion (see Chap. 13, Hypoglycemia).

7. **Defibrillation.** The most common dysrhythmia in pediatric patients requiring resuscitation is severe bradycardia or asystole (which occurs in 90% of cases). Defibrillation is rarely required. Children most likely to fibrillate are postoperative cardiac patients, and cold water drowning victims who have been warmed from less than 30°C. Availability of pediatric sized paddles (4.5-cm diameter in infants, 8

**Table 3-3. First-line medications**

| Drug | Dose | Interval | Quantity preparation | Route |
|------|------|----------|----------------------|-------|
| Oxygen | 100% | | | |
| Epinephrine | 0.01 mg/kg | q5min | 0.1 ml/kg (1:10,000) | IO, IV, ETT |
| Sodium bicarbonate | 1 mM/kg (1 mEq/kg) in children, 0.5 mM/kg in infants initially, then 0.5 mM/kg subsequently | For use in prolonged arrest or documented metabolic acidosis, up to q10min | 1 ml/kg (8.4%) | IO, IV |
| Dextrose | 25% 0.25 mg/kg (child), 10% 0.25 mg/kg (neonate) | prn<br>prn | 1 ml/kg (25%)<br>2.5 ml/kg (10%) | IO, IV |

Key: IO = intraosseous, IV = intravenous, ETT = endotracheal cm in children) and familiarity with the machine are essential. Arcing of the charge through or across the surface of the skin is prevented by ensuring that the electrode jelly from the two sites is not in contact and that the paddles are not too close together on the chest wall. All persons should be well clear of the child and bed before defibrillation is attempted. Paddle placement is similar to that in the adult, with one paddle positioned below the right clavicle and the other in the anterior axillary line, lateral to the left nipple.

   **a.** For **ventricular fibrillation** the dose is 2 joule/ kg in **nonsynchronized** mode. If this is unsuccessful, give a bolus of lidocaine and repeat with 2–4 joules/kg. Bretylium may be tried in refractory cases.

   **b.** For **ventricular tachycardia** the initial dose is 0.2 joule/kg in **synchronized** mode. If this is unsuccessful, give a bolus of lidocaine and increase the dose to a maximum of 1.0 joule/kg (see Chap. 9).

**8. Monitoring.** Following each intervention, stop cardiac massage and briefly examine the patient for signs of spontaneous cardiac output. Electrical rhythm, pulse, heart sounds, and perfusion should be assessed. If cardiac output returns, measure the blood pressure. A child who is moving or has return of color to the periphery has an adequate spontaneous cardiac output; cardiac massage should be stopped even if a pulse cannot be felt. The child who is gasping is not breathing adequately; positive pressure ventilation should be continued. As soon as it is convenient in the resuscitation process, measure the core (rectal) temperature and obtain blood for measurement of arterial gases, electrolytes, glucose, calcium, potassium, and toxic screening.

**9. Medications—second line** (Table 3-4)

   **a. Atropine.** Atropine may be useful for the treatment of bradycardia. It is rarely effective if there is concurrent acidosis or hypotension.

   **b. Lidocaine.** Lidocaine should be given to all children with ventricular fibrillation, runs of ventricular tachycardia, or frequent multifocal ventricular ectopic beats. If the bolus dose is ineffective, it should be followed with a constant infusion.

   **c. Calcium chloride.** The only real indication for calcium is hypocalcemia (obtain a measurement of ionized calcium if possible). It may be given to try to convert fine ventricular fibrillation to coarse fibrillation, which is more amenable to defibrillation. Do not administer by means of a push directly into a central line because severe bradycardia may result.

   **d. Dopamine.** Dopamine may be used as an inotropic agent to treat persistently low cardiac out-

**Table 3-4. Second-line medications**

| Drug | Dose | Route |
|------|------|-------|
| Calcium chloride | 15–30 mg/kg prn (0.15–0.30 ml/kg of 10% solution). Use only for documented (by ionized specimen if possible) hypocalcemia | IV, IO |
| Atropine | 0.02 mg/kg, minimum dose 0.1 mg | ETT, IV, IO |
| Lidocaine | 1 mg/kg bolus, then 10–30 µg/kg/min by infusion | ETT, IV, IO |
| Dopamine | 2–20 µg/kg/min by infusion | IV, IO |
| Isoproterenol | 0.10–1.0 µg/kg/min by infusion | IV, IO |
| Bretylium | 5 mg/kg; if ineffective, repeat with 10 mg/kg | IV, IO |

Key: IO = intraosseous, IV = intravenous, ETT = endotracheal

put that is refractory to fluid administration. It should not be mixed with an alkaline solution.

    **e. Isoproterenol.** Isoproterenol is used to increase cardiac rate. It may be useful for treatment of symptomatic third-degree heart block or severe bradycardia until a pacemaker is available. It may cause hypotension due to peripheral vasodilation; this can be corrected with volume infusion.

    **f. Bretylium.** Bretylium is given for treatment of ventricular fibrillation or ventricular tachycardia that is resistant to direct current (DC) shock and lidocaine.

**10. Stabilization.** When cardiac output has returned, it is essential to prevent secondary or ongoing asphyxial injury by maintaining ventilation and perfusion. Give high-flow oxygen, order a chest x ray and blood gas measurements, and secure all tubes and lines. Identifiable causes of cardiorespiratory arrest should be treated and intensive support maintained to minimize central nervous system damage. Thorough sequential charting of the patient's condition, treatment, and response must follow the resuscitation procedure with clear documentation of any problems that were encountered.

11. **Stopping resuscitation.** Termination of resuscitative efforts should be considered if no return of cardiac output is achieved after adequate airway control, ventilation, and resuscitative drugs have been administered. Children are unlikely to respond to CPR after three "rounds" of medication despite optimal resuscitation efforts—usually 25–30 minutes after resuscitation commenced. Signs of brain death are helpful but pupillary response may not be completely reliable during resuscitation, as it is influenced by drugs and neurologic events that may have precipitated the arrest. Exceptional situations, when more prolonged resuscitative efforts are justified, include patients with toxic or hypothermic arrest. Following unsuccessful resuscitation, attend to the psychologic needs of the relatives (see Chap. 25, Sudden Unexpected Death).

II. **Choking.** Most cases of fatal foreign body aspiration occur in toddlers who inhale hot dogs, round candies, nuts, grapes, or small toys.

    A. **Management**

        1. The choking victim who is **conscious and able to maintain the airway** despite coughing or stridor should immediately be referred to a surgeon for laryngoscopy or bronchoscopy (see Chaps. 7 and 14). **No attempt should be made to dislodge the foreign body while the child remains conscious.**

        2. The victim with signs of **airway obstruction leading to apnea or unconsciousness** requires immediate resuscitation (also see Chaps. 1 and 14).

            a. **Choking in the child**

                (1) **Heimlich maneuver.** Apply up to eight abdominal thrusts using the Heimlich maneuver until the foreign body is expelled.

                    (a) **The child less than age 7** should be placed on his back with the rescuer kneeling beside him (see Fig. 3-3). Position the heel of one hand on the abdomen in the midline between the umbilicus and the rib cage and perform rapid inward and upward thrusts.

                    (b) **In the older and larger child,** the maneuver can be performed with the child in the standing, sitting, or recumbent (supine) position. In the standing or sitting position, the rescuer should stand behind the victim, wrap his arms around the waist, and make a fist with one hand. Place the thumb side of the fist against the abdomen in the midline, slightly above the navel and well below the tip of the xiphoid process. Grasp the fist with the other hand and press the fist into the abdomen with a quick upward thrust. Each new thrust should be a separate distinct movement.

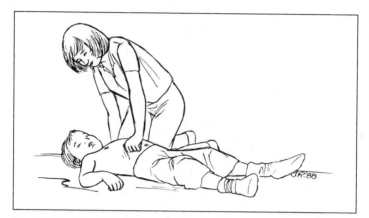

**Fig. 3-3. Kneeling Heimlich maneuver. Age 1 to 7 years. One hand only.**

   (2) **Jaw lift and inspection.** If the obstruction
       is not relieved by using the Heimlich maneu-
       ver, open the mouth and lift the jaw forward
       (see Chap. 1). A foreign body that is seen
       should be manually extracted by a finger
       sweep or, if available, Magill forceps. Blind
       sweeps should be avoided; they may increase
       the obstruction.
   (3) **Ventilation.** If there is no spontaneous res-
       piration, attempt mouth-to-mouth or bag-
       mask ventilation. If unsuccessful, alternate
       abdominal thrusts with mouth-to-mouth or
       bag-mask ventilation. Intubation or crico-
       thyroidotomy may be attempted (see Chaps.
       1 and 32).
 b. **Choking in the infant** (Fig. 3-4). **Abdominal
    thrusts in infants are associated with liver
    trauma and should be avoided.**
   (1) **Back blows.** Place the infant face down on
       the rescuer's forearm in a 60-degree head-
       down position, with the head and neck sta-
       bilized. The infant's forearm is rested firmly
       against the rescuer's body (often the knee)
       for additional support. Rapidly administer
       four back blows between the scapulae with
       the heel of the hand.
   (2) **Chest thrusts.** If the obstruction is not re-
       lieved, turn the infant to a supine position
       on a firm surface. Deliver four rapid chest
       thrusts similar to external cardiac compres-
       sions, using two fingers on the sternum.
   (3) **Jaw lift and inspection.** If breathing has
       not resumed, open the airway using the jaw
       lift technique to determine if the foreign

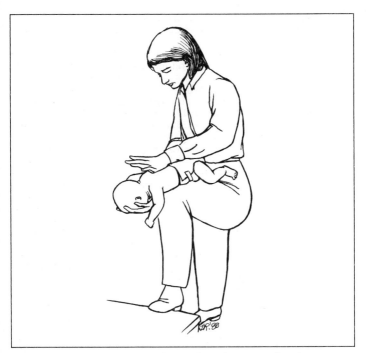

**Fig. 3-4. Back blows in the choking infant. Age 1 month to 1 year.**

body is visible (see Chap. 1). Blind finger sweeps should not be used.

(4) **Ventilation.** If there is still no spontaneous breathing, attempt ventilation with the mouth-to-mouth or bag-mask technique. Repeat the above steps if ventilation cannot be established. Intubation and cricothyroidotomy may also be attempted.

**III. Disposition.** Admit all resuscitated patients to an intensive care unit.

**IV. Key points**

A. Most children suffering cardiac arrest have had a preceding respiratory arrest; anticipation and treatment of respiratory failure may prevent respiratory or cardiac arrest.

B. After each intervention, briefly stop CPR and determine cardiac output.

C. Do not perform abdominal thrusts in the choking infant.

**Bibliography**

Barker, G. A. Cardiopulmonary resuscitation in the child—a physiological approach. *Med. North Am.* (3rd ser.) 3:484, 1986.

Eisenberg, M., Bergner, L., and Hallstrom, A. Epidemiology of cardiac arrest and resuscitation in children. *Ann. Emer. Med.* 12:672, 1983.

Friesen, R., Duncan, P., Tweed, W., et al. Appraisal of pediatric cardiopulmonary resuscitation. *Can. Med. Assoc. J.* 1–6: 1055, 1985.

Krause, G., Kumar, K., White, B., et al. Ischemic resuscitation and perfusion mechanism of tissue injury and prospects for protection. *Am. Heart J.* 111:768, 1986.

Orlowski, J. P. Pediatric cardiopulmonary resuscitation. *Emer. Med. Clin. North Am.* 1:3, 1985.

Rogers, M. New developments in cardiopulmonary resuscitation. *Pediatrics* 71:655, 1983.

Standards and guidelines for cardiopulmonary resuscitation (CPR) and emergency cardiac care (E.E.C.). *J.A.M.A.* 225:2905, 1986.

Wolf Creek 111 Conference on Cardiopulmonary Resuscitation. *Crit. Care Med.* 13:881, 1985.

# 4

# Shock

Robert White

Shock is a state in which tissue perfusion is inadequate or inappropriate, resulting in cellular hypoxia, abnormal cellular metabolism, and a breakdown in microcirculatory homeostasis. In children, shock is commonly associated with trauma, acute severe dehydration, and overwhelming sepsis. Early diagnosis is the key to successful resuscitation. For diagnosis and management of toxic shock, see Chap. 21.

## I. Classification

A. **Hypovolemic shock.** Hypovolemic shock is the most common type of shock occurring in children. Hypovolemia is caused by direct circulating fluid volume loss from hemorrhage, sequestration, or dehydration.

B. **Distributive shock.** In distributive shock there is a decrease in peripheral vascular resistance that is not fully compensated for by an increase in cardiac output. **Septic shock** may occur during the course of any infective process that releases lipopolysaccharides or other toxic molecules into the circulation, and it is characterized by altered capillary flow and permeability, decreased tissue oxygenation, and disseminated intravascular coagulation (DIC).

C. **Cardiogenic shock.** Cardiogenic shock is the least common type of shock presenting to the emergency room. Cardiogenic shock occurs when the cardiac output fails to meet the body's metabolic requirements despite an adequate cardiac filling pressure. Most cases are due to congenital heart disease and present in the neonatal period (see Chap. 8).

## II. Diagnosis and assessment

A. **General signs** (Table 4-2). Assessing the adequacy of cardiac output on clinical grounds alone can be difficult and misleading. Children in shock often present with subtle signs (Table 4-2). The absence of hypotension does not rule out shock in a pediatric patient; when hypotension intervenes, the shock is severe. If shock is untreated, multiple organ dysfunction develops, including renal failure (acute tubular necrosis [ATN]), cardiac failure, gastrointestinal bleeding, and adult-type respiratory distress syndrome (ARDS).

B. **Signs of distributive shock**

1. In distributive shock a high cardiac output state may not be recognized when it is associated with renal and peripheral vasoconstriction and arteriovenous shunting.

a. The early presentation is that of **"warm shock,"** with intense vasodilatation and a flushed, well-perfused appearance. These children have full bounding pulses, wide pulse pressures, and delayed capillary refill. Early changes in mental status are characteristic, including restlessness, irritability, and decreased level of consciousness.

**Table 4-1. Some causes of shock**

| Type | Examples |
|------|----------|
| Hypovolemic shock | Trauma, diarrhea and vomiting, burns, diabetes, third-space losses (bowel, peritoneum), adrenal insufficiency |
| Cardiogenic shock | Left-sided outflow tract lesions: critical aortic stenosis, hypoplastic left heart syndrome, coarctation of the aorta<br>Nonstructural cardiogenic shock: asphyxia, enteroviral infection in the newborn, cardiomyopathy, myocarditis, dysrhythmia, tamponade |
| Distributive shock | Septic shock, toxic shock, spinal injury, anaphylaxis, toxic ingestion |

**Table 4-2. Signs and symptoms of shock**

Tachycardia

Weak pulses

Cool or mottled extremities

Decreased capillary refill (> 2 sec)

Disturbed level of consciousness

Temperature instability

Poor urine output

Tachypnea

Hypotension (severe shock)

    **b.** When **"cold shock"** intervenes, the child has a high heart rate, hypotension, and a narrowed pulse pressure. In this stage the prognosis is dismal.

  **2. Septic shock** frequently occurs in the child with a predisposition to infection such as immune deficiency or congenital anomalies of the urinary tract (pyelonephritis) or bowel (Hirchsprung's colitis). There may be a history of fever, upper respiratory tract infection (URI), rash, or other symptoms of infectious disease. DIC is common in patients with septic shock and presents with bleeding and purpura.

  **3. Other causes** of distributive shock include spinal injury, anaphylaxis, and toxic shock (see Chaps. 21, 30, 38 for diagnosis and treatment).

**C. Signs of cardiogenic shock.** Cardiogenic shock usually presents in infancy with symptoms and signs of pump failure (see Chap. 8). The liver is often massively enlarged, and the chest x ray shows plethoric lung fields and cardiomegaly. On auscultation a gallop is usually heard, but there may be no murmur. In general, congenital heart lesions causing shock are not cyanotic. Instead, the child appears grey with absent or poor pulses. In patients with coarctation of the aorta, there are differential pulses in the legs and arms.

## III. Investigations

### A. Arterial blood gas.
Arterial blood gas and plasma bicarbonate determination is necessary to assess oxygenation and acid-base balance.

1. Hypoxemia (arterial $PaO_2 < 60$ mm Hg) is common owing to ventilation-perfusion mismatch from pulmonary edema, pulmonary infection, ARDS, or cellular factors such as poor perfusion and circulating toxins.

2. The child in shock invariably has a metabolic acidosis (pH < 7.35). In general, correction of metabolic acidosis should be achieved by improving perfusion, not by bicarbonate administration. Inappropriate administration of bicarbonate can cause metabolic alkalosis with severe consequences. Bicarbonate administration is indicated when there is severe acidosis (pH < 7.20) resulting in organ dysfunction (hypotension, dysrhythmia, or cardiac failure). The dose is calculated to correct half of the base deficit. Following bicarbonate administration, obtain repeat blood gas and plasma bicarbonate measurements.

$NaHCO_3$ dose (mEq) = Base deficit *or* (desired $HCO_3$ − actual $HCO_3$) × 0.3 × wt (kg)

See Chap. 23, Acid-Base Disturbances and Chap. 1 for details on normal values, blood gas interpretation, and bicarbonate administration.

### B. Hemodynamic Assessment.
Pulmonary capillary wedge pressure (PCWP) monitoring by means of a Swan-Ganz catheter is the most accurate method of hemodynamic monitoring, although it is rarely feasible in the emergency room setting. Endeavor to keep the PCWP between 10 and 18 mm Hg. Central venous pressure monitoring is less accurate in the child who has myocardial dysfunction. Nonetheless, it is useful in the assessment and therapy of most children with shock. The normal range is 5–12 mm Hg.

### C. Other investigations.
Obtain blood for measurement of electrolytes, calcium (ionized if possible), glucose, BUN, creatinine, blood culture, cross-match, complete blood count (CBC), peripheral smear, and a screen for DIC including platelet count, PT, partial thromboplastin time (PTT), fibrinogen, and fibrin degradation products (FDPs). Baseline liver function tests and serum albumin level should also be checked. Send a sample of urine for urinalysis and culture. A urine sample sent for measurement of electrolytes and osmolality will help to determine whether there is renal or prerenal failure in the child with decreased urine output (see Chap. 23).

## IV. Management

**A. Resuscitation.** Give maximum flow oxygen by partial rebreathing mask. The child with shock and signs of respiratory failure (see Chap. 1 and Table 1-2) requires immediate intubation and ventilation with 100% oxygen. Care should be taken with the use of any anesthetic agent because a sudden decrease in blood pressure may result following its administration. Avoid high peak inspiratory and end-inspiratory pressures, and use a rapid ventilation rate to prevent impairment of cardiac filling.

**B. Fluids.** Place the child in the Trendelenburg position. In trauma victims, bleeding should be controlled with point pressure and vessel ligation while attempts are made to secure vascular access. Establish two large-bore intravenous lines (see Chap. 2). Initially give a bolus of normal saline or Ringer's lactate, 10 ml/kg, and repeat as necessary, frequently assessing the child's perfusion (Table 4-2) for signs of improvement. In general, subsequent fluid therapy should be based on the pattern of fluid depletion: crystalloid such as Ringer's lactate or normal saline is given in patients with dehydration, 5% albumin is given in children with burns or third-space losses, and whole or reconstituted blood is given in trauma patients.

**C. Stabilization and monitoring**

1. Monitor vital signs, capillary filling, and urine output to measure the response to therapy. Try to achieve a minimum urine output of 1 ml/kg/hour (normal 2–4 ml/kg/hour).

2. Start arterial and central lines (see Chap. 2). Rapid infusion of fluids should be continued until the central venous pressure is within the range of 5–12 mm Hg. In addition, give maintenance IV fluid therapy with 5% or 10% DW plus 20–40 mEq NaCl/liter. Maintain the hematocrit at 30–35% with packed red cell transfusions to achieve optimal oxygen-carrying capacity and blood viscosity. If there is evidence of DIC treat the child as outlined in Chap. 19.

3. Insert a nasogastric tube (orogastric in patients with suspected basilar skull fracture) and Foley catheter (use caution in patients with urethral trauma). Continue to monitor blood measurements, as listed in sec. **III.D.** When the child is stable, order a chest x ray, electrocardiogram (ECG), and, if indicated, an echocardiogram.

**D. Medications.** The child who does not respond to volume replacement usually requires pharmacologic therapy. This is especially likely in cases of septic shock. At times, there is value in combining two agents in the critically ill child: for instance, a low-dose dopamine infusion to maintain renal perfusion in conjunction with a dobutamine or epinephrine infusion as an inotropic agent. When possible, these medications should be given through a central line.

1. **Dopamine.** Dopamine has a variety of dose-related

effects. It is inactivated in alkaline solutions and should not be given with bicarbonate.

   **a.** When given at a rate of 2–5 µg/kg/minute, it acts on dopaminergic receptors to increase renal and splanchnic circulation. Mean arterial pressure may fall with reduction of afterload, and an infusion of volume expanders or an increase in the dopamine rate may be necessary.

   **b.** At a rate of 5–10 µg/kg/minute there is an inotropic effect.

   **c.** Above a rate of 10 µg/kg/minute the alpha-adrenergic effect of vasoconstriction increases and may decrease tissue oxygen supply. Above a rate of 20 µg/kg/minute dopamine can be arrhythmogenic.

**2. Dobutamine.** Dobutamine is an effective inotropic agent with minimal effects on heart rate and peripheral vasoconstriction. Children often require high doses to achieve demonstrable changes in mean arterial pressure or cardiac output. Begin at a rate of 5 µg/kg/minute and increase in increments of 2–5 µg/kg/minute to a maximum of 40 µg/kg/minute.

**3. Isoproterenol.** This drug is useful for the treatment of shock with heart failure: It has only beta-adrenergic effects, and it decreases the pulmonary vascular resistance. Isoproterenol is not a pressor; blood pressure may decrease with its administration, and a rapid fluid infusion may be required. Begin at a rate of 0.1 µg/kg/minute and gradually increase the dose by increments of 0.1 µg/kg/minute until the desired effect is achieved or there is tachycardia over 200/minute or other dysrhythmia. It should not be given in an alkaline solution or in the child who has had epinephrine.

**4. Epinephrine.** This drug has both alpha- and beta-adrenergic effects, increasing myocardial contractility, heart rate, and cardiac output. Because epinephrine increases myocardial oxygen demand and pulmonary vascular resistance, it is less desirable than dopamine or dobutamine. It is infused at a rate of 0.1–0.5 µg/kg/minute. Do not give in an alkaline solution.

**E. Treat the cause**

   **1. Sepsis.** If sepsis is suspected or the cause of shock is unknown, begin antimicrobial therapy as soon as intravenous access is established. When possible, anticipate organisms that are most likely to be causative—for example, gram-negative bacteria in the child with pyelonephritis. When the cause of shock or sepsis is unknown, give the following medications according to age:

      **a.** Under 4 weeks: Ampicillin 200 mg/kg/day IV divided q6h, and gentamicin 7.5 mg/kg/day IV divided q8h.

      **b.** 4 weeks to 3 months: Ampicillin 200–400 mg/kg/day IV divided q6h, and cefotaxime 150 mg/kg/day IV divided q8h.

      **c.** 3 months to 6 years: Ampicillin 200–400 mg/kg/ day IV divided q6h, and chloramphenicol 100 mg/ kg/day IV divided q6h *or* cefotaxime, as above.

      **d.** Over 6 years: Cefotaxime 150 mg/kg/day IV divided q8h.

    **2. Cardiogenic shock.** (See Chap. 8.) Avoid excessive fluid administration in the child with cardiogenic shock.

      **a. Nonstructural heart disease** (cardiomyopathy, myocarditis). Nonstructural cardiogenic shock requires early treatment with pressor agents (dopamine, dobutamine, or epinephrine) in addition to other medications combating heart failure.

      **b. Structural heart disease. Neonates** with cardiogenic shock may have severe left-sided obstructive lesions such as coarctation of the aorta or critical aortic stenosis. These children may improve dramatically with an intravenous infusion of prostaglandin $E_1$. Prostaglandin $E_1$ acts by maintaining patency of the ductus arteriosus and is given at a rate of 0.05–0.10 µg/kg/minute. An important side effect is apnea, which may be transient and respond to stimulation, or may require intubation and ventilation. Other side effects are fever, jitteriness, and a cutaneous flush along the course of the vein. When the drug is effective, improvement is apparent almost immediately.

    **3. Other causes.** These include anaphylaxis, adrenal crisis, diabetic ketoacidosis, toxic ingestion, hypothermia, and trauma. (See Chaps. 13, 27, 29, 30, and 32–34.)

  **F. Steroids.** Aside from cases of adrenal insufficiency, there is no conclusive evidence that steroids are of benefit in the treatment of shock. Mortality may be increased in patients given steroids who suffer from septic shock.

**V. Disposition.** All children with shock should be admitted to an intensive care unit.

**VI. Key points**

  **A.** Children in shock may have a normal blood pressure.

  **B.** Patients with septic shock may initially have a flushed appearance, giving the false impression of adequate perfusion.

### Bibliography

Crone, R. K. Acute circulatory failure in children. *Pediatr. Clin. North Am.* 27:525, 1980.

Houston, M. C., Thompson, W. L., and Robertson, D. Shock: Diagnosis and management. *Arch. Intern. Med.* 144:1433, 1984.

Zimmerman, J. J., and Dietrich, K. A. Current prospectus on septic shock. *Pediatr. Clin. North Am.* 34:131, 1987.

# 5

# Newborn Resuscitation

Alfonso J. Solimano

During labor, delivery, and the first minutes of life the risk of asphyxia is considerable. This risk is increased when birth occurs before arrival at the hospital. When delivery takes place in the emergency room, there is little time to prepare for the care of the mother or the newborn child. Prompt, skillful intervention can prevent the sequelae of asphyxia, minimizing neonatal morbidity and mortality. (For information on the diagnosis and management of head injury in the newborn see Chap. 41.)

## I. Preparation for delivery

**A. History.** If there is time prior to delivery, take an obstetric history. Inquire about gestational age, maternal illness, fever, bleeding, and the time of rupture of membranes. The need for resuscitation can often be anticipated prior to or during labor (Table 5-1). Communication with the delivering physician is essential to determine the needs of the newborn requiring resuscitation. When possible, discuss plans for therapy and transport with the parents.

**B. Equipment.** Prior to delivery, the following equipment should be made ready. Check that all items are functioning.

   1. **Overhead warmer.** Commercially manufactured infant resuscitators are fully contained units that increase the efficiency of neonatal resuscitation. Turn the warmer on prior to delivery. Make sure that a skin probe is available and that the temperature control is set to the automatic mode. Check the temperature alarm function. If a commercial infant warmer is not available, warm towels and blankets and a thermometer should be available.

   2. **Resuscitation equipment.** Check the oxygen source for adequate flow. If an oxygen blender is available, set it to provide 100% oxygen. In all cases, gases should be obtained from a reliable central wall source, not from tanks. When using Kreiselman valves, the intermittent positive pressure ventilation (IPPV) pressure should be set at 20–30 cm $H_2O$. If Jackson-Reese anesthetic or self-inflating bags are employed, an anaeroid manometer should be connected in parallel to monitor the pressure being delivered. A neonatal size 0 mask should be attached to the ventilation equipment.

   3. **Oxygen.** Oxygen flow delivered to the bag-mask system should be set at 5 liters/minute. Connect self-inflating bags to an appropriate reservoir to provide a sufficient $FIO_2$. Have full oxygen tanks available for transport to the nursery.

   4. **Suction.** Attach a No. 10 Argyle catheter to suction with a vacuum pressure of 80–100 mm Hg. Bulb sy-

**Table 5-1. Disorders in newborns that often require resuscitation**

Problems prior to labor:
  Prematurity
  Multiple pregnancy
  Severe intrauterine growth retardation (IUGR)
  Severe oligohydramnios
  Infant of diabetic mother
  Severe hemolytic disease
  Suspected hemolytic disease
  Suspected serious congenital anomalies
  Severe perinatal infection
Problems during labor:
  Fetal distress
  Meconium
  Prolapsed cord
  Emergency cesarean section

ringes do not provide continuous or reliable suction and are inadequate.

5. **Intubation equipment.** Prepare a laryngoscope. Ensure that blades of size 0 (for premature infants) and size 1 (for term infants) are available—Wisconsin, Miller, or Welch Allyn-fiberoptic blades are preferred. Test the light source. Magill forceps, adhesive tape, and straight or Cole-type endotracheal tubes in sizes 2.5 and 3.0 with guides and connectors should also be available.

6. **Resuscitation drugs and IV equipment.** In situations where full resuscitation is anticipated (see Table 5-1), drugs should be drawn up in syringes, ready to be injected through an umbilical venous catheter (see Table 5-4).

7. **Other equipment.** An umbilical vessel cannulation tray and a paracentesis tray may be required and should be available on short notice. If an umbilical vessel tray is unavailable, a cutdown tray with umbilical tape may be substituted. Wear gloves, mask, and gown for protection against infection.

II. **Resuscitation.** The primary objectives of resuscitation in the newborn are to maintain body temperature and establish cardiorespiratory function. When possible, obtain assistance from specialists in neonatology or anesthesia.

A. **Maintenance of body temperature.** Immediately after birth, place the naked infant under the radiant warmer and briefly dry the skin with prewarmed absorbent towels. Attach a skin probe to a clean dry area of the abdomen to activate the servocontrol heater. When the cardiorespiratory status of the baby is stable, wet towels should be changed for dry ones, and the skin temperature should be checked and recorded.

**Table 5-2. APGAR evaluation of a newborn infant**

| Score | 0 | 1 | 2 |
|---|---|---|---|
| Sign | | | |
| Heart rate | Absent | $<100$ | $>100$ |
| Respiratory effort | Absent | Slow, irregular | Good crying |
| Muscle tone | Limp | Some flexion of extremities | Active motion |
| Reflex irritability | No response | Grimace | Cough or sneeze |
| Color | Blue, pale | Body pink, extremities blue | Completely pink |

**B. Establishing cardiorespiratory function**
   **1. Assessment**
      **a. APGAR score.** Heart rate, respiratory effort, color (oxygen requirement), muscle tone, and reflex activity are determined and recorded as an APGAR score (Table 5-2). Heart rate is estimated by counting the number of heartbeats while saying "one–one thousand, two–one thousand," which is roughly 2 seconds in duration. Two counted beats in this time equals a rate of 60, three beats equals 90, four beats equals 120, and so on. The other four parts of the score are evident on summary observation. For an infant in distress, the APGAR assessment should be done as early as possible after birth and should be repeated as frequently as needed to determine whether further resuscitation is necessary.
      **b. Apnea.** If the baby is apneic the APGAR parameters may help (Table 5-3) to determine whether apnea is primary or secondary in type.
         **(1) Primary apnea** occurs soon after asphyxial insult and is easily reversed with stimulation and oxygen administration.
         **(2) Secondary apnea** is associated with unresponsiveness, flaccidity, profound bradycardia (heart rate $< 80$), shock, and acidosis; death follows if resuscitation is not initiated immediately. In these infants, artificial respirations should be started without delay, preferably using endotracheal intubation.
   **2. Airway.** Patency of the airway must be established. This procedure includes suctioning the oropharynx and placing the infant on his back with a slightly hyperextended neck in the "sniffing" position. Avoid excessive hyperextension or flexion of the neck because this can obstruct the airway. The tongue may cause significant obstruction in infants who are depressed

**Table 5-3. Primary and secondary apnea—evaluation**

| Apgar parameter | Primary apnea | Secondary apnea |
|---|---|---|
| Heart rate | 80–100/min | <80/min |
| Respiratory effort | Absent/weak | Absent |
| Muscle tone | Hypotonic | Flaccid |
| Reflex irritability | Quickly responds to tactile stimulation or bagging | Unresponsive |
| Color | Blue (cardiac output maintained) | Pale/grey (cardiac output decreased) |

Source: Adapted from Dawes G. *Foetal and Neonatal Physiology.* Chicago: Year Book Publishers, 1968.

or who have a hypoplastic mandible. Babies with choanal atresia have a characteristic clinical presentation, with respiratory distress that occurs when the child stops crying.

Vigorous deep suctioning should be avoided because severe bradycardia may result. If a patent airway cannot be established by suctioning and positioning, endotracheal intubation and ventilation must be performed.

3. **Breathing.** If the airway is patent but respiratory effort is insufficient, artificial respiration should be commenced with a face mask and bag, using inspiratory pressures of 20–30 cm $H_2O$ at a rate of 40–60 breaths/minute. The mask should cover both the mouth and the nose. Observe the baby's chest for symmetric chest wall movement and auscultate to ensure equal breath sounds bilaterally. With effective ventilation the heart rate should be more than 100, and the child's color should improve from blue or pale to pink. If this does not occur, intubate and provide IPPV with 100% oxygen until the baby is pink (see Chap. 1 for details). The stomach may become distended after prolonged IPPV with the face mask; a nasogastric tube should be inserted and aspirated intermittently to prevent regurgitation.

4. **Circulation.** The most common cause of severe persistent bradycardia in the newborn is hypoxia. Establishment of an adequate airway and ventilation is mandatory to improve circulatory status. If the heart rate is below 60 or fails to rise to over 80 in response to IPPV, cardiac massage is necessary.

Cardiac massage should not be performed during intubation (for technique see Chap. 3). The operator's hands should encircle the chest, and the thumbs should depress the sternum 1–2 cm (½–¾ in.) in depth at a rate of 120/minute (two compressions per each "one–one thousand")—see Fig. 3-2. The compression and relaxation phases are given equal time, with a compression-to-ventilation ratio of 3 : 1. Effectiveness of cardiac massage is assessed by palpating the femoral or umbilical pulse.

5. **Drugs.** Drugs (Table 5-4) are rarely needed during resuscitation of the newborn. There is no evidence that atropine or calcium is helpful in the acute phase of neonatal resuscitation. Ventilatory assistance should always precede the administration of naloxone.

6. **Evaluation.** Continued evaluation of the infant's status and response to therapy is important. If the baby does not respond to resuscitation, evaluation of airway patency and ventilation should be repeated. If the endotracheal tube is in the trachea and there are no mechanical problems with ventilation, complicating factors such as pneumothorax and diaphragmatic hernia should be excluded.

7. **Stabilization.** Following resuscitation and detailed assessment, the infant should be transferred to an appropriate facility for further monitoring. If transfer to a neonatal intensive care unit is required, obtain a chest x ray and blood sample for measurement of glucose, blood gases, complete blood count (CBC), differential count, and blood culture. If sepsis is suspected, perform a blood culture and lumbar puncture, obtain a urinalysis and urine culture, and treat the patient with intravenous ampicillin 200 mg/kg/day divided q8h, and gentamicin 5 mg/kg/day divided q12h. Early management of metabolic derangements such as metabolic acidosis and hypoglycemia or sequelae of asphyxia such as seizures and hypoventilation is important.

III. **Meconium aspiration.** Meconium is passed in 15% of deliveries. Aggressive intervention at birth has reduced the incidence and severity of meconium aspiration syndrome and associated asphyxia, pneumothorax, pneumonitis, pneumonia, and persistent fetal circulation.

A. **Management. Watery, meconium-stained** amniotic fluid does not require endotracheal intubation.

1. **Immediate suction.** In the presence of **thick, particulate meconium,** the physician delivering the baby must suction the pharynx at the perineum before the rest of the body is born. Use a 10F catheter connected to 80–100 mm Hg pressure wall suction. A bulb syringe is inadequate.

2. **Tracheal suction.** As soon as the baby is delivered, perform endotracheal intubation and then apply 80–100 mm Hg wall suction on the tube, while withdrawing it. The use of a connector such as the Neotech Meconium Aspirator (Neotech Products, Inc.) allows direct connection of endotracheal tube adapter to suction line connecting tube. Suction catheters inserted through the endotracheal tube are

**Table 5-4. Medications used in neonatal resuscitation**

| Drug | Indication | Dose | Route | Response | Complications |
|---|---|---|---|---|---|
| "Baby" sodium bicarbonate (4.2%) | Metabolic acidosis | 4 ml/kg (2 mEq/kg) per dose, over 2 min | IV | Increases pH, requires adequate ventilation | Hypernatremia, hypocalcemia, cerebral hypoxia |
| Epinephrine (1:10,000) | Asystole or severe bradycardia | 0.1–0.3 ml/kg | IV ETT | Increases heart rate, blood pressure, CO | Hypertension, ventricular fibrillation |
| Glucose (10%) | Hypoglycemia | 2.5 ml/kg, then infuse 5 mg/kg/min | IV | Increases blood glucose | |
| Dopamine | Low CO shock | 5–15 μg/kg/min to maintain blood pressure | IV | Increases CO, PVR | Dysrhythmias Decreases renal perfusion at >12–15 μg/kg/min |
| 5% Albumin FFP or normal saline | Hypovolemic shock | 10 ml/kg over 5–10 min and repeat prn | IV | Increases perfusion | Circulatory overload in cardiogenic shock |
| Group O-Rh negative blood | Acute blood loss | 10 ml/kg and repeat prn | IV | Increases perfusion and oxygen-carrying capacity | Cross-match against mother's serum |
| Narcan neonatal (0.02 mg/ml) | Narcotic depression (administration to mother within past 4 hours) | 0.01 mg/kg (0.5 ml/ kg); repeat prn | IV, IM, SC, ETT | Improved respiratory effort | Do not use in infants of narcotic-addicted mothers |

Key: CO = Cardiac output, PVR = peripheral vascular resistance, ETT = endotracheal tube, FFP = fresh frozen plasma.

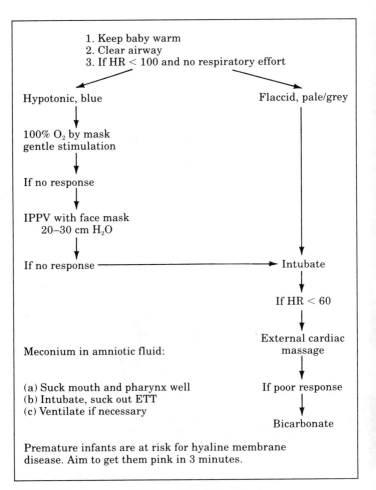

1. Keep baby warm
2. Clear airway
3. If HR < 100 and no respiratory effort

Hypotonic, blue                    Flaccid, pale/grey

100% O$_2$ by mask
gentle stimulation

If no response

IPPV with face mask
    20–30 cm H$_2$O

If no response ──────────────→ Intubate

                                If HR < 60

                                External cardiac
                                massage

Meconium in amniotic fluid:

(a) Suck mouth and pharynx well    If poor response
(b) Intubate, suck out ETT
(c) Ventilate if necessary
                                Bicarbonate

Premature infants are at risk for hyaline membrane
disease. Aim to get them pink in 3 minutes.

**Fig. 5-1. Newborn resuscitation algorithm.**

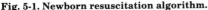

inadequate unless the baby has been intubated with
a minimum 3.5 size endotracheal tube and a No.10F
suction catheter is used.

If meconium is obtained from below the vocal
cords, suctioning may be repeated if the baby's condition allows it. Suctioning twice is usually sufficient. It is likely that the infant will require IPPV for
adequate oxygenation. Remember that the stomach
may be full of meconium.

**B. Procedure**

**1. Umbilical vein catheterization.** The umbilical
vein is the preferred site for vascular access during
delivery room resuscitation: it is easily located and

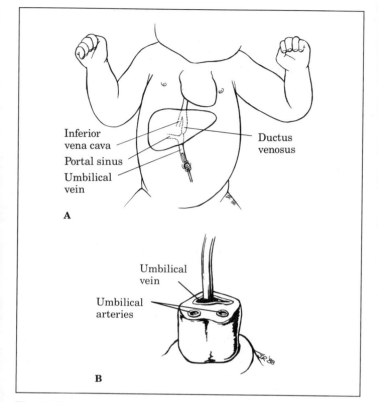

Inferior
vena cava

Portal sinus

Umbilical
vein

Ductus
venosus

**A**

Umbilical
vein

Umbilical
arteries

**B**

**Fig. 5-2. In an emergency, optimal catheter placement is 1 cm below skin level in order to avoid bifurcation into the portal system. A, B. Umbilical vein catheterization.**

is large enough to allow rapid catheter insertion (Fig. 5-2).

    **a. Indications.** Emergency vascular access in the newborn.

    **b. Equipment**

       **(1)** To ensure aseptic technique, use

         **(a)** Gown, mask, cap, and gloves

         **(b)** Sterile drapes

         **(c)** Two medicine cups, tincture of chlorhexidine 0.5%

         **(d)** Sterile normal saline, 2- × 2- in. gauze

       **(2)** To insert line, use

         **(a)** Two straight mosquito hemostats

         **(b)** Umbilical catheters (3.5F or 5F Argyle)

         **(c)** 10- in. umbilical tape

         **(d)** Two curved mosquito hemostats

         **(e)** One lacrimal forceps (smooth, deep, curved Iris forceps)

(**f**) Scalpel blade and handle
(**g**) Scissors
(**h**) Needle driver and 3–0 silk suture
(3) To maintain line, use
    (**a**) One stopcock
    (**b**) Syringes
    (**c**) IV solution: 5% DW or saline
**c. Method**
    (1) Use sterile technique and mask, gloves, and gown.
    (2) Attach catheter to syringe via stopcock and flush with IV solution.
    (3) Tie an umbilical tape around the base of the cord for hemostasis.
    (4) Cut the cord horizontally with a scalpel blade, 1–2 cm above skin level.
    (5) Use chlorhexidine to clean the cord and the abdomen around the cord.
    (6) Identify the umbilical vein.
    (7) Insert the catheter so that it is just below skin level.
    (8) If free flow of blood is present, medication may be administered.
    (9) Secure the catheter in place on the umbilical stump with suture.
    (10) Flush the catheter intermittently to maintain patency of the lumen.

**IV. Disposition.** Admit all resuscitated newborns to a neonatal intensive care unit.

**V. Key points.** Successful neonatal resuscitation depends on
  **A.** Anticipation of the need for resuscitation by identifying infants at risk before birth.
  **B.** Preparation of equipment and supplies well in advance of delivery.
  **C.** Management appropriate to the infant's condition, following these steps:

    A— assessment
    A— airway
    B— breathing
    C— circulation
    D— drugs
    E— evaluation
       and
    W— warmth.

  **D.** The most common cause of severe persistent bradycardia in the newborn is hypoxia.

**Bibliography**

Barker, G. Cardiopulmonary resuscitation in the child—A physiologic approach. *Med. North Am.* 3:484, 1986.

Bloom, R., and Copley, C. *Textbook of Neonatal Resuscitation.* American Heart Association, 1987.

Carson, B., Losey, R., Bowes, W., et al. Combined obstetric and pediatric approach to prevent meconium aspiration syndrome. *Am. J. Obstet. Gynecol.* 126:712, 1976.

Fisher, D., and Patton, J. Resuscitation of the Newborn Infant. In Klaus and Fanaroff (eds.), *Care of the High Risk Neonate* (3rd ed.). Philadelphia: Saunders, 1986.

Gage, J. E. Suctioning of upper airway meconium in newborn infants. *J.A.M.A.* 246:2590, 1981.

Gregory, G., Gooding, C., Phibbs, R., et al. Meconium aspiration in infants: A prospective study. *J. Pediatr.* 85:848, 1974.

Phibbs, R. Delivery Room Management of the Newborn. In G. Avery (ed.), *Neonatology: Pathophysiology and Management of the Newborn* (3rd ed.). Philadelphia: Lippincott, 1986.

Scanlon, J., and Daze, A. (eds.). *Code Pink: A Practical System for Neonatal/Perinatal Resuscitation.* Baltimore: University Park Press, 1981.

Solimano. A. Resuscitation of the depressed neonate. *B.C. Med. J.* 28:107–109, 1986.

Standards for cardiopulmonary resuscitation (CPR) and emergency cardiac care (ECC). Part IV: Neonatal advanced life support. *J.A.M.A.* 255:2969, 1986.

# Cardiac and Pulmonary Emergencies

# 6

# Acute Upper Airway Obstruction

Gregory A. Baldwin

Acute upper airway obstruction is a medical emergency requiring rapid diagnosis and therapy. The child with stridor, with or without respiratory distress, may have croup, epiglottitis, foreign body aspiration, or food impaction in the upper esophagus. Rare causes of upper airway obstruction include bacterial tracheitis, angioneurotic edema, retropharyngeal abscess, massive tonsillar hypertrophy secondary to infectious mononucleosis, and other disorders as listed in Table 6-1. When there is severe acute upper airway obstruction, notify anesthesiology, ENT surgery, and the intensive care unit immediately (Fig. 6-1).

I. **Acute Epiglottitis (Supraglottitis).** Acute epiglottitis is a life-threatening infection of the supraglottic tissues, mainly involving the epiglottis and aryepiglottic folds. *Haemophilus influenzae* type b is the pathogen in nearly all cases. Airway obstruction can occur suddenly and may lead to respiratory arrest. Acute epiglottitis is more common in young children (2–6 years of age) but it can occur at any age: 25–30% of patients are less than 2 years old, 5–10% are less than 1 year old, and cases occur in adults.

A. **Diagnosis and assessment**

1. **History.** Classic epiglottitis is characterized by acute onset of inspiratory stridor, high fever, dysphagia, drooling, and refusal of food. In contrast to patients with croup, these children do not cough. Infants and young children may present with stridor, fever, poor feeding, and "toxicity."

2. **Examination**

a. **Children.** Children with epiglottitis appear toxic, anxious, and usually sit rigidly in the tripod position (neck extended forward into "sniffing" position, leaning back on hands with arms extended) or other position to maintain the airway.

b. **Infants.** Infants or children who are unable to sit will not adopt the tripod position. Their presentation is often subtle, with stridor and signs of systemic infection or toxicity. There is often an increase in both inspiratory and expiratory sounds that may lead to a mistaken impression of wheezing.

B. **Management**

1. **Comfort.** Agitation may increase respiratory distress and precipitate laryngospasm. Do not move the child from his preferred position, often in the mother's lap. The physical examination should be cautious and gentle. Avoid distressing procedures such as venipuncture. Do not lay the child down or look in the mouth. Humidified oxygen may be given by mask if it does not disturb the child. Never leave a patient with a suspected case of epiglottitis unattended by a physician. Do not use narcotics or sedatives (includ-

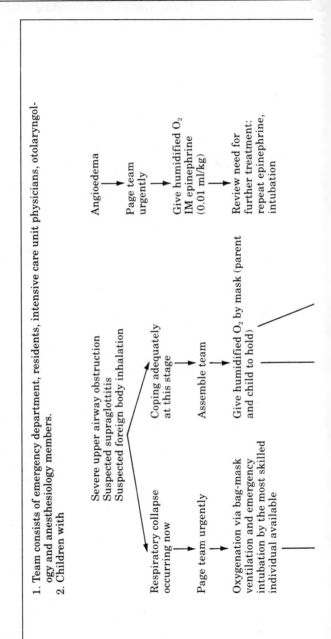

1. Team consists of emergency department, residents, intensive care unit physicians, otolaryngology and anesthesiology members.
2. Children with

Angioedema → Page team urgently → Give humidified $O_2$ IM epinephrine (0.01 ml/kg) → Review need for further treatment: repeat epinephrine, intubation

Severe upper airway obstruction
Suspected supraglottitis
Suspected foreign body inhalation

Coping adequately at this stage → Assemble team → Give humidified $O_2$ by mask (parent and child to hold)

Respiratory collapse occurring now → Page team urgently → Oxygenation via bag-mask ventilation and emergency intubation by the most skilled individual available

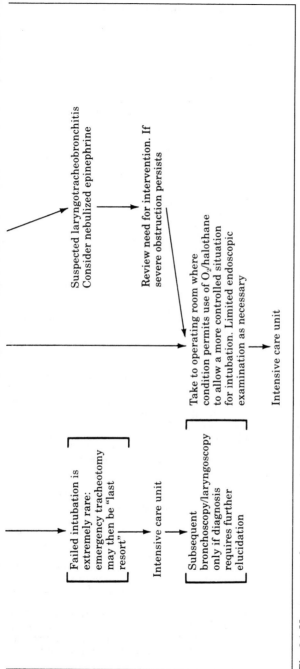

**Fig. 6-1.** Management of severe upper airway obstruction. (From H. Kilham, J. Gillis, and B. Benjamin. Severe upper airway obstruction. *Pediatr. Clin. North Am.* 34:1, 1987.)

**Table 6-1. Serious acute upper airway obstruction in the infant and child**

| Type | Example |
| --- | --- |
| Infection | Supraglottitis (epiglottitis) |
| | Acute laryngotracheobronchitis (croup) |
| | Bacterial tracheitis |
| | Pharyngeal abscesses (e.g., retropharyngeal) |
| | Tonsillitis/tonsillar hypertrophy |
| | Diphtheria |
| Accidents/trauma | Glottic, subglottic, or esophageal foreign body |
| | External trauma to the neck |
| | Burns to the upper airway |
| | Iatrogenic (postintubation) injury |
| Others | Angioedema |
| | Spasmodic croup |
| | Tumors |
| Newborn causes | Nose (choanal atresia, tumor, trauma) |
| | Facial/skeletal anomaly (Pierre-Robin syndrome, Treacher-Collins syndrome) |
| | Mouth and oropharynx (tumor, ectopic thyroid tissue, macroglossia) |
| | Larynx (laryngomalacia, vocal cord paralysis, laryngeal web, subglottic stenosis) |
| | Trachea (vascular ring) |

Source: Modified from H. Kilham, J. Gillis, and B. Benjamin. Severe upper airway obstruction. *Pediatr. Clin. North Am.* 34: 1, 1987.

ing antihistamines) in children with acute upper airway obstruction.

2. **Anticipate.** Have appropriate equipment ready for bag-mask ventilation and intubation (see Chap. 1).
3. **Notify.** A team composed of specialists in ear-nose-and-throat (ENT) surgery, anesthesia, and intensive care should be summoned to the emergency department. The operating room should be requested to prepare for possible rigid bronchoscopy or tracheostomy.
4. **Definitive treatment.** The preferred method of airway management is inhalational anesthesia with halothane and oxygen, followed by nasotracheal intubation in the operating room. Following intubation, take cultures of the blood (positive in 85% of cases) and epiglottis surface (positive in 35% of cases) and treat the patient with cefuroxime 75–100 mg/kg/day IV divided q8h OR ampicillin 200 mg/kg/day IV divided q6h and chloramphenicol, 50–75 mg/kg/day IV divided q6h, until culture results are available. Treatment is usually continued for 5–7 days, unless additional sites of infection warrant longer treatment. Appropriate contacts of the patient require prophylaxis with rifampin when the di-

agnosis has been verified (see Chap. 21, Infectious Meningitis).

**5. Acute respiratory arrest**

   **a.** Most children with acute respiratory arrest from epiglottitis can be adequately ventilated with a bag and mask and 100% oxygen. Forceful ventilation with high pressures may be required.

   **b.** Always ensure that the child is preoxygenated with bag-mask ventilation prior to endotracheal intubation. If orotracheal intubation is attempted, suction secretions gently. See Chap. 1, **III.A.,** for method.

   **c.** If the vocal cords cannot be seen because of tissue swelling, have an assistant press gently on the chest; air bubbles may be visible at the site of the vocal cords.

   **d.** Cricothyroidotomy and tracheostomy are difficult, time-consuming procedures that should be avoided if possible (see Chap. 1).

**6. X rays.** X rays may be ordered in doubtful cases when airway obstruction is mild. Never order x rays in the presence of moderate or severe obstruction. Always have a physician capable of establishing an airway in attendance. Key features of the x-ray diagnosis of epiglottitis can be remembered by the mnemonic HEAT (Fig. 6-2).

   **a.** H—Hypopharynx: An increased volume of air is present.

   **b.** E—Epiglottis: enlarged. The epiglottis may be located:

      **(1)** By noting that the base of the epiglottis intercepts the plane of the wing of the hyoid bone, which is calcified at birth.

      **(2)** By following the surface of the tongue back to the vallecula; the epiglottis is posterior to the vallecula.

   **c.** A—Aryepiglottic folds:

   **d.** T—Tracheoesophageal air column: interrupted. Normally, the hypopharyngeal and tracheal air columns abut on each other, and the aryepiglottic folds are thin lines. In epiglottitis, the folds are markedly thickened, separating the air columns.

**7. Stabilization.** The child's elbow joints should be immobilized with elbow splints or plaster casts to prevent self-extubation. Provide regular pulmonary toilet with hourly saline instillation and suctioning to prevent atelectasis. In some children, relief of upper airway obstruction leads to postobstructive pulmonary edema, and ventilation or continuous positive airway pressure is required. Look for and treat other foci of infection such as otitis media, pneumonia, and meningitis.

**II. Croup.** Viral croup (laryngotracheobronchitis, laryngotracheitis) is most often due to parainfluenza types 1 or 2. It is most common in late fall and early winter, although it

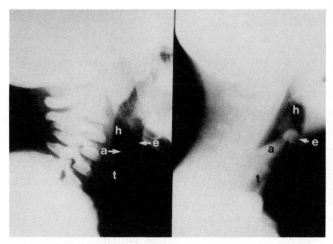

Fig. 6-2. Radiological diagnosis of epiglottitis. X ray on the left shows normal patient. X ray on the right shows features of epiglottitis. (*h* = increased air in the hypopharynx; *e* = enlarged epiglottis; *a* = thickened aryepiglottic folds; *t* = interruption of tracheoesophageal air column.)

can present at any time of year. Severe airway obstruction can occur; 5% of children seen in the emergency room with croup require admission to the intensive care unit, and 2% need airway support. In cases of severe croup, consider the diagnosis of bacterial tracheitis (see sec. **III** below).

**A. Diagnosis and assessment**

   **1. History.** Initially there is a short (few days) history of cough, coryza, and mild fever. Subsequently, patients develop the classic symptom complex of hoarse voice, brassy cough, and stridor, which is both inspiratory and expiratory. Feeding is usually normal. Severity of the condition may vary greatly from moment to moment, the child appearing relatively well between episodes of respiratory distress. Symptoms are usually worse at night.

   **2. Examination.** In contrast to the anxious, immobile child with epiglottitis, the child with croup is often agitated and restless. Fever is usually mild, though occasionally it may be as high as 39°C. Children with moderate croup have tachypnea, tachycardia, and inspiratory indrawing with use of accessory muscles of respiration. Expiratory rhonchi are commonly heard on auscultation. Rocking respirations, restlessness, cyanosis, or fatigue may indicate impending respiratory failure; these children need urgent treatment and transfer to an intensive care unit.

   **3. X rays.** X rays may be useful when the symptoms are

mild and the diagnosis is in doubt. A lateral neck film reveals subglottic narrowing, whereas the "steeple" sign with loss of normal shouldering of the trachea may be seen on the anteroposterior view.

B. **Management**
1. **Mild croup (no stridor at rest).** Children with mild croup can usually be managed at home. Parents should be advised of the signs of severe respiratory distress and encouraged to return to the hospital if there is deterioration in the child's condition. A cool mist vaporizer placed in the room may be helpful. Admission to hospital is warranted in the following cases:
   **a.** Significant stridor at rest
   **b.** Tachycardia (heart rate >160) or tachypnea (>60)
   **c.** Suprasternal, intercostal, or subcostal chest retractions, or use of accessory muscles of respiration
   **d.** Signs of respiratory failure (see Chap. 1)
2. **Moderate or severe croup**
   **a.** Comfort. In general, avoid distressing procedures that may antagonize the patient. If the child is drinking adequately and is not in need of an artificial airway, an intravenous line is unnecessary. Mist tents and oxygen masks may be of help, but they are useless if they upset the child. The best place for a child with moderate or severe croup is usually his mother's lap.
   **b. Monitoring.** Blood gas measurements are rarely indicated; respiratory distress and the need for intubation are usually determined clinically (see Chap. 1). However, pulse oximetry and a transcutaneous $PCO_2$ electrode monitor can be valuable for continuous monitoring of respiratory status.
   **c. Treatment**
      **(1)** Racemic epinephrine given by nebulizer is often effective in reducing airway obstruction in patients with croup. The dose is 0.50 ml in the child older than 1 year and 0.25 ml in the child younger than 1 year, diluted up to 2.5 ml with normal saline. This solution may be given as often as necessary, even continuously in the severely ill child. If treatment is required more than q2h, transfer to the intensive care unit is advised. Children who have received epinephrine should be observed for 4 to 6 hours before discharge because rebound swelling and airway obstruction may occur.
      **(2)** Children who require admission to a hospital should be given dexamethasone 0.6 mg/kg IM once.
   **d. Airway support.** Up to 2% of children with croup may require an artificial airway. The pro-

cedure should be performed in the operating room because tracheostomy is necessary if subglottic swelling is severe and intubation is impossible. The size of the endotracheal tube should be reduced (internal diameter decreased by 0.5 mm in children under 2 years of age and by 1.0 mm if over 2 years of age).

III. **Bacterial tracheitis.** Bacterial tracheitis is a rare and severe cause of rapidly progressive upper airway obstruction and is due to bacterial infection of the trachea by *Staphylococcus aureus, Haemophilus influenzae* type b, and rarely, *Branhamella catarrhalis*. Sudden occlusion of the trachea by sloughed mucosa or thick secretions can result in death.

Initially, the presentation is identical to that of croup. Subsequently, patients develop high fever, toxicity, and inspiratory stridor that is characteristically soft, low pitched, and unresponsive to racemic epinephrine. There may be a low-pitched cough with expectoration of purulent sputum. Coughing paroxysms may lead to cyanosis and severe distress. X rays may be normal or identical to those with croup with evidence of subglottic narrowing. Secretions or sloughed mucosa may indent the tracheal air column. Often the diagnosis is uncertain until tracheal intubation is required, whereupon copious purulent secretions are encountered distal to the glottis.

Diagnosis is made by endoscopy in the operating room, and treatment is with airway management and intravenous cloxacillin or oxacillin, 150 mg/kg/day divided q6h, and cefuroxime, 150 mg/kg/day divided q8h. When intubation is required, repeated vigorous suctioning of the endotracheal tube may be necessary to clear the trachea of necrotic membrane and other material. Tracheal secretions should be obtained for Gram's stain and culture, and treatment should be revised on the basis of these culture results.

IV. **Disposition.** Admit all patients with severe acute upper airway obstruction. For a list of indications for admitting children with croup see sec. **I** above. Children with epiglottitis, severe croup, and bacterial tracheitis require urgent airway management in the operating room.

V. **Key points**
   A. When children present with severe upper airway obstruction, ENT surgery, anesthesia, and intensive care specialists should be summoned immediately.
   B. Most children with acute respiratory collapse due to epiglottitis can be ventilated initially with a bag and mask.
   C. Children who have received racemic epinephrine treatment must be observed for a minimum of 4 hours prior to discharge.

**Bibliography**

Bains, D. M. D., Wark, H., and Overton, J. H. Acute epiglottitis in children. *Anaesth. Intens. Care* 13:25, 1984.

Benjamin, B., and O'Reilly, B. Acute epiglottitis in infants and children. *Ann. Otol.* 85:565, 1976.

Blackstock, D., Adderley, R. J., and Steward, D. J. Epiglottitis in young infants. *Anaesthesiology* 67:97, 1987.

Blanc, F., Webber, M. L., Leduc, C., et al. Acute epiglottitis in children: Management of 27 consecutive cases of nasotracheal intubation with special emphasis on anaesthetic considerations. *Can. Anaesth. Soc. J.* 24:1, 1977.

Diaz, K. H., and Lockhart, C. H. Early diagnosis and airway management of acute epiglottitis. *South. Med. J.* 75:399, 1982.

Kilham, H. K., Gillis, J. G., and Benjamin, B. Severe upper airway obstruction. *Pediatr. Clin. North Am.* 34:1, 1987.

Liston, S. L., Gehrz, R. C., Segal, L. G., et al. Bacterial tracheitis. *Am. J. Dis. Child.* 137:764, 1983.

# Lower Airway Obstruction

David Smith and John M. Dean

The hallmark of lower airway obstructive disease is cough, wheezing, and a prolonged expiratory phase. In the older child, acute onset of wheezing is most commonly due to asthma. In the wheezing infant and toddler, the likely causes are bronchiolitis, early onset asthma, and pneumonia. Other causes requiring consideration are foreign body aspiration, intraluminal and extraluminal masses, upper airway obstruction, and congestive heart failure with pulmonary edema.

## I. Approach to the wheezing child
### A. Determine the severity of distress
1. **Mild distress.** When respiratory impairment is mild, there is wheezing, tachypnea, and tachycardia. Auscultation of the chest usually reveals good air entry, rhonchi, and fine crepitant rales.
2. **Moderate distress.** As respiratory impairment increases, the child becomes anxious and breathes with expiratory grunts, nasal flaring, and use of the accessory muscles of respiration, including the strap muscles of the neck, abdominal muscles, diaphragm, and intercostal muscles. There is indrawing of supraclavicular, substernal, or intercostal tissues. Beware of the "silent chest" on auscultation—this usually represents severe obstruction. Occasionally, children with prolonged severe attacks will be dehydrated from increased insensible fluid losses and decreased intake.
3. **Severe distress (respiratory failure).** Children with severe obstruction may present with restlessness, somnolence, cyanosis, dysrhythmia, decreased breath sounds despite vigorous effort, weakening respiratory effort, or limpness. Consider the possibility of concomitant pneumothorax or pneumonia in such cases. In young infants, prolonged apneic spells may be a prominent feature of bronchiolitis with respiratory syncytial virus (RSV) infection, especially during the 48–72 hours after the onset of symptoms.

### B. Laboratory investigations.
Blood gas measurements, arterial if possible, should be obtained in all children with moderate or severe respiratory distress with wheezing. If available, pulse oximetry is invaluable for continuous assessment of respiratory status. When obstruction is marked, there is impaired gas exchange resulting in hypoxemia and hypercapnia. A rapidly rising or high $PCO_2$ indicates respiratory failure (see Chap. 1).

### C. X rays.
A chest x ray need not be done in all children with an episode of wheezing. X rays should be ordered when there is doubt about the diagnosis, when moderate to severe symptoms are present, or when there is suspicion of pneumothorax, pneumonia, or foreign body aspiration.

**II. Bronchiolitis.** Bronchiolitis is a common respiratory tract infection in the first 2 years of life, with a peak incidence in the winter and spring in North America. The infection is usually caused by RSV but may also be due to adenovirus, influenza, or parainfluenza viruses. Viral invasion of the bronchial tree produces reactive edema and narrowing of the airway lumen, causing air trapping, overinflation, and atelectasis.

   **A. Diagnosis and assessment.** Symptoms begin with coryza and progress to cough and wheezing with respiratory distress. Fever, if present, is low grade. The severity of the presentation can vary from an undistressed child with mild wheeze and cough to respiratory failure. Infants with cardiac or pulmonary disease, premature infants, and immune-compromised children are prone to severe infection with respiratory failure. Apneic spells can occur in young infants. A chest x ray usually indicates air trapping, thickening of bronchial walls, interstitial pneumonia, and atelectasis. Definitive diagnosis is made from nasopharyngeal washings for RSV culture and rapid fluorescent antibody testing for RSV antigen. In general, the child under the age of 2 with these symptoms has bronchiolitis. The symptoms of asthma can be identical. Suspect asthma in the child with a personal or family history of atopy, previous episodes of wheezing, or a dramatic response to bronchodilator therapy.

   **B. Management**

      **1. Resuscitation.** Give oxygen to all children. Those with repeated apnea or imminent respiratory failure should be intubated and ventilated. Obtain baseline blood gas measurements and a chest x ray in all cases, and, if available, monitor with pulse oximetry. If fluid intake is inadequate, intravenous therapy is necessary.

      **2. Bronchodilators.** If the child is older than 6 months, a trial of therapy with a nebulized bronchodilator such as albuterol (Ventolin) is indicated. The dose of albuterol is 0.02 ml/kg of nebulizer solution (maximum dose 1 ml) in 2–3 ml of isotonic saline. For dosages of other nebulized bronchodilators see Table 7-1.

      **3. Ribavirin.** Ribavirin, an antiviral agent, should be given to critically ill patients, expremature infants, immune-compromised children, and those with underlying cardiac or pulmonary disease. It is administered as an aerosol, 1 vial for 22 hours/day for 5–7 days either through an endotracheal tube (ETT) or directly into a mist tent or head box through a small-particle aerosol generator (SPAG). When given through an ETT precautions must be taken to ensure that the drug does not circulate through the ventilator; otherwise, serious damage may result due to precipitation of medication.

      **4. Mild disease.** Children without respiratory distress or a history of cardiopulmonary disease, immune compromise, or prematurity may be dis-

**Table 7-1. Nebulized bronchodilators**

| Drug | Dose | Comments |
|------|------|----------|
| Fenoterol (Berotec) | 0.03 ml/kg | Dilute in 2–3 ml normal saline |
| Salbutamol, albuterol (Ventolin) | 0.02 ml/kg | Dilute in 2–3 ml normal saline. Max. dose 1 ml |
| Orciprenaline (Alupent) | 0.01–0.03 ml/kg | Dilute in 3 ml normal saline |
| Terbutaline | 0.03–0.05 ml/kg | Dilute in 2–3 ml normal saline |

charged home with follow-up arranged 24–48 hours later.

III. **Asthma.** Asthma is a common condition characterized by respiratory distress and expiratory wheezing associated with reversible airway obstruction. It can affect all age groups, including infants in the first 6 months of life (though this is uncommon). Airway obstruction occurs owing to smooth muscle spasm (albuterol, theophylline responsive), edema, and accumulation of mucus and cellular debris (steroid responsive). The severity of obstruction varies throughout the lung fields, causing ventilation-perfusion mismatch.

A. **Diagnosis and assessment.** If the child is a known asthmatic, determine the number of times he has been hospitalized (including admissions to the intensive care unit) and the medications he is currently taking or has recently taken. Obtain baseline blood gas measurements in children who are moderately or severely distressed and a serum theophylline level in those taking medication. Measurements of electrolytes, complete blood count (CBC), and a blood culture may be ordered as indicated. The characteristic blood gas pattern of adult asthmatics is early hyperventilation and decreased $PCO_2$, progressing to hypercarbia as obstruction increases. This pattern is not always seen in children. Spirometry assessment with a Wright peak flow meter is a good method of determining the severity of the acute attack in the older child, particularly in asthmatics who have a poor subjective sense of dyspnea (see Table 7-2). If available, pulse oximetry is an excellent method for continuous monitoring. Order a chest x ray if pneumothorax or pneumonia is suspected. The classic x-ray findings of asthma include hyperinflation and patchy atelectasis.

B. **Management**

1. **Resuscitation.** A child who uses accessory muscles to breathe or has retractions, pulsus paradoxus $\geq 10$ mm Hg, restlessness, or increasing fatigue needs immediate therapy (see sec. III.B.4). Consider transfer-

Table 7-2. Normal peak flow values for age

| Age (years) | Peak flow (liters/min) | |
|---|---|---|
| | Males | Females |
| 5 | 120 | 145 |
| 6 | 175 | 175 |
| 7 | 210 | 190 |
| 8 | 235 | 230 |
| 9 | 260 | 255 |
| 10 | 285 | 285 |
| 12 | 335 | 348 |
| 14 | 385 | 460 |
| 16 | 530 | 470 |

Note: These are approximations only. Values assume correct use of the peak flow meter.

ring such a child to the intensive care unit for treatment and monitoring.

2. **Mild distress.** Occasionally, mild asthma can present with severe unremitting cough and minimal or no wheezing. These children often respond dramatically to treatment with nebulized bronchodilators and beta agonists (see below, sec. **III.B.2.b and d.(1)**).

   a. **Oxygen.** Give 30–40% humidified oxygen by mask or nasal prongs.

   b. **Nebulized bronchodilators** (see Table 7-1). In children over the age of 6 months, nebulized bronchodilators such as albuterol may be given. The dose of albuterol is .02 ml/kg, given in a 2- to 3-ml dose of isotonic saline. The maximum dose is 1.0 ml. If there is little or no response, repeat a second dose in 15 minutes. In patients with severe asthma, nebulized albuterol can be administered q15min. Alternative nebulized agents include fenoterol, orciprenaline, and terbutaline (see Table 7-1).

   c. **Epinephrine.** If albuterol or other beta-adrenergic agonists are unavailable, epinephrine 1 : 1000 solution can be given, 0.01 mg/kg SC stat and q10min prn 2 times. Epinephrine can result in extreme tachycardia, increased myocardial oxygen demand, and hypertension and should be used with caution in severely compromised or hypoxemic children.

   d. **Outpatient therapy.** If there is complete resolution of symptoms with no evidence of respiratory distress following treatment, the child may be discharged home. Advise parents to return if the child's condition deteriorates. In children who present with minimal or no respiratory distress, outpatient therapy is often unnecessary. In other children who are currently taking no regular medications, the following may be prescribed:

(1) **Beta agonists.** Once the acute phase is over, older children who are able to use an inhaler can be discharged on a beta-adrenergic metered dose inhaler such as albuterol 1–2 puffs q4h prn. In younger children a syrup such as orciprenaline (Alupent), 2 mg/kg/day PO divided q8h, may be given instead.

(2) **Theophylline.** When compared with the beta agonists, theophylline and associated agents are weaker bronchodilators and usually have more side effects. These medications are suitable for children over 1 year of age. In children less than 1 year, use an oral beta agonist (see (1) above).

   (a) **Loading dose.** In the child not previously taking theophylline, begin with a loading dose of 6–7 mg/kg PO of a short-acting preparation such as Palaron or Slo-phyllin.

   (b) **Maintenance dosage.** Short-acting preparations given q6h may be continued on a maintenance dosage as follows: Over age 16: 15 mg/kg/day; 12–16 years: 18 mg/kg/day; 9–12 years: 20 mg/kg/day; 1–9 years: 24 mg/kg/day. Patients in need of chronic maintenance therapy are best treated with a long-acting preparation such as Somophylline 12 or Theodur Sprinkle, given q8–12h.

   (c) In all cases, the dosage should be tailored to the individual by monitoring predose serum blood levels. These samples must be taken 48–72 hours after initiating therapy. The therapeutic range is 55–110 μmol/liter (10–20 μg/ml).

   (d) Advise parents of the side effects, including diarrhea and vomiting. Theophylline clearance may be decreased in children with viral illness, congestive heart failure, hypoalbuminemia, or hepatic dysfunction and in those taking cimetidine, erythromycin, or propranolol. Clearance may be increased in patients who smoke or who are taking phenytoin or phenobarbital.

(3) **Steroids.** Children who have recently been taking prednisone or inhaled steroids and those with repeated visits for nebulized medication may benefit from a 5-day course of oral prednisone, 2 mg/kg/day PO divided

q12h. Unless there is an ongoing need for steroids, these medications should be tapered rapidly over 3 to 4 days once the attack has resolved.

(4) Follow-up and other treatment. Any intercurrent bacterial infection should be treated with antibiotics. Arrange follow-up in 48–72 hours for reassessment, monitoring of theophylline levels, and advice on prevention and treatment of subsequent attacks. Attempts should be made to determine the triggering event.

3. **Moderate or severe distress**
    a. **Oxygen and nebulized bronchodilators.** Nebulized bronchodilators should be administered as outlined above (see sec. **III.B.2.b**).
    b. **Intravenous aminophylline.** Aminophylline should be given by intravenous infusion if there is a limited response to albuterol or at the outset of therapy if the child is in severe distress. Theophylline should be avoided in the treatment of bronchospasm in children under 6 months of age because the response is poor and metabolism is slow and variable.
        (1) **Loading dose.** If the child is not currently taking a theophylline medication, give an IV loading dose of 6 mg/kg, administered in 30 ml of fluid over 30 minutes. If the child is taking a theophylline preparation, give an IV loading dose of up to 3 mg/kg depending on the time of the last dose.
        (2) **Maintenance infusion.** Follow the loading dose with a maintenance infusion dose of 0.9 mg/kg/hour in adolescents and 1.0 mg/kg/hour in younger children. To make up a standard infusion of aminophylline, add 500 mg of aminophylline to 500 ml of 5% DW; the intravenous rate in milliliters per hour equals the child's weight in kilograms for an infusion of 1.0 mg/kg/hour.
        (3) **Monitor and maintain level.** Check the serum theophylline level 30 minutes and 4–6 hours after the loading dose has been given. The therapeutic range is 55–110 μmol/liter (10–20 μg/ml). If the child is in respiratory distress and the level is less than 80 μmol/liter (15 μg/ml), give a repeat bolus of 2 mg/kg over 30 minutes IV and check the level again. Theophylline toxicity may affect the gastrointestinal system (diarrhea, vomiting), central nervous system (CNS, seizures), and cardiovascular system (dysrhythmias) severely. See Chap. 27.
    c. **Steroids.** Systemic steroids—hydrocortisone 20 mg/kg/day IV divided q6h, or predisone 2 mg/kg/

day (maximum daily dose 40 mg) PO divided q12h—should be given to severe asthmatics who meet one or more of the following criteria:

(1) They are taking inhaled steroids currently.
(2) They required steroids previously.
(3) They did not respond adequately to other therapy, remaining wheezy and distressed despite 2–3 hourly nebulized bronchodilators.

4. **Status asthmaticus.** If there is moderate or severe distress despite treatment with three doses of epinephrine or nebulized bronchodilators, the child is in status asthmaticus.

a. **Immediate therapy.** Place the child on a cardiac monitor, give high-flow oxygen by mask, and start an intravenous line.

b. **Nebulized medication.** Give albuterol or another bronchodilator by oxygen-powered nebulizer every 15 minutes.

c. **Intravenous medication.** Give loading and maintenance doses of intravenous aminophylline and administer intravenous steroids as outlined above. If there is an inadequate response to these measures, consider treatment with intravenous infusions of isoproterenol, epinephrine, or albuterol (see Infusion section of Appendix V for dosage and administration).

d. **Ventilation.** Intubation and ventilation with general anesthetic agents using volume-cycled ventilators may be required in children who are resistant to other forms of therapy. Arrange transfer to an intensive care facility.

IV. **Foreign body aspiration**

A. **Diagnosis and assessment.** The most common sites of aspiration are the right and left main stem bronchi in that order. A history of choking or gagging on food or a small toy should not be ignored in the child with symptoms or signs of foreign body aspiration. Initially, a foreign body in the bronchus may be asymptomatic, may cause mild distress with cough and wheeze, or may result in more severe symptoms of obstruction with hemoptysis. Auscultation of the chest may be normal, but there are usually inspiratory and expiratory rhonchi and diminished or absent breath sounds on one side. If **partial** obstruction of a bronchus is suspected, obtain inspiratory and expiratory chest x rays; look for obstructive emphysema with shifting of the mediastinum away from the foreign body during expiration. If there is **complete** obstruction of a bronchus there may be collapse of the lung with ipsilateral shift of the mediastinum. A normal chest x ray does not rule out the diagnosis of foreign body aspiration. Fluoroscopy can be invaluable in locating a radiolucent object (see Chap. 14).

B. **Management.** When foreign body aspiration is suspected, consult an ENT surgeon for rigid bronchoscopy under general anesthesia. Do not tip the stable child upside down or try to remove the foreign body; this may convert a partial to a complete obstruction. Initial treatment of the child with respiratory distress includes oxygen and bronchodilators by nebulizer (see Table 7-2). There may be infection distal to the foreign body; if there is fever, obtain blood samples, for CBC and culture and treat with intravenous ampicillin 100 mg/kg/day IV divided q6h or cefuroxime 75–150 mg/kg/day divided q8h.

**V. Disposition.** Admit all patients with respiratory distress who do not completely respond to therapy with nebulized adrenergic agonists. Children in status asthmaticus should be transferred to an intensive care unit. All children with foreign body aspiration require admission and bronchoscopy.

**VI. Key points**
   **A.** Asthma and bronchiolitis may be life threatening and require immediate therapy. Bronchiolitis is the result of a specific infection, whereas asthma has a multifactorial etiology.
   **B.** Bronchodilators may be useful for either condition in children over the age of 6 months. Early use of steroids is important in the treatment of severe asthma.
   **C.** Children with severe respiratory distress should be managed in a pediatric intensive care unit.

### Bibliography

Behrman, R. E., and Vaughan V. C., (eds.). *Nelson's Textbook of Pediatrics.* Philadelphia: Saunders, 1983.

Patterson, R. (ed.). *Allergic Diseases: Diagnosis and Management.* Philadelphia: Lippincott, 1980.

Seibert, R. W. Foreign Bodies. In J. Y. Suen and S. J. Wetmore (eds.), *Emergencies in Otolaryngology.* New York: Churchill Livingstone, 1986.

Weinberger, M., et al. Clinical pharmacology of drugs used for asthma. *Pediatr. Clin. North Am.* 28:47, 1981.

Wright, P. F. Bronchiolitis. *Pediatr. Rev.* 7(7):219–222, 1986.

# Congestive Heart Failure

George G. S. Sandor

Cardiac failure occurs when the heart is unable to deliver adequate oxygen to the tissues. The majority of children present with respiratory distress, gallop rhythm, cardiomegaly, and hepatomegaly.

I. **Causes.** Most cases of congestive heart failure are due to congenital lesions and present in infancy. Acquired heart disease is seen in all age groups. Diseases causing heart failure can be classified according to the pathophysiologic mechanism: (1) abnormalities causing volume load; (2) abnormalities causing pressure load; (3) abnormalities of the cardiac muscle; (4) abnormalities of heart rate.

   A. **The older child.** Causes of cardiac failure in the older child include viral myocarditis, rheumatic carditis, congestive cardiomyopathies, and palliated congenital cardiac malformations. In children with existing heart disease, the stress of respiratory infections such as bronchiolitis or influenza can induce heart failure. Severe anemia from any cause can lead to high-output heart failure.

   B. **The infant.** Heart failure in infancy is usually due to congenital disease or myocarditis. Congenital disease that presents in the first weeks of life is usually due to a left-sided obstructive lesion such as aortic stenosis, coarctation, or hypoplastic left heart syndrome.

   C. **Hemodynamic classification.** See Table 8-1.

II. **Diagnosis**

   A. **History**

      1. **Infants.** Neonates and infants with heart failure frequently fail to thrive. Feeding is often slow (>15–20 minutes) and may be associated with shortness of breath, sweating, pallor, cyanosis, cough, or vomiting.

      2. **Children.** Respiratory symptoms predominate in the older child (see sec. **II.B**). In addition, patients may be tired, anorexic, and pale and show poor growth. Other symptoms include nonspecific chest pain and palpitations. Orthopnea, paroxysmal nocturnal dyspnea, and syncope are rare. In the previously well child with recent viral infection, consider the etiology of viral myocarditis, which is one of the most common forms of acquired congestive heart failure. In children with known congenital heart disease determine whether intercurrent infection or noncompliance with medication is the cause of decompensation.

   B. **Examination.** Look for signs of poor perfusion and systemic or pulmonary congestion and determine the pathophysiologic mechanism (volume, pressure, muscle, rate).

      1. **General signs**

         a. The child responds to cardiac failure with **in-**

**Table 8-1. Hemodynamic classification of heart failure**

| Pathophysiologic mechanism | Examples |
| --- | --- |
| Volume load | |
|    Left-to-right shunts | VSD, PDA, AV canal, AV malformation |
|    Regurgitant valve lesions | Truncus arteriosus |
|    Other | Severe anemia |
| Pressure load | |
|    Left-sided obstruction | Hypoplastic left heart, coarctation, AS |
|    Other | Severe hypertension |
| Myocardial disease | |
|    Intrinsic | Myocarditis, endocardial fibroelastosis, cardiomyopathies |
|    Metabolic | Pompe's disease, hypoxia, hypocalcemia, hypoglycemia |
| Heart rate | |
|    Tachyarrhythmia | |
|    Bradyarrhythmia | |

Key: VSD = ventricular septal defect, PDA = patent ductus arteriosus, AV = atrioventricular, AS = aortic stenosis

      creased **sympathetic tone** causing tachycardia and sweating.

    **b. Cardiomegaly** may be detected by noting a lateral and downward displacement of the apex. There is a gallop rhythm, heard best at the apex with the bell of the stethoscope.

    **c. Pulmonary edema** or pulmonary congestion often mimics bronchiolitis, asthma, or pneumonia with wheezing, tachypnea, respiratory retractions, and cough. There may be rhonchi on auscultation. Inspiratory rales due to pulmonary edema are rare in the young child with heart failure.

    **d. Systemic venous congestion** secondary to cardiac failure causes hepatomegaly with an increase in the liver span. This is the most consistent sign of early failure in infancy. Peripheral edema and neck vein distention are difficult to detect in the infant and young child. When cardiac output is severely impaired, the child has cool peripheries and a rapid pulse.

    **e. Cyanosis and hypotension** are signs of extreme distress in the child with heart failure. Cyanosis may also be due to a congenital lesion with right-to-left shunting (see Chap. 20).

  **2. Signs of volume overload.** With volume overload the precordium is usually hyperactive, and there is cardiomegaly. *Left* ventricular overload results in an active apical impulse. *Right*-sided overload results in an active right ventricular impulse felt at the parasternal area or epigastrium. Shunts at the great vessel level, such as patent ductus arteriosus (PDA), cause bounding pulses. Auscultation of a continuous machinery murmur may help confirm the diagnosis of PDA.

   **3. Signs of pressure overload.** Poor peripheral pulses indicate a left ventricular outflow obstruction. Pressure load can cause ventricular dilatation, but, in contrast to volume overload, the apex is not vigorous. Careful auscultation may help to locate the lesion.

   **4. Signs of myocardial dysfunction.** Myocardial dysfunction frequently results in poor pulses, quiet heart sounds, and a dilated heart with a weak apex beat.

**C. X rays.** Chest x-ray findings of cardiomegaly and pulmonary congestion often aid in the diagnosis of heart failure in the child who presents to the emergency room with respiratory distress.

**III. Management.** See Table 9-1 for drug dosages.

  **A. General measures**

    **1.** Give oxygen to all children with heart failure and obtain blood gas measurements, electrocardiogram (ECG), chest x ray, and an echocardiogram. Obtain blood for measurement of blood urea nitrogen (BUN), electrolytes, glucose, and complete blood count (CBC). Repeated blood gas determinations are crucial when respiratory distress is increasing.

    **2.** Start an intravenous line, restrict fluid intake to two-thirds of the maintenance amount, and stop feeding until the condition is stable. Indications for ventilation of the child with cardiac failure include a $PaCO_2$ greater than 60 mm Hg, increasing fatigue, or hypoxia with an $FIO_2$ of 0.6 or greater (see Chap. 1).

    **3.** The child with congestive heart failure should be positioned sitting upright. In the infant this is achieved by using a Cuddle Seat or by raising the head of the bed with the child held in place by a sling around the diaper area.

    **4.** A cardiologist should be consulted immediately.

**B. Correct the cause.** Correction of the cause is the best approach when cardiac failure is secondary to hypoglycemia, acidosis, anemia, or dysrhythmia (see Chaps. 9, 13, 19, and 23). When possible, the clinical status of patients with surgical congenital lesions should be improved prior to surgery.

**C. Diuretics.** Diuretic therapy is beneficial to most children with heart failure. In the emergency room setting, furosemide (Lasix) is the agent of choice; give 1 mg/kg intravenously.

**D. Digoxin.** In nearly all cases, digoxin is the inotropic drug of choice. After a diuretic has been given, the child should be digitalized with three doses given q8h over a period of 16 hours. Rule out hypokalemia prior to administration. See Table 9-1 for details regarding digoxin therapy.

**E. Other medications** (see Table 9-1 for dosages)
    **1. Inotropic agents**
        **a. Dopamine.** An intravenous infusion of dopamine can be used in cases of severe cardiac failure when collapse is imminent (see Chap. 4).
        **b. Isoproterenol.** Isoproterenol may be helpful in children with heart failure and severe bradycardia. Isoproterenol increases myocardial irritability and predisposes to dysrhythmia and hypotension (see Chap. 4).
    **2. Prostaglandin E.** This drug should be given to the sick newborn with an obstructive (pressure load) or cyanotic heart lesion (see Chaps. 4 and 20, Cyanosis in the Infant).

**IV. Disposition.** All children presenting with heart failure should be admitted. Severely ill infants should be cared for in an intensive care unit.

**V. Key points**
    **A.** Congestive heart failure in children usually presents with signs of pulmonary congestion, hepatomegaly, and a gallop rhythm.
    **B.** Correction of the cause when identified, as well as careful use of oxygen, diuretics, and digoxin will ameliorate severe congestive heart failure in the majority of children.
    **C.** Prostaglandin $E_1$ may be useful for temporary treatment of severe obstructive congenital heart disease.

**Bibliography**

Adams, F. and Emmanuellides, G. *Heart Disease in Infants, Children and Adolescents.* Baltimore: Williams & Wilkins, 1983.

Keith, J., Rowe, R., and Vlad, P. *Heart Disease in Infancy and Childhood.* New York: Macmillan, 1978.

# Dysrhythmias

George G. S. Sandor

Dysrhythmias may be primary electrophysiologic phenomena or secondary to such conditions as acquired or congenital heart disease, hypothermia, electrolyte disturbance, toxic ingestion, or systemic disease (such as systemic lupus erythematosus). For normal heart rates for age see Appendix II.

I. **Electrocardiographic recognition.** Diagnosis is achieved by systematic analysis of the surface electrocardiogram (ECG), including examination of the R-R interval and rate, the QRS duration (normally $\leq$ 0.08–0.10 seconds, depending on age), and the interrelationship of the P and QRS waves (Fig. 9-1).

II. **Commonly observed dysrhythmias that do not require treatment**
   A. **Supraventricular**
      1. Atrial ectopic beats
      2. Junctional ectopic beats
      3. Sinus pause
      4. First-degree heart block
      5. Type 1 second-degree heart block
   B. **Ventricular.** Ventricular dysrhythmias that do not require treatment include:
      1. Ventricular ectopic beats (Fig. 9-3)
      2. Ventricular bigeminy
      3. Ventricular escape beats following a sinus pause of less than 3 seconds' duration (in the absence of bradycardia)

III. **Tachyarrhythmias.** The approximate definitions of tachycardia by age are: > 180 beats/minute in the newborn and infant, > 150 beats/minute in the toddler, and > 120 beats/minute in children over 6 years of age.
   A. **Principles of management of tachyarrhythmias.** For drug dosages see Table 9-1.
      1. Assess and control problems in the airway, breathing, or circulation.
      2. Give oxygen by mask, start an intravenous line, and obtain blood gas measurements. In the child taking digoxin, determine the digoxin level present in the blood. If the cause of dysrhythmia is unknown, draw blood for measurement of electrolytes, glucose, and toxic screen.
      3. Children with tachyarrhythmia are considered **hemodynamically unstable** if any of the following are present: (1) heart failure, (2) evidence of poor perfusion, including cool peripheries, reduced capillary filling, and decreased urine output, or (3) hypotension. If the child is **unstable,** use synchronized DC cardioversion beginning with a dose of 0.2 joule/kg. If this is unsuccessful, repeat cardioversion, increasing the dose in increments of 0.2 joule/kg to a maximum of 1.0 joule/kg (see Chap. 3).

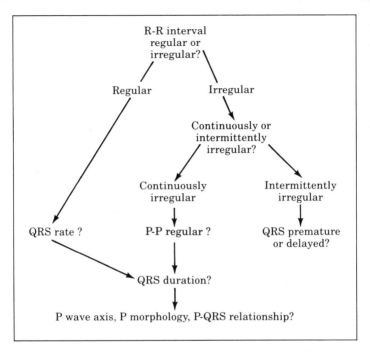

Fig. 9-1. ECG recognition algorithm. (From Garson, A., Jr., Gillette, P. C., and McNamara, D. G. *A Guide to Cardiac Dysrhythmias in Children*. Philadelphia: Saunders, 1981.)

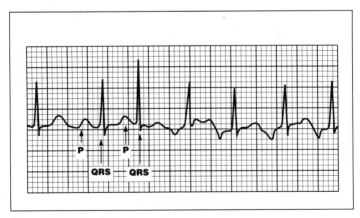

Fig. 9-2. SVT ectopic beats.

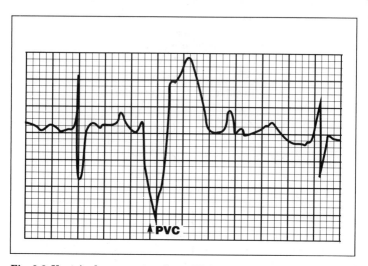

**Fig. 9-3. Ventricular premature beat (PVC).**

4. If the child with a tachyarrhythmia is hemodynamically **stable,** a trial of vagal maneuvers or drug therapy is in order.

**B. Supraventricular tachycardia** (SVT). SVT is one of the most common tachyarrhythmias in children. SVT is a group of disorders that includes paroxysmal atrial tachycardia (PAT), atrial flutter, atrial fibrillation, and aberrantly conducted supraventricular tachyarrhythmias. In the absence of intrinsic cardiac disease, these disturbances can usually be tolerated for 24 hours or more before the child becomes unstable.

**Dysrhythmias due to increased automaticity** (paroxysmal junctional reciprocating tachycardia, atrial ectopic tachycardia) are less common. They tend to "warm up and slow down" rather than having a sudden onset or termination. P waves are absent or abnormal, and the rate is slower than in SVT. They are usually well tolerated and are resistant to treatment.

1. **Paroxysmal atrial tachycardia** (Fig. 9-4). Usually of sudden onset and termination, PAT is often due to reentrant phenomena such as Wolfe-Parkinson-White (WPW) syndrome, the most common identifiable cause of reentrant tachycardia.

   a. **ECG findings**

      (1) The R-R interval is regular, although it may be irregular with concurrent atrioventricular (AV) block.

      (2) The QRS rate is increased to 160–200/minute in cases of sinoatrial node reentry, and 240–300/minute in AV node reentry.

**Table 9-1. Cardiac medications**

| Drug | Dose | Route | Caution |
|---|---|---|---|
| Atropine | 0.02 mg/kg (minimum dose 0.1 mg) | IV | |
| Bretylium | Initially: 5 mg/kg | IV (over 10 min) | |
| | Maintenance: 5–10 mg/kg q6–8h | IV | |
| Digoxin | *Loading:* Give 50% of load as first dose IV, then 25% q8h for two subsequent doses: | | Add 25% for PO |
| | Neonate: see Appendix V | | |
| | 1 mo–2 yr: 30–40 μg/kg | IV | Assess $K^+$, BUN, and creatinine in serum |
| | Over 2 yr: 25–30 μg/kg | IV | |
| | *Maintenance:* | | |
| | Neonate: see Appendix V | | |
| | 1 mo–2 yr: 10–12 μg/kg/day | IV | Divide dose q12h. Start maintenance dose 12 hours after last portion of loading dose |
| | Over 2 yr: 6–8 μg/kg/day | IV | |
| Dopamine | 2–25 μg/kg/min | IV | May cause necrosis if it extravasates. Use central IV if possible |
| Isoproterenol | 0.025–1.0 μg/kg/min | IV | Ventricular irritability |
| Lidocaine | Initially: 1 mg/kg and may repeat once | IV | Seizures |
| | Maintenance: 10–50 μg/kg/min | IV | |
| Propranolol | Initially: 0.05–0.20 mg/kg | IV (over 10 min) | Myocardial depression |
| | Maintenance: 0.05–5.00 mg/kg/day | PO | |
| Verapamil | 0.15–0.40 mg/kg; may repeat once | IV | Myocardial depression, avoid in neonates |

   **(3)** The QRS duration is normal unless there is concurrent AV block.
   **(4)** The P wave is not visible.
   **b. Treatment.** The majority of cases revert spontaneously to sinus rhythm.
      **(1)** If the patient is hemodynamically **unstable,** use synchronized DC cardioversion with 0.2–1.0 joule/kg.
      **(2)** If the child is hemodynamically **stable:**
         **(a) Vagal maneuvers** such as the diving reflex may be tried, using an ice water-soaked cloth applied to the face.
         **(b) Digoxin** may be used but only if the QRS complexes are narrow ($\leq 0.10$ seconds).
         **(c) Verapamil** can be effective. It should be used with caution, especially if other myocardial depressants have been given. Verapamil is contraindicated in infancy and in patients with myocardial disease.
         **(d) Propranolol** can be administered. It is contraindicated in the child who has been given verapamil.
         **(e) Overdrive pacing** can be used if it is available.
   **2. Atrial flutter** (Fig. 9-5). In children, atrial flutter may be associated with atrial enlargement, sick sinus syndrome, and electrolyte abnormalities.
      **a. ECG findings**
         **(1)** The R-R interval is regular (irregular when there is concurrent AV block).
         **(2)** The QRS rate is increased (may be slow when there is concurrent AV block).
         **(3)** A sawtooth configuration of flutter waves is seen.
         **(4)** The atrial rate is 250–500/minute, and the ventricular rate varies with AV conduction (one-half the atrial rate in 2 : 1 heart block, one-third in 3 : 1 heart block).
      **b. Treatment**
         **(1)** If the child is hemodynamically **unstable,** cardioversion with synchronized DC shock (0.2–1.0 joule/kg) may be used.
         **(2)** If the patient is hemodynamically **stable,** digitalization is the treatment of choice.
         **(3)** Quinidine, procainamide, and propranolol may also be used; these are contraindicated in sinus node disease—see sec. **IV.B.**
         **(4)** Overdrive pacing may be used.
   **3. Atrial fibrillation** (Fig. 9-6). This is a rare dysrhythmia in children. Atrial fibrillation is seen with atrial enlargement, electrolyte abnormalities, hyperthyroidism, certain myocardial diseases, and following cardiac surgery. It can occur simultaneously with atrial flutter.

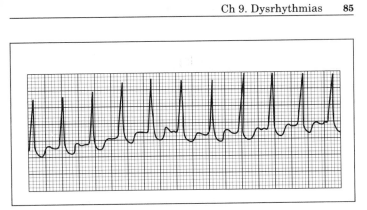

**Fig. 9-4. SVT rate 160.**

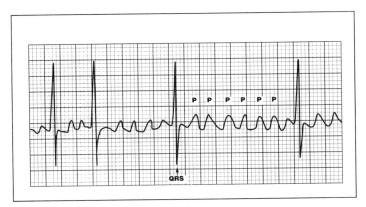

**Fig. 9-5. Atrial flutter, variable block.**

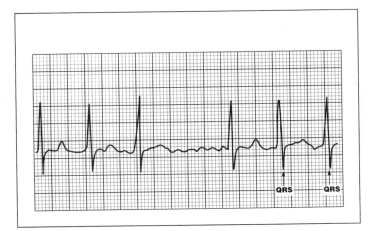

**Fig. 9-6. Atrial fibrillation, variable block.**

### a. ECG findings
   (1) The R-R interval is irregularly irregular.
   (2) The atrial rate is irregular with a jagged baseline.
   (3) There are no P waves.
### b. Treatment. Treatment is the same as that used for atrial flutter. Chronic therapy with digoxin is recommended.
## C. Ventricular tachycardia (Fig. 9-7). This rare dysrhythmia occurs in children with congenital heart disease, electrolyte abnormalities, hypoxia, poisoning, tumors, long QT and WPW syndromes, and following cardiac surgery. **Ventricular tachycardia (VT) must be differentiated from SVT associated with aberrant conduction, bundle branch block, or conduction down an accessory bundle.**

### 1. ECG findings. Use the ECG to differentiate SVT from VT:
   **a.** In SVT the rate is usually 170–350 beats/minute; in VT the rate is slower (although in some instances VT may be in excess of 200/minute).
   **b.** In SVT a P wave is often seen, and there is a triphasic QRS complex in lead $V_1$; these are absent in VT.
   **c.** The regularity of tachycardia, the QRS configuration, the presence of fusion beats, and the position of the initial QRS vector are unreliable for use in differentiating between SVT and VT in children.

### 2. Treatment
   **a.** If the patient is hemodynamically **unstable,** use cardioversion with synchronized DC shock, 0.2–1.0 joule/kg. This should be followed with a lidocaine infusion.
   **b.** Intravenous lidocaine infusion can be used before or after attempting DC cardioversion.
   **c.** Overdrive pacing may be used in refractory cases.

## IV. Bradyarrhythmias. The approximate definitions of bradycardia by age are: < 90 beats/minute in the newborn, < 110 in the infant, < 80 in the toddler, and < 60 in the child over 6 years (Appendix II). Normal neonates and infants may have asymptomatic and transient decreases in heart rate while asleep—to 70/minute and occasionally to 50/minute. Healthy children and adults have been found to have heart rates of 40/minute during deep sleep.

Symptomatic bradycardia may result in syncope, seizures, heart failure, or shock; in these cases the cause is usually an underlying structural or myocardial disease. In the previously well child, suspect hypothermia or drug ingestion (cyclic antidepressants, narcotics, digoxin, barbiturates, cholinergics). For drug dosages used in treatment, see Table 9-1.

### A. Management of the child with symptomatic bradyarrhythmia
   **1.** Assess and control problems relating to the airway, breathing, or circulation.

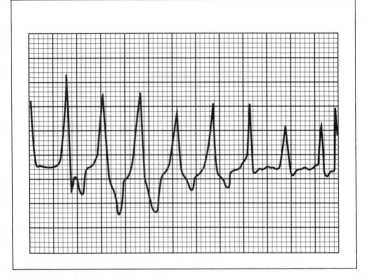

**Fig. 9-7. Ventricular tachycardia.**

2. Give oxygen by mask, start an intravenous line, and check blood gas measurements. In the child taking digoxin, determine the digoxin level present in the blood. If the cause of dysrhythmia is unknown, draw a blood sample for measurement of electrolytes, glucose, and toxic screen.

3. Symptomatic bradycardia usually requires treatment with a pacemaker; atropine and isoproterenol may be used to temporize if a pacemaker is not immediately available.

4. Children with ventricular fibrillation require advanced life support and immediate defibrillation with 2 joule/kg in **nonsynchronized** mode (see Chap. 3).

B. **Sinus node disease.** Often termed "sick sinus syndrome," this entity may present with syncope, brady- or tachyarrhythmias, or heart failure. Severe sinus node disease results in decreased perfusion and hypotension.

1. **ECG findings**

a. Severe sinus bradycardia can occur.

b. There may be a loss of P waves and a very low ventricular rate.

2. **Treatment**

a. The **asymptomatic** child with stable vital signs should be placed on a cardiac monitor and admitted for observation.

b. If the child is **symptomatic:**

(1) Atropine may be given intravenously, intramuscularly, or through an endotracheal tube.

(2) If atropine is ineffective, start an intrave-

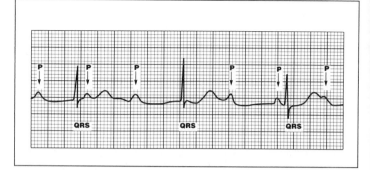

**Fig. 9-8. Complete heart block.**

nous infusion of isoproterenol and arrange
for insertion of a temporary cardiac pacemaker.

(3) Temporary pacing is required in most children with symptomatic bradycardia. Exceptions to this rule are children in whom the
arrhythmia is due to a noncardiac cause—
such as drug ingestion or severe hypothermia—that responds to medical therapy.

**C. Heart block**

1. Congenital heart block may be associated with neonatal lupus or structural malformations such as ventricular inversion.

2. Acquired heart block may be due to myocarditis,
drug ingestion (cyclic antidepressants, digoxin), cardiac surgery, or cardiac catheterization.

3. Patients with first- and second-degree block are usually asymptomatic. Children with third-degree or
complete heart block are often symptomatic and require emergency treatment (Fig. 9-8).

4. **ECG findings in third-degree heart block**

   a. The R-R interval is regular.

   b. The QRS rate is decreased.

   c. The duration of the QRS complex is normal.

   d. There is dissociation between the P wave and the
   QRS complex.

   e. Note: Third-degree heart block can occur simultaneously with any supraventricular rhythm.

5. **Treatment.** The treatment is the same as that used
for sinus node disease.

**D. Ventricular fibrillation.** Ventricular fibrillation originates from ventricular tachycardia. This is an end-
stage dysrhythmia that results in little or no cardiac
output. Full resuscitation with chest compression, intubation, and ventilation is required (see Chap. 3).

1. **ECG findings.** The ECG shows low voltage, irregular, polymorphous complexes.

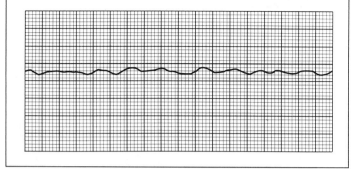

**Fig. 9-9. Ventricular fibrillation.**

    **2. Treatment** (see Chap. 3)
      **a.** Defibrillate with **nonsynchronized** DC shock, 2–4 joules/kg.
      **b.** If defibrillation is unsuccessful, give lidocaine, first as a bolus and then by infusion.
      **c.** Bretylium may be tried in refractory cases.
**V. Disposition.** Admit all patients with serious dysrhythmias. Children who have unstable hemodynamic status should be transferred to an intensive care unit.
**VI. Key points**
    **A.** A systematic approach to the surface ECG, determining the R-R interval and rate, the P-P interval, and the relationship between the P and QRS waves will lead to the diagnosis in most cases.
    **B.** SVT is the most common serious dysrhythmia in children. It can be treated with vagal maneuvers or digoxin in the hemodynamically stable child, whereas **synchronized** cardioversion is the treatment of choice in the patient who is hemodynamically unstable.

**Bibliography**

Adams, F., and Emmanuellides, G. *Heart Disease in Infants, Children and Adolescents.* Baltimore: Williams & Wilkins, 1983.

Keith, J., Rowe, R., and Vlad, P. *Heart Disease in Infancy and Childhood.* New York: Macmillan, 1978.

Roberts, N., and Gelbland, H. *Cardiac Arrhythmias in the Infant, Neonate and Child.* Norwalk: Appleton-Century-Crofts, 1983.

Gillette, P., and Garson, A., Jr. *Pediatric Cardiac Dysrhythmias.* New York: Grune & Stratton, 1981.

Garson, A., Jr., Gillette, P., and McNamara. *A Guide to Cardiac Dysrhythmias in Children.* New York: Grune & Stratton, 1981.

# Syncope, Chest Pain, and Hemoptysis

Gregory A. Baldwin

**I. Syncope.** Sudden loss of consciousness in the child is usually due to a vasovagal episode or orthostatic hypotension. In most instances, the diagnosis can be made by the history alone.

  **A.** Diagnosis and assessment

    **1. History**

      **a. Fainting.** Fainting or vasovagal syncope is preceded by a prodrome with a sensation of numbness, sweating, lightheadedness, vertigo, and visual disturbance. Fainting spells occur while the person is standing upright after extreme emotion or after prolonged standing or fasting, often on a hot, humid day. There is complete recovery on waking.

      **b. Orthostatic hypotension.** Children with orthostatic hypotension often have a history of postural dizziness and are dehydrated or anemic.

      **c. Seizures.** Seizures may be preceded by an aura. Incontinence, abnormal movements, and post-episode confusion or sleepiness support the diagnosis of seizure.

      **d. Hysterical syncope.** Hysterical syncope is seen primarily in older children and adolescent females. It occurs in front of witnesses, and there is often a background of emotional stress. There is no prodrome, and there may be associated moaning or unusual body movements.

      **e. Hyperventilation.** Hyperventilation per se rarely causes real syncope but is often described by victims as a "blackout."

      **f. Drug ingestion or abuse.** Causative agents include CNS depressants, cocaine, and amphetamines.

      **g. Metabolic disease.** Diabetes mellitus or any disease that predisposes to hypoglycemia, hypocalcemia, or hypoxia can result in syncope.

      **h. Cough/swallowing syncope.** Rare cases of syncope induced by paroxysmal cough or swallowing have been reported in children.

      **i. Cardiac syncope.** Cardiac syncope is suggested by a history of sudden loss of consciousness during exercise or exertion. Previous cardiac disease, palpitations, or other cardiac symptoms support the diagnosis.

      **j. Syncope in infants.** Syncope in the infant should never be regarded as simple or benign; it is invariably due to neonatal apnea, seizure, or cardiac dysrhythmia.

    **2. Examination.** Assess the vital signs, including postural changes in blood pressure and heart rate. In

**Table 10-1. Causes of syncope in childhood**

| | |
|---|---|
| Vascular/reflex | Simple syncope (faint), orthostatic hypotension, anemia/volume loss, hyperventilation, cough, micturition, swallow, migraine, Takayasu disease, pregnancy |
| Cardiac | Obstruction, dysrhythmia, heart block, myocarditis, cardiomyopathy, mitral valve prolapse, pericardial effusion, long QT syndrome, coronary anomaly, pulmonary artery hypertension, right ventricular dysplasia, indwelling central venous catheter, tumor |
| Neurologic | Seizures, vertigo, autonomic instability (central) |
| Psychologic | Hysteria, hyperventilation |
| Metabolic | Hypoglycemia, hypocalcemia, hypomagnesemia, hypoxia, abnormal values for sodium, potassium, chloride |
| Drugs | Cyclic antidepressants, antihypertensives, diuretics, barbiturates, phenothiazines, quinidine, nitrates, cocaine, and other substances of abuse |

Source: Adapted from R. N. Ruckman. Cardiac causes of syncope. *Pediatr. Rev.* 9: 100, 1987.

moving from a lying to a standing position, the drop in systolic blood pressure should be less than 15 mm Hg, and the increase in heart rate should be less than 20 beats/minute. A full cardiovascular and neurologic examination should be performed, noting any murmurs, dysrhythmia, decrease in the level of consciousness, or focal neurologic signs.

3. **Electrocardiogram.** Obtain an electrocardiogram (ECG) and examine it for evidence of dysrhythmia, prolonged QT interval, or signs of Wolfe-Parkinson-White (WPW) syndrome such as a wide QRS, a delta wave upstroke, or short PR interval.

4. **Laboratory tests.** Obtain blood for measurement of complete blood count (CBC), electrolytes, and glucose. Calcium and magnesium measurements may be ordered when indicated by the history or physical examination.

B. **Disposition.** Admit children with true loss of consciousness due to organic disorders, infants, and patients with a history that suggests a cardiac cause of syncope. Continuous ECG monitoring is mandatory.

C. **Key points.** Most cases of syncope are benign fainting spells. Syncope associated with cardiac symptoms or exercise or that occurring in young children or infants is more likely to be cardiac in etiology.

**Table 10-2. Causes of chest pain in children**

| | |
|---|---|
| Musculoskeletal | Chest wall strain, costochondritis, direct trauma, slipping rib syndrome |
| Cardiac disease | Dysrhythmia, outflow obstruction, Kawasaki's syndrome, Friedreich's ataxia, coronary artery anomalies, myocardial infarction or ischemia |
| Pulmonary disease | Chronic cough, pneumonia, asthma, pleural effusion, pneumothorax, pneumomediastinum |
| Gastrointestinal disorders | Esophagitis, esophageal foreign body, caustic ingestion |
| Miscellaneous disorders | Sickle cell crisis, precordial catch, cigarette smoking, shingles, pleurodynia, thoracic tumor, breast mass |

Source: Adapted from S. M. Selbst. Evaluation of chest pain in children. *Pediatr. Rev.* 8: 57, 1986.

**II. Chest pain.** Chest pain is unusual before late childhood or adolescence. It is rarely cardiac in origin (Table 10-2). The diagnosis can usually be made by the history and physical examination alone, without the aid of x rays, ECGs, or other investigations.

**A. Diagnosis and assessment**

    **1. History.** In general, chest pain of long standing is less likely to have an organic etiology, whereas pain of acute onset needs a more thorough investigation.

        **a. Pleuritic pain.** Pleuritic pain is sharp and increases with coughing or deep breathing. It may arise from the musculoskeletal chest wall, lung, pleura, or pericardium. Musculoskeletal disorders are the most commonly diagnosed causes of chest pain in children; question the child about recent trauma or activities causing muscle strain. Pain that is relieved in a particular position suggests a diagnosis of chest wall trauma, muscle strain, or pericarditis. Costochondritis causes pleuritic pain at the costochondral junction. It occurs following coughing fits associated with upper respiratory tract infection or exercise and is more common in females. Spontaneous pneumothorax presents with sudden onset of pain and shortness of breath and usually occurs in adolescents and young adults.

        **b. Esophageal pain.** Esophageal disorders such as esophagitis, foreign body lodged in the esophagus, or caustic ingestion can cause chest pain. Esophagitis may be accompanied by burning epigastric discomfort that radiates into the chest and is related to meals.

**c. Functional disturbance.** Children with pain due to psychologic stress often have a history of anxiety and emotional disturbance. The pain is usually pleuritic and may be associated with psychogenic hyperventilation.

**d. Cardiac pain.** Suspect cardiac chest pain in the child with a history of heart disease, Kawasaki's syndrome, or Friedreich's ataxia. The older child may describe a squeezing, aching, retrosternal discomfort, often with radiation into the left arm, jaw, or back. Pain that is made worse by exercise or is accompanied by syncope or palpitations is highly suggestive of cardiac disease.

**2. Examination.** Check the vital signs; if dysrhythmia or tachypnea is present, suspect cardiac or pulmonary disease. On chest examination, listen for wheeze, rales, or alteration in breath sounds suggesting a pulmonary etiology. A friction rub may be due to pulmonary or pericardial disease. In the cardiovascular examination, listen for murmurs and dysrhythmia. A midsystolic click and late systolic murmur may be due to mitral valve prolapse, which is believed to cause chest pain and dysrhythmia in children.

Palpate the chest wall. Crepitus over the neck and upper chest due to subcutaneous emphysema suggests a diagnosis of mediastinal emphysema and/or pneumothorax. Musculoskeletal pain may be reproduced or altered by direct pressure over the painful area or by movement of the arms or chest. When pain from esophagitis is suspected, the diagnosis can often be confirmed if relief is gained with a dose of antacid.

**3. X rays and ECG.** X rays and ECG are rarely needed in the evaluation of the child with chest pain and are unlikely to be helpful unless the history or physical examination suggests a cardiac or pulmonary cause.

**B. Disposition.** Children with chest pain need hospitalization if there is evidence of serious chest trauma, associated cardiac symptoms, a history of Kawasaki's syndrome, cardiac disease, or Friedreich's ataxia. Patients with pain on exertion or pain due to pleural effusion, pneumothorax, foreign body, or caustic ingestion also require admission.

**C. Key points.** Chest pain is nearly always musculoskeletal in origin.

**III. Hemoptysis.** In most instances, hemoptysis is **apparent** and is secondary to nasopharyngeal or gastrointestinal bleeding. Most cases of **true** hemoptysis are due to infection with pneumonia, laryngotracheobronchitis, or cystic fibrosis. Foreign body aspiration, neoplasm, tuberculosis, trauma, and cardiac or arteriovenous malformations are other causes of this rare symptom in childhood. **Massive**

hemoptysis is primarily seen in children with bronchiectasis and, in particular, in cystic fibrosis (CF) patients.

**A. Management**

1. All children with significant (more than blood-tinged), true hemoptysis require admission to hospital. Cystic fibrosis patients with only "streaking" in the sputum can be treated as outpatients with vitamin K, 5 mg PO twice a week, instructing parents to return if bleeding increases or chest symptoms worsen.

2. A chest x ray should be ordered to look for lung pathology, although a normal x ray does not rule out disorders such as foreign body aspiration.

3. Massive hemoptysis ($>$ 300 ml over 24 hours in the adolescent, $>$ 10 ml/kg/24 hours in the child) may lead to asphyxiation and shock and must be attended to urgently. These children require intravenous access, cross-match, and admission to an intensive care unit for resuscitation and investigation with endoscopy.

4. CF patients with massive hemoptysis should be treated with vitamin K 5 mg PO daily. Physiotherapy should be withheld. Obtain blood for cross-match, CBC, platelet count, prothrombin time (PT), and partial thromboplastin time (PTT), and start treatment with intravenous antibiotics.

**B. Key points**

1. The most common causes of hemoptysis are infection and foreign body aspiration.

2. Patients with massive hemoptysis ($>$ 10 ml/kg or 300 ml in 24 hours) require immediate IV line placement, cross-match, and admission to an intensive care unit.

**Bibliography**

Rowland, T. W., and Richards, M. M. The natural history of idiopathic chest pain in children. *Clin. Pediatr.* 25:612, 1986.

Ruckman, R. N. Cardiac causes of syncope. *Pediatr. Rev.* 9:101, 1987.

Selbst, S. M. Evaluation of chest pain in children. *Pediatr. Rev.* 8:56, 1986.

Tom, L. W. C., et al. Hemoptysis in children. *Ann. Otol. Rhinol. Laryngol.* 89:419, 1980.

Trento, A. Massive hemoptysis in patients with cystic fibrosis: Three case reports and a protocol for clinical management. *Ann. Thorac. Surg.* 39:254, 1985.

# Diagnostic Categories

# 11

# Dental Disorders

Karen Wardill and Gary D. Derkson

## I. Examination of the dental patient
### A. Extraoral examination
1. **Inspection**
   a. **Symmetry.** Observe the symmetry of the facial outline anteriorly, in profile, and with the child's head raised to look at the ceiling. Asymmetry of the jaw may be due to a fracture or a dental infection. Swelling or deformity of the face or neck should also be noted.
   b. **Skin.** Note the color of the facial skin and look for hematoma, bruising, and ulcers. A fistulous tract from a dental abscess may present with a skin "pimple."
   c. **Mouth.** Observe the range and symmetry of mandibular movement as the patient opens the mouth. Deviation of the jaw may be due to weakness of the jaw muscles. Trismus is due to masseter muscle spasm and may indicate peritonsillar abscess, dental infection, or tetany. Inspect the lips for color, swelling, or ulceration. The child who is unable to cover the teeth with the lips may have tooth displacement or cellulitis of a maxillary anterior tooth.
2. **Palpation.** Palpate the temporomandibular joint (TM joint) as the child opens and closes the mouth. Pain and tenderness over the condyles may be due to subcondylar fracture (see Chap. 37). Feel the maxilla and nose for mobility, crepitus, subcutaneous emphysema, and discontinuity. The mandible should be palpated from the TM joint to the chin. Note the size and tenderness of any neck nodes or masses. Test the sensation of the facial skin. Numbness or paresthesia usually indicates trigeminal nerve disruption. Palpate the lips for swelling; chipped teeth and other foreign bodies may embed in the lips and must be removed.

### B. Intraoral examination
1. **Inspection.** Use a good light source to examine the mouth. Halitosis may be a sign of infection or poor oral hygiene.
   a. **Soft tissues.** Note any swelling, inflammation, ulcers, or bleeding. Foreign bodies or loose chips of teeth should be removed. Look at the gums, mucosa, palate, tongue, floor of the mouth, and teeth. The gums should appear pink, firm, and stippled. Note any gingival swellings or color changes. The mucosa of the mouth should be pink, moist, and glassy. Inspect the tongue, lifting it with a gauze pad to examine its underside and the floor of the mouth. The floor of the mouth is normally grey-blue and flat; a hematoma may be due to a fracture.

**Table 11-1. Normal chronological development of teeth**

**Primary teeth**

| Tooth | Eruption (mo) | Shedding (yr) |
|---|---|---|
| Central incisor | 6–9 | 7–8 |
| Lateral incisor | 7–10 | 7–9 |
| Canine | 16–20 | 10–12 |
| First molar | 12–16 | 9–11 |
| Second molar | 20–30 | 11–12 |

**Secondary teeth**

| | Eruption | |
|---|---|---|
| Tooth | Lower | Upper |
| Central incisor | 6–7 | 7–8 |
| Lateral incisor | 7–8 | 8–9 |
| Canine | 9–11 | 11–12 |
| First premolar | 10–12 | 10–11 |
| Second premolar | 11–12 | 10–12 |
| First molar | 6–7 | 6–7 |
| Second molar | 11–13 | 12–13 |
| Third molar | 17–25 | 17–25 |

Note: The lower teeth erupt before the corresponding upper teeth, and teeth usually erupt earlier in girls than in boys. There is a wide variation in the eruption schedule.

Source: Adapted from R. J. Gorlin, J. J. Pindborg, and M. M. Cohen, Jr. *Syndromes of the Head and Neck* (2nd ed.), New York: McGraw-Hill, 1976.

**b. Teeth.** When examining a child's teeth, it is important to distinguish between a normal primary exfoliated tooth and a traumatic injury (see Table 11-1 for the time of normal eruption and shedding). Observe the teeth for movement as the child opens and closes the mouth. When the teeth are traumatically displaced the patient often complains that they "do not feel right" when the mouth is closed. Inspect all four quadrants for missing, chipped, displaced, or fractured teeth. The presence of a bloody socket may indicate a traumatic injury. Exposure of the **dentin** is indicated by its yellow color. With **pulp** exposure, redness of the pulp chamber is visible, and there is often bleeding from the tooth. Grossly decayed teeth may be associated with a fistulous tract that opens onto the gum.

**2. Palpation.** Maxillary fracture results in crepitus and deformity of the palate. Using the thumb and index finger, palpate the base of the alveolar ridge in

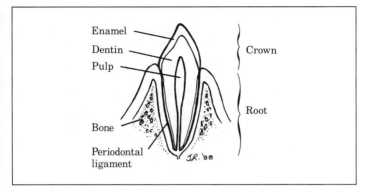

**Fig. 11-1. Dental anatomy.**

all four quadrants. Loose or floppy alveolar bone suggests fracture. In children who are unable to localize pain, infection may be diagnosed by finding inflammation and tenderness apical to the involved tooth. All teeth should be examined for mobility, tenderness, and fragmentation. Abscessed teeth are often mobile, and purulent exudate may be discharged when the tooth is moved.

3. **Percussion.** Tap each tooth using the end of a mouth mirror or tongue depressor. Decayed, abscessed, or vertically fractured teeth are often hypersensitive to percussion. Pain on percussion of the posterior maxillary teeth on one side is suggestive of ipsilateral maxillary sinusitis.

II. **Dental injury.** Dental injury occurs most commonly in toddlers who are learning to walk and in adolescents playing contact sports.

A. **Diagnosis and assessment.** A complete history of the injury should be taken including when, where, and how it took place. A past history of dental problems and treatment can also be helpful. Ask about temperature sensitivity, spontaneous pain, reactions to sweet and sour foods, and mobility of the tooth. Paresthesia of the lips may indicate a fractured mandible.

The risk of cervical spine and head injury is high in patients with facial fracture; the neurologic status of the patient should be assessed (see Chap. 41). Consider nonaccidental injury when the history is inconsistent or implausible; child abuse often presents with maxillofacial or dental injury.

B. **Initial management of facial or dental injury.** Assess and control the airway, breathing, and circulation. Airway obstruction can occur secondary to profuse bleeding, aspiration of a tooth, or fracture of the mandible with posterior displacement of the tongue.

1. The mouth should be suctioned and the child placed prone or on the side. If the mandible is fractured and

displaced, the airway can be cleared by performing the jaw-thrust maneuver (see Chap. 1).

**2.** If the tongue is causing obstruction, an oropharyngeal or nasopharyngeal airway can be placed (see Chap. 1).

**3.** Bleeding should be controlled by direct pressure or vessel ligation.

**4.** Determine tetanus immunization status and treat those at risk (see Appendix).

**5.** In children with congenital or acquired heart disease or immune compromise consider antibiotic prophylaxis against endocarditis (see recent American Heart Association guidelines [*Med. Lett. Drugs Ther.* reference in Bibliography]).

**C.** Specific dental and facial injuries

  **1. Tooth injury**

    **a. Uncomplicated tooth fracture.** This fracture involves the hard dental tissue but does not extend into the pulp. The tooth may be jagged and the fracture line often appears deep, but there is no bleeding from the central core of the tooth.

      **(1) Management.** The pulp must be protected from exposure and necrosis with a dressing of calcium hydroxide. Refer to a dentist as soon as is convenient for treatment.

    **b. Complicated tooth fracture.** This fracture involves the pulp and presents with bleeding from the central core of the tooth. The prognosis depends on the amount of the pulpal exposure, the position of the fracture, and the time lapsed until treatment.

      **(1) Management.** Complicated fractures should be referred immediately to a dentist.

  **2. Injury to the periodontal structures.** The tooth is held in the socket by the periodontal ligament—a collection of elastic and collagen fibers. Trauma can produce various degrees of damage to the ligament with resulting mobility or loss of the tooth. Because the disrupted tooth is sensitive, the older child is usually able to demonstrate which tooth is affected. Periodontal injury is classified as follows:

    **a. Sensitive tooth—concussion.** The affected tooth is very sensitive to percussion. There is no displacement or excessive mobility.

      **(1) Management.** No treatment is indicated.

    **b. Mobile tooth—subluxation** (Fig. 11-2). There is excessive movement in the vertical or horizontal direction (Fig. 11-2). Bleeding may be seen at the gum line, indicating damage to the periodontal ligament. The tooth is very sensitive to percussion.

      **(1) Management.** Refer the patient to a dentist at his convenience.

    **c. Displacement.** The most common displacement injury is a downward and inward movement of an

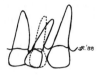

**Fig. 11-2. Subluxated tooth.**

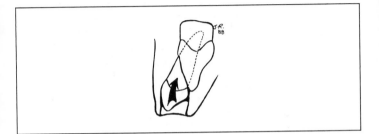

**Fig. 11-3. Intrusive injury.**

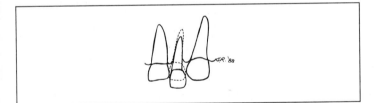

**Fig. 11-4. Extrusive injury.**

anterior maxillary tooth with fracture of the labial wall of the alveolar socket.

(1) Intrusion (Fig. 11-3) occurs when the tooth is pushed into the socket. X rays are often required to make the diagnosis, to rule out avulsive injury, or to assess the position of a primary tooth in relation to an unerupted permanent tooth. Intrusive injuries have a poor prognosis due to damage to the cellular component of the root.

(2) Extrusion (Fig. 11-4) occurs when teeth are displaced vertically out of the socket. The prognosis of extruded teeth is usually good if treatment is prompt.

(3) Lateral luxation is displacement in a lateral direction. Fracture of the alveolar bone is commonly associated.

(4) **Management.** Children with displacement injuries should be referred to a dentist immediately for splinting. Extruded primary teeth are usually extracted to prevent damage to the permanent teeth during realignment.

d. **Complete displacement of the tooth—exarticulation/avulsion.** When teeth are missing from the jaw, it is important to account for all of them; rule out aspiration, intrusion, or ingestion by x ray if necessary. **Primary teeth** are not reimplanted. **Secondary teeth** should be reimplanted as soon as possible; the best results are obtained if the tooth is replaced within 30 minutes, but reimplantation may be successful up to 12 hours after avulsion. If the parent phones the emergency room following avulsion of a secondary tooth, give the following advice:

(1) Gently rinse the tooth with cool tap water to remove any debris. **Do not scrub the tooth.**

(2) Reimplant the tooth into the socket, holding it by the crown and taking care not to disturb the root area. Do not be concerned if the tooth extrudes slightly.

(3) If the parent cannot reimplant the tooth, have the child or parent put the tooth under his tongue. Alternatively, place the tooth in a cup of milk or collect saliva from the patient and use it as the transport medium.

(4) Send the patient directly to the dentist for treatment by immobilization. Dental follow-up is mandatory to initiate pulp therapy.

3. **Injury to the supporting bone**

a. **Comminution of the alveolar socket.** This injury occurs with intrusive and lateral luxation of the teeth. Other than management of any disrupted teeth, treatment is usually not required.

b. **Other types of mandible and maxillary fractures.** See Chap. 37.

D. **Disposition.** An avulsed tooth should be immediately reimplanted by the parents. Immediate referral to a dentist is required for tooth displacement, avulsion, or complicated fracture. Elective follow-up with a dentist should be arranged for uncomplicated fracture or subluxation injury.

E. **Key points**

1. Children with pulp exposure—suggested by bleeding from an injured tooth—require immediate dental referral.

2. A permanent tooth that has been completely dislodged from the socket should be reimplanted as soon as possible.

III. **Dental infection**

A. **Classification.** Infection in children may be classified as follows:

   1. Simple toothache—pulpitis
   2. Dentoalveolar abscess
   3. Soft tissue infection of dental origin (see Chap. 37)
   4. Osteomyelitis secondary to an infected tooth or bony
      fracture (see Chap. 37)
B. **Specific disorders**
   1. **Simple toothache.** Simple toothache may be due to
      a carious lesion—the tooth has a discolored area and
      may be sensitive to sweets and changes in tempera-
      ture. Extension of caries into the pulp may cause se-
      vere toothache with pain on percussion, but the tooth
      is not unduly mobile. Mobility or surrounding swell-
      ing occurs when pulpitis spreads to the periodontal
      ligament and alveolar bone.
      a. **Management.** A few drops of eugenol (oil of
         cloves) placed on a cotton pledget and inserted
         into the carious lesion can provide temporary re-
         lief. Acetaminophen or codeine can be prescribed
         for analgesia, with dental follow-up arranged in
         1–2 days.
   2. **Dentoalveolar abscess.** This infection begins at
      the apex of the tooth root but may spread rapidly
      into the surrounding soft tissues. Pain is often se-
      vere. The involved tooth is very tender to percussion
      and may be abnormally mobile or slightly extruded
      from the socket. The soft tissue around the tooth is
      often swollen and fluctuant. Children with severe in-
      fection may have fever and lymphadenopathy. A
      chronic abscess may result in fistula formation with
      a 'pimplelike' lesion on the gum or, rarely, on the
      face. Spread of infection may result in sinusitis, cel-
      lulitis, or bacteremia.
      a. **Management.** A primary abscessed tooth must
         be treated aggressively before the infection leads
         to enamel defects in the underlying permanent
         tooth.
         (1) Phenoxymethyl penicillin is the antibiotic of
             choice. Erythromycin is a suitable alterna-
             tive.
             (a) In the child weighing $\geq 27$ kg, treat with
                 an initial dose of penicillin of 1 gm fol-
                 lowed by 500 mg PO q6h.
             (b) In the child under 27 kg (60 lb) the pen-
                 icillin dosage is 50 mg/kg/day PO di-
                 vided q6h.
         (2) Warm saline rinses may be used to encour-
             age drainage. Do not treat with extraoral hot
             compresses because these promote external
             drainage and may lead to formation of a fa-
             cial fistula.
         (3) If a fluctuant area is palpable around the
             tooth, incision and drainage can provide re-
             lief. Using a scalpel blade, make a small in-
             cision over the fluctuant area on the **buccal**
             side of the tooth. Incision on the **lingual** side
             of the mandibular tooth can result in sali-

vary duct disruption. For deeper abscesses that are not superficially palpable, local anesthesia will be required; refer the patient to a dentist.

**(4)** Provide analgesia with acetaminophen 10 mg/kg PO q4h prn, or codeine, 0.5–1.0 mg/kg PO q6–8h prn.

**(5)** Refer all patients to a dentist as soon as possible for drainage or tooth extraction.

**(6)** The child with high fever, toxicity, or facial cellulitis should be admitted for intravenous antibiotic therapy with penicillin G, 50,000–100,000 units/kg/day IV divided q6h. Erythromycin and cefuroxime are suitable alternatives.

**C. Disposition.** Hospital admission is required if the child is not able to take in oral fluids or if parental compliance with follow-up treatment cannot be ensured. Children with symptoms of toxicity, facial cellulitis, sinusitis, or spread of infection to other soft tissues should be admitted for treatment with intravenous antibiotics (see Chaps. 13, 15).

**D. Key points.** Most dental abscesses can be managed with oral phenoxymethyl penicillin and outpatient dental referral.

## IV. Postextraction complications

**A. Bleeding.** Oozing commonly occurs up to 12 hours after extraction. If bleeding is prolonged, rule out bleeding disorders; order a CBC, platelet count, prothrombin time (PT), and partial thromboplastin time (PTT).

**1. Management.** Proceed through the following steps until the bleeding is controlled.

**a.** Instruct the child to bite down for 30 minutes on gauze sponges placed over the socket.

**b.** Tannic acid, from a teabag placed over the socket, may control the bleeding. Dip the teabag in hot water and allow to cool before applying to the socket. Repeat step a.

**c.** Suture the socket edges together under local anesthesia using 3–0 silk. Repeat step a.

**d.** Remove the sutures, pack the socket with ¼-in. gauze and resuture the socket. Repeat step a.

**B. Infection.** Infection of the socket following extraction is rare. Treat with warm saline rinses and antibiotics (see sec. III.B.2).

**C. Key points.** Local pressure is usually effective in managing postextraction bleeding.

## Bibliography

Castaldi, C. R., and Brass, G. A. *Dentistry for the Adolescent.* Philadelphia: Saunders, 1988.

Braham, R. L., and Morris, M. E. *Textbook of Pediatric Dentistry* (2nd ed.). Baltimore: Williams & Wilkins, 1985.

Fleisher, G., and Ludwig, S. (eds.). *Textbook of Pediatric Emergency Medicine.* Baltimore: Williams & Wilkins, 1984.

Markowitz, M., Rheumatic Fever. In R. E. Behrman and V. K. Vaughan, *Nelson Textbook of Pediatrics.* Philadelphia: Saunders, 1983. P. 593.

*Med. Lett. Drugs Ther.* 26:3, 1984.

# 12

# Dermatology

Loretta Fiorillo

## I. Infection

**A. Impetigo.** Impetigo is a superficial skin infection caused by *Staphylococcus aureus* or group A beta-hemolytic streptococcus. Staphylococcal infection is frequent in children with atopic dermatitis.

**1. Diagnosis and assessment. Impetigo** is characterized by vesicles, often grouped, that quickly become pustules and then rupture and become covered with a honey-colored crust. There is a surrounding erythema and edema. In **bullous impetigo,** vesicles enlarge into flaccid bullae containing straw-colored or cloudy yellow fluid. There is no surrounding erythema. **Systemic infection** is rare and usually occurs in immune-compromised children or neonates.

**2. Management**

**a.** Obtain a swab from bullous fluid or beneath crusts for Gram's stain and culture before starting therapy. Take a nasal swab to determine staphylococcal carrier status in children with a history of recurrent infection.

**b.** Treat with cloxacillin, 50 mg/kg/day PO divided q6h, erythromycin, 40 mg/kg/day PO divided q6h, or cephalexin, 25–50 mg/kg/day PO divided q6h.

**c.** In older children with limited nonbullous lesions, use mupirocin (Bactroban) ointment topically twice daily. Instruct the parent to remove any crusts with twice daily cool compresses and then cleanse the area with an antiseptic solution such as Betadine.

**d.** Neonates and children with severe generalized infections should be hospitalized for intravenous therapy with cloxacillin or oxacillin, 100–200 mg/kg/day divided q6h, or another suitable antistaphylococcal drug.

**B. Scalded skin syndrome.** This is a life-threatening infection caused by exfoliation-producing isolates of *S. aureus*. It is most common in infancy and rarely occurs after age 5.

**1. Diagnosis and assessment.** Onset is abrupt with diffuse erythema, marked skin tenderness, and fever. Within 12–24 hours superficial flaccid bullae develop and then rupture almost immediately, leaving a beefy, red, weeping surface. Exfoliation is extensive and may affect most of the body. There is usually a positive Nikolsky's sign, with separation of the epidermis on light rubbing. The focus of staphylococcal infection may be minor or inapparent. Unruptured bullae usually contain sterile fluid.

**2. Management**

**a.** Perform a skin swab for Gram's stain and culture. Obtain a urinalysis and draw blood for culture, complete blood count (CBC), electrolytes, blood urea nitrogen (BUN), and creatinine measurements.

**b.** Start an intravenous line. Children with scalded skin syndrome should be treated similarly to patients with second-degree burns (see Chap. 26), including meticulous fluid and nutritional management. Give intravenous cloxacillin or oxacillin 100 mg/kg/day divided q6h, or another suitable antistaphylococcal drug.

**C. Cellulitis.** Cellulitis is an acute inflammation of the skin and subcutaneous tissue, commonly due to group A streptococcus, *S. aureus,* or *Haemophilus influenzae type b* (less common). Occasionally, *Pseudomonas aeruginosa* infection is seen following puncture wounds of the foot.

**1. Diagnosis and assessment.** In most cases there is a history of recent minor skin trauma. The skin is red, swollen, hot, hard, and painful. There is often accompanying lymphangitis, fever, and malaise.

**2. Management**

**a.** Obtain cultures of blood and, when indicated, the involved tissue, urine, or other suspected sites.

**b.** Older children with limited minor infections can be treated with cloxacillin, cephalexin, or erythromycin, 30–50 mg/kg/day PO divided q6h for 10 days.

**c.** Patients with large areas of cellulitis, systemic symptoms (fever, chills, toxicity), or facial involvement require admission for intravenous antibiotics. Cefuroxime, 100–150 mg/kg/day divided q8h, is preferred for its coverage of *H. influenzae type b,* staphylococci, and streptococci. Confirmed streptococcal infection should be treated with penicillin G, 50,000–100,000 units/kg/day IV divided q6h.

**d.** Perform incision and drainage of focal collections, and elevate and immobilize involved limbs. Cellulitis of the orbit and eyelids is a serious disease requiring ophthalmologic consultation and intravenous antibiotics (see Chap. 15, Orbital Cellulitis).

**D. Scabies.** This is an extremely pruritic eruption caused by the mite *Sarcoptes scabiei var. hominis.*

**1. Diagnosis and assessment.** Although multiple inflammatory papules and vesicles are the most common manifestations of scabies, burrows are pathognomonic. Burrows are linear or arcuate intraepidermal tunnels dug by the female mite and are commonly found on the wrist, finger and toe webs, elbows, abdomen, and genitalia. Often overlooked sites of involvement in the infant include the scalp, face, palms, and soles. There is extreme pruritus that is maximal at night, leading to excoriation. Bacterial superinfection is frequent, especially in the infant. In the majority of cases, one or more family members are infected. Microscopic diagnosis is made by placing a drop of mineral oil on a burrow, scraping the roof of the burrow with a No. 15 scalpel blade, and then placing the scrapings in a drop of oil on a glass slide with a coverslip and viewing under low power. Look for mites, ova, and feces.

2. **Management**

a. The child and all family members must be simultaneously treated with lindane (gamma benzene hexachloride, Kwellada) in two applications, 7 days apart. Lindane is applied to the skin from the neck down, covering the entire skin surface, and is washed off after a variable period of time: (1) 8 hours in children over 1 year of age, (2) 4–6 hours in children 6 months to 1 year old, (3) 2 hours for babies under 6 months, and (4) up to 8 hours for the soles of the feet of infants (due to the thick stratum corneum). Lindane should not be applied immediately after a hot bath because skin irritation may result. Neurotoxicity with vomiting, headaches, dizziness, and seizures may follow prolonged topical exposure, especially in infants; thumb-sucking children should wear impermeable mittens during treatment. Lindane is contraindicated in pregnancy; instead, prescribe crotamiton (Eurax) 10% given in two applications 24 hours apart, then rinsed off 48 hours later. Resistance to lindane has been reported; permethrin, a safe and effective alternative, will soon be available.

b. All family bedlinen and clothes should be thoroughly washed in hot water. Parents should be warned that pruritus can persist for 1–2 weeks after infestation has resolved. Symptomatic relief may be obtained from diphenhydramine (Benadryl) or hydroxyzine (Atarax).

E. **Pinworm infestation.** In the United States pinworm infestation is the most common helminthic infestation in humans. Occasionally, irritation from pruritus may be severe, and the child presents with severe agitation or episodes of screaming. Pinworm infestation should be suspected when there is anal pruritus or if worms have been visualized. The diagnosis can be made with the Scotch tape test: Gently apply tape to the perianal region, apply the adhesive side to a glass slide, and examine under the light microscope for ova. This test is more likely to be positive when it is performed at night. Treat pinworms with mebendazole, 100 mg PO once, or pyrantel pamoate, 11 mg/kg (maximum dose 1 gm) PO once. In both cases, a second dose of medication should be administered after 2 weeks.

F. **Herpesvirus infection**

1. **Chickenpox (varicella).** This is the primary infection caused by the varicella-zoster virus. The incubation period is 11–20 days. Children are contagious

from the day preceding the rash until all the lesions are crusted.

**a. Diagnosis and assessment.** Highly pruritic lesions appear in successive crops that begin as vesicles, progress to pustules, and crust in a few days. Vesicles (2–4 mm diameter) surrounded by a red halo first appear on the face, neck, or upper trunk and spread to the rest of the body. Common systemic symptoms include fever, headache, malaise, and myalgia. Oral lesions may also be seen. Complications include bacterial superinfection (common), encephalitis with cerebellar ataxia, pneumonia, and hepatitis (rare unless the host is immune compromised). Hemorrhagic varicella is a form of immune thrombocytopenic purpura, characterized by bleeding into the vesicles and the mucous membranes.

The diagnosis is usually made clinically—the development of crops of vesicles is characteristic. Laboratory diagnosis may be made from vesicle fluid examined under the electron microscope or using fluorescent antibody methods (this result takes a few hours) or from viral culture (slow) of vesicle fluid. The Tzanck smear, taken from a vigorous swab of the base of a deroofed vesicle and showing multinucleated giant cells, is a sensitive but nonspecific test.

**b. Management**

   **(1) In healthy children** the treatment is symptomatic. Tepid baths followed by application of calamine lotion help to decrease pruritus. Oral antihistamines (diphenhydramine, hydroxyzine) may be used, and cloxacillin, 50 mg/kg/day PO divided q6h, should be given when bacterial superinfection is suspected. Advise against salicylate use because of its association with Reye's syndrome.

   **(2) Immune-compromised susceptible children** exposed to varicella and newborns delivered to mothers who developed rash from 5 days before to 2 days after birth must be treated with varicella-zoster immune globulin (VZIG), 1 vial/10 kg (maximum dose 5 vials) IM within 96 hours of exposure.

   **(3)** Admission and treatment with intravenous acyclovir, 30 mg/kg/day IV divided q8h for 7 days, is necessary for the following patients.

     **(a)** Children with varicella infection who are immune compromised, including oncology patients who have received chemotherapy within the preceding year (see Chap. 19).

     **(b)** Those with an atypical course suggesting immune compromise (prolonged vesicle stage, increasing numbers of new vesicles beyond 5 days).

(c) Patients with varicella encephalitis, hepatitis, or pneumonia.

(4) In children in categories (2) or (3) above, obtain blood for liver function tests and order a chest x ray.

2. **Herpes zoster.** Herpes zoster results from reactivation of varicella-zoster virus and often occurs years after chickenpox infection. Children present with nonpruritic vesicular lesions in a dermatome distribution. There may be discomfort, but severe pain is unusual. Laboratory diagnosis is identical to that used for chickenpox (see sec. **I.F.1.a**). Immunecompromised children with herpes zoster may require therapy with acyclovir, 30 mg/kg/day IV divided q8h for 7 days.

3. **Eczema herpeticum.** This is a widespread severe cutaneous infection caused by herpes simplex virus 1 (HSV 1) in children with preexisting skin disease, commonly atopic dermatitis. Patients develop a myriad of small vesicles that often break, leaving extensive areas of weeping erosions. Secondary staphylococcal infection is common.

   a. **Management.** Swab the affected area for Gram's stain and culture. Confirmation of HSV infection is made by immunofluorescence, microscopy, Tzanck smear, or viral culture from a vesicle (see sec. **I.F.1** above).

   Treat with cloxacillin orally or cloxacillin, oxacillin, or another suitable antistaphylococcal agent IV, depending on severity. Children with extensive rash should be hospitalized and treated with intravenous acyclovir, 15 mg/kg/day divided q8h for 5–7 days.

G. **Disposition.** Admit the child when cellulitis involves the face or large areas of skin or when there are systemic signs and symptoms. Admit all neonates and children with severe generalized impetigo and children with complicated varicella-zoster infection (neonates, or children who are immune compromised or have encephalitis, hepatitis, or pneumonitis). Children with extensive scalded skin syndrome should be transferred to a burn unit.

H. **Key points**

1. Cellulitis that involves large areas or the face, or that is associated with systemic symptoms requires intravenous antibiotic therapy.

2. Often overlooked sites of scabies in the infant include the scalp, face, palms, and soles.

3. Immune-compromised patients with herpes virus infection require intravenous acyclovir therapy.

II. **Hypersensitivity reactions**

A. **Urticaria** is the most common type of hypersensitivity reaction in the skin. **Immunologic** or **IgE-mediated** urticaria is a hypersensitivity reaction that occurs in children previously exposed to the offending agent.

Common causes include drugs (especially penicillin), foods such as fish, eggs, nuts, tomatoes, and chocolate, physical factors such as cold, light, and heat, blood and blood products, and infections (EBV, hepatitis, streptococcus).

**Nonimmunologic** urticaria can occur after first exposure to such agents as acetylsalicylic acid (ASA), opiates, or contrast media.

1. **Diagnosis and assessment.** Urticaria is manifested as wheals: raised, pale and pink pruritic areas of edema of the upper dermis that may continue to appear for several days. The diagnosis is clinical and is based on the characteristic appearance and, when possible, a history of exposure.

2. **Management.** Avoiding the precipitating cause is the key to prevention. Cold compresses can be applied to pruritic areas, and the child may be given antihistamines (diphenhydramine, hydroxyzine) by mouth. A cream made of 1% hydrocortisone cream, 0.25% menthol, and camphor may help alleviate the itch and settle the itch. For management of anaphylaxis, see Chap. 30.

B. **Erythema multiforme and serum sickness.** Erythema multiforme is an acute self-limited hypersensitivity eruption that is most commonly seen in children over age 3, with a peak incidence in the second decade. Common precipitating events include viral infection (herpesvirus, adenovirus, Epstein-Barr virus), *Mycoplasma pneumoniae* infection, and drug ingestion, especially long-acting sulfonamides.

1. **Diagnosis and assessment.** The rash may be pleomorphic with macular, vesicular, and urticarial components, but target lesions are pathognomonic. Target lesions are dull red macules, 1–2 cm in diameter that rapidly develop a purpuric, cyanotic, or occasionally bullous center. Around this center is a clear halo, giving the lesion a bull's eye appearance. Successive crops may appear during a period of 1–2 weeks, often healing with mild hyperpigmentation over 3–4 weeks. The rash is symmetric and characteristically involves the extensor surfaces of the limbs. The diagnosis can be confirmed by skin biopsy. The presence of concurrent arthritis and fever suggests the diagnosis of serum sickness.

2. **Management.** In general, symptomatic treatment and reassurance of the parents are all that are required. Lesions usually resolve over 1–2 weeks. Arthralgia or arthritis can be treated with ASA 20–30 mg/kg/dose PO q6h.

C. **Stevens-Johnson Syndrome.** This is an extreme form of erythema multiforme with systemic symptoms and involvement of the mucous membranes. Untreated, the mortality is 5–15%. For more information, see Chap. 24, Acute Arthritis.

1. **Diagnosis and assessment.** Stevens-Johnson syndrome is preceded by a prodromal phase of 1–14 days

**Table 12-1. Major exanthems**

| Disease | Agent | Exanthem | Associated findings |
|---|---|---|---|
| Measles | Measles virus | Purple red papules starting on face move down to trunk in 3 days, coalesce | Koplik spots, high fever, toxicity, conjunctivitis, photophobia, coryza, cough, adenopathy |
| Rubella | Rubella virus | Discrete, pink-red papules start on face, spread downward rapidly | Mild fever, malaise, occipital and postauricular adenopathy |
| Roseola | Herpes virus | Discrete, pink, noncoalescent macules with central distribution appear as fever decreases | High fever 3–5 days; Patient seems well despite fever |
| Enterovirus | Coxsackie virus A, B Echovirus | Highly variable: macular, papular, rubelliform, petechial | Nonspecific fever, headache, myalgias |
| Erythema infectiosum | Human parvovirus | "Slapped cheeks," pink-red lacy reticular eruption on trunk and extremities. Recrudescent up to weeks | Patient appears well. Occasional mild flulike symptoms |
| Varicella | Varicella-zoster virus | Pruritic papulovesicles at different stages of development. Central distribution, spreads peripherally. Mucous membranes commonly involved | Fever, malaise, myalgias |

| | | | |
|---|---|---|---|
| Scarlet fever | Group A beta-hemolytic streptococci | Tiny red papules, rough sandpaper feel. More lesions in skin folds and areas of warmth. Pastia's lines in flexion creases | Pharyngitis. Strawberry tongue, adenopathy, late desquamation |
| Staphylococcal scalded skin syndrome | Phage group 1 *S. aureus* | Diffuse tender erythema. Positive Nikolsky's sign. Large flaccid bullae, then sheets of desquamation | Upper respiratory infection symptoms, fever, focus of staphylococcal infection |
| Toxic shock syndrome | Phage group 2 *S. aureus* | Sunburned appearance, late desquamation | Fever, hypotension; involves three or more organ systems |
| Rocky Mountain spotted fever | *Rickettsia rickettsii* | Maculopapular, becomes petechial, begins at wrists and ankles, spreads centrally | Fever, chills, malaise, headache, myalgia, arthralgia |
| Meningococcemia | *Neisseria meningitidis* | Petechiae and purpura; affects trunk and extremities, palms and soles | Variable from mild to profound shock |
| Kawasaki's syndrome | Unknown | Polymorphous: morbilliform, urticarial, scarlatiniform, petechial, target lesions in generalized distribution | Fever, conjunctivitis, oral cavity changes, hand and foot changes, lymphadenopathy |

Source: Adapted from A. H. Hartley, and J. E. Rasmussen. Infectious exanthems. *Pediatr. Rev.* 9:322, 1988.

of fever, malaise, sore throat, vomiting, arthralgia or arthritis, and myalgia. Dermatologic manifestations begin abruptly with erythema multiforme and painful, red, bullous lesions of the mucous membranes, particularly the mouth and conjunctivae. The bullae rupture easily, forming hemorrhagic crusts or grey pseudomembranes. In severe cases there may be involvement of most of the gastrointestinal, respiratory, or genitourinary tracts. Diagnosis can be confirmed by skin biopsy.

  **2. Management.** Start an intravenous line; most children will be dehydrated from poor fluid intake, and severe cases require parenteral nutrition. Urethritis may lead to urinary retention requiring catheterization. An ophthalmologist should be consulted to check for corneal ulceration, uveitis, and panophthalmitis.

**D. Drug eruptions.** Drug eruptions are more common after parenteral administration of medications, although any exposure—including topical exposure—may result in a generalized eruption. In children not previously sensitized, the onset may occur as late as 1–2 weeks after receiving the medication. Eruptions may worsen after the medication has been stopped.

  **1. Diagnosis and assessment.** The clinical presentation may vary from a mild rash to anaphylaxis. The most frequent rashes are maculopapular, morbilliform, and urticarial, usually bright red and often pruritic. Patients may feel remarkably well in spite of the eruptions. Diagnosis may be made by skin testing or the radioallergosorbent (RAST) test for specific IgE.

  **2. Management.** Management depends on the severity of the reaction. If possible, the drug(s) should be stopped and rechallenge avoided, especially if the rash is urticarial. Symptomatic treatment with cold compresses, emollients, topical steroids, or oral antihistamines often helps.

**E. Toxic epidermal necrolysis (TEN).** TEN is the most severe form of cutaneous hypersensitivity, considered by some to be a variant of Stevens-Johnson syndrome. Although the occurrence in children is rare, morbidity and mortality are high. The pathogenesis is not well understood, but most cases are secondary to medications, especially sulfonamides, anticonvulsants, and nonsteroidal anti-inflammatory agents.

  **1. Diagnosis and assessment.** Onset is acute, sometimes preceded by a burning sensation in the mucous membranes, and often heralded by oral and conjunctival erythema and erosions. The presentation resembles that of scalded skin syndrome with widespread erythema, tenderness, blister formation, detachment of the epidermis causing denudation, and a positive Nikolsky's sign (see sec. **I.B**). A skin biopsy is diagnostic.

Toxicity, leukocytosis, and high fever are common. Mucous membrane involvement is severe, and the nails may be shed. Systemic complications include elevated liver enzyme levels, renal failure, and fluid and electrolyte imbalance. Sepsis and shock are frequent causes of death. Granulocytopenia is associated with a poor prognosis.

   2. **Management.** These children require management similar to that used for patients with widespread second-degree burn injury, including immediate intravenous access and fluid therapy. Transfer to a burn unit should be arranged as soon as possible (see Chap. 26).

**F. Poison ivy/oak dermatitis (rhus dermatitis).** Poison ivy is the most common cause of allergic contact dermatitis in North America, affecting 90% of people exposed.

   1. **Diagnosis and assessment.** Shortly after contact the patient develops an acute, intensely pruritic, vesicular, and exudative dermatitis.

   2. **Management**

      a. **Immediate.** Thoroughly wash the skin with soap and water to eliminate the allergin. Contaminated clothes must be removed and laundered.

      b. **Subsequent.** Apply cold tap water compresses for 15 minutes every 4–6 hours. Cool baths are indicated for widespread rash. Clobetasol ointment or another potent fluorinated steroid can be applied topically bid until vesiculation subsides. Antihistamines such as diphenhydramine (Benadryl) or hydroxyzine (Atarax) help to relieve itching. Severe cases should be treated with oral prednisone, 1–2 mg/kg/day PO divided q12h, gradually tapering the dose over 2 weeks. Early discontinuation of steroids may result in flare-up.

**G. Disposition.** Admit patients with Stevens-Johnson syndrome and those with anaphylactic drug reactions. All children with toxic epidermal necrolysis should be transferred to a burn unit after stabilization.

**H. Key points**

   1. Consult an ophthalmologist in all cases of suspected Stevens-Johnson syndrome.

   2. Treat severe cases of poison ivy or poison oak with steroids, topically or PO.

   3. Acute onset of bullous lesions may be due to a severe hypersensitivity reaction such as TEN or Stevens-Johnson syndrome.

**Bibliography**

Habif, T. P. (ed.). *Clinical Dermatology.* St. Louis: C. V. Mosby, 1985.

Fitzpatrick, T. B. (ed.). *Dermatology in General Medicine* (3rd ed.). New York: McGraw Hill, 1987.

# 13

# Endocrinology

## Acute Adrenal Insufficiency
Robert M. Couch

Acute adrenal insufficiency results when the adrenal cortex is unable to respond to stress by increasing cortisol production. In secondary or tertiary adrenal insufficiency (of pituitary or hypothalamic origin), glucocorticoid production is impaired. In primary adrenal insufficiency, mineralocorticoid (aldosterone) production is also affected.

I. **Diagnosis and assessment.** The presentation can be variable; a high index of suspicion is important. Adrenal insufficiency should be considered in any child with shock of unknown etiology.

A. **The infant.** In the newborn, adrenal crisis is rare before 5–7 days of life. Congenital adrenal hyperplasia (CAH), especially 21-hydroxylase deficiency, is the most likely cause. Suspect CAH in infants with ambiguous genitalia. Rarer causes are adrenal aplasia or hypoplasia, adrenal hemorrhage, and hypothalamic or pituitary lesions.

In the classic presentation, the infant's symptoms are failure to thrive, vomiting, dehydration, and eventually deterioration into shock. Hyperpigmentation of the nipples, axillae, or genitalia may be present, but is often difficult to detect in the newborn. Laboratory investigations reveal hyponatremia, hyperkalemia, metabolic acidosis, and occasionally hypoglycemia. Urinary sodium excretion is increased. The main differential diagnosis is a congenital salt-losing renal anomaly.

B. **The child.** In the older child, the most common cause of adrenal crisis is autoimmune adrenalitis. The onset is usually prolonged and insidious, but acute crises may be precipitated by an intercurrent illness. Adrenal crisis may also follow sudden withdrawal of glucocorticoid therapy, hypothalamic or pituitary lesions, or an overwhelming infection such as meningococcemia. Most children present to the emergency room with shock. There is usually a history of fatigue, weakness, anorexia, and weight loss over a period of months. Nausea, vomiting, and abdominal pain are common. Hyperpigmentation (gums, knuckles, sun-exposed areas) is easily detected in children with primary adrenal failure. The laboratory findings are identical to those in the infant (see sec. **I.A**).

II. **Management.** When adrenal insufficiency is suspected, do not wait for laboratory results before initiating treatment.

A. **Resuscitation.** Assess and control airway, breathing, and circulation problems. Start two large-bore intravenous lines, administer oxygen by mask, and place the child on a cardiac monitor.

B. **Investigations.** Obtain 5–10 ml of blood for measurement of cortisol and aldosterone levels (plain tube, clotted sample) and 5 ml of plasma for adrenocorticotropic hormone (ACTH) and renin levels (EDTA tube, placed on ice). When enzyme defects are suspected, save an extra sample of serum for measurement of other adrenal steroid metabolites (e.g., 17-hydroxyprogesterone in cases of 21-hydroxylase deficiency). In clinically stable patients, a 1-hour ACTH stimulation test should be done prior to commencing hydrocortisone replacement therapy. This test is performed by giving cortrosyn, 0.25 mg IV, and then measuring serum cortisol levels at 0, 30, and 60 minutes after the dose.

C. **Fluids.** Initially, give a bolus of 10 ml/kg of intravenous fluid and repeat this dose prn until the patient is stable (see Chap. 4). In infants use 10% dextrose normal saline; in children use 5% dextrose normal saline. Following this initial fluid bolus, replace one-half of the total estimated fluid deficit over 8 hours and the remaining half during the following 16 hours. Assume a minimum deficit of 10% of expected body weight. See Chap. 23, Fluid and Electrolyte Disorders.

D. **Hyperkalemia.** Hyperkalemia usually corrects itself spontaneously following saline infusion. For management of children with severe or refractory hyperkalemia, see Chap. 23.

E. **Steroids.** Intravenous hydrocortisone is essential.
   1. **Infants** should receive a bolus dose of 25 mg IV followed by a continuous infusion of 50–100 mg/m$^2$/24 hours.
   2. The initial hydrocortisone bolus dose in **children** is 50–100 mg IV followed by a continuous infusion of 50–100 mg/m$^2$/24 hours.
   3. Once the child is able to tolerate **oral medication,** start therapy with fludrocortisone acetate (Florinef), 0.1–0.2 mg PO per day in infants and 0.05–0.1 mg PO per day in children.

F. **Consultation.** All children with suspected adrenal insufficiency should be seen by an endocrinologist.

G. **Disposition.** Admit all children with acute adrenal insufficiency. Patients with severe hyperkalemia should be transferred to the intensive care unit.

H. **Key points**
   1. Most cases of adrenal insufficiency present in infancy. Suspect the diagnosis in newborns with ambiguous genitalia.
   2. Treat with intravenous fluids and hydrocortisone.

**Bibliography**

Bongiovanni, A. M. The Adrenal Cortex. In S. A. Kaplan (ed.). *Clinical Pediatric and Adolescent Endocrinology,* Philadelphia: W. B. Saunders, 1982.

Hughes, I. A. Congenital and acquired disorders of the adrenal cortex. *Clin. Endocrinol. Metab.* 11:83, 1982.

**Table 13-1. Causes of hypoglycemia**

| Age group | Class | Examples |
|---|---|---|
| Neonates | Decreased production | |
| | Transient | Prematurity, growth retardation, asphyxia, sepsis |
| | Persistent | Enzyme defects of glycogen synthesis, glycogenolysis, and gluconeogenesis; counter-regulatory hormone deficiency |
| | Increased utilization (hyperinsulinism) | |
| | Transient | Infant of diabetic mother |
| | Persistent | Nesidioblastosis |
| Children | Decreased production | Ketotic hypoglycemia, counter-regulatory hormone deficiency, enzyme defects of glycogen synthesis, glycogenolysis, and gluconeogenesis, hepatic failure, drugs (salicylates, alcohol) |
| | Increased utilization | Hyperinsulinism |

# Hypoglycemia
Robert M. Couch

## I. Definitions
   **A.** In children over 24 hours of age, hypoglycemia is defined as a blood glucose concentration below 2.2 mmol/liter (40 mg/dl).
   **B.** In the first 24 hours of life it is defined as below 1.7 mmol/liter (30 mg/dl) in full-term infants and 1.1 mmol/liter (20 mg/dl) in premature infants.
   **C.** Blood glucose values in hypoglycemia are 15% higher than those in serum or plasma; the plasma or serum level defining hypoglycemia is therefore 2.5 mmol/liter (45 mg/dl).
## II. Diagnosis and Assessment (Table 13-1). In the **newborn** the common causes of persistent hypoglycemia are hyperinsulinism, hepatic enzyme deficiency, and counterregulatory hormone (i.e., glucagon, cortisol, growth hormone) deficiency. In the **child,** hypoglycemia is usually secondary to insulin administration in the patient with diabetes mellitus.
## III. Diagnosis. The symptoms of hypoglycemia result from glucodeprivation of the central nervous system (CNS) and increased adrenergic activity. Since hypoglycemia in children

is more likely to occur with fasting, a history of nutritional intake in the previous 24 hours is vital.

**A. Symptoms in the newborn.** In the newborn the symptoms can be subtle, and a high index of suspicion is needed. There may be irritability, jitteriness, respiratory distress, cyanosis, apnea, hypotonia, or seizures.

**B. Symptoms in the child.** Hypoglycemia must be ruled out in any child with coma or convulsions. Presenting symptoms and signs can also include confusion, irritability, sweating, pallor, and tachycardia.

**C. Diagnostic methods.** A quick assessment of blood glucose level can be obtained by using a Dextrostix or glucose monitor and strip (Glucometer), but a laboratory measurement must also be obtained. A plasma glucose (heparinized blood) specimen enables a more rapid determination than a serum sample.

**IV. Management.** Immediate diagnosis and treatment are essential. Children with convulsions or prolonged recurrent episodes are most likely to suffer brain damage.

**A. Investigation.** Start an intravenous line. When the cause of hypoglycemia is unknown, obtain 5–10 ml of blood in a heparinized tube for measurements of glucose, lactate, beta-hydroxybutyrate, insulin, cortisol, and growth hormone **before commencing treatment.** If possible, blood for glucagon and catecholamine levels and a toxic screen should also be obtained. The first voided urine specimen should be tested for ketones (negative in hyperinsulinism).

**B. Treatment. When hypoglycemia is suspected, do not wait for the results of blood or plasma glucose tests before starting treatment.**

   **1. Newborn.** In neonates, intravenous 10% dextrose, 2.5 ml/kg, should be administered as a rapid bolus followed by a continuous infusion of 3–5 ml/kg/hour (5–8 mg glucose/kg/minute).

   **2. Children.** Fifty percent dextrose diluted to 25% with water is given at a dose of 1 ml/kg initially, followed by an infusion of 10% dextrose at 2–3 ml/kg/hour (3–5 mg glucose/kg/minute). The clinical response to the bolus of glucose is always dramatic and helps to confirm the diagnosis.

   **3. Intramuscular therapy.** If there is difficulty in establishing an IV, give glucagon 0.03 mg/kg IM (maximum dose 1 mg). Glucagon therapy has a transient effect and must be followed by an intravenous dextrose infusion.

   **4. Stabilization.** Frequent blood or plasma glucose monitoring is required until the patient is stable. Oral intake should be commenced as soon as the child is able to drink.

**V. Disposition.** The patient with hypoglycemia of unknown etiology requires admission to hospital for investigation and treatment.

**VI. Key points**

   **1.** When possible draw blood for investigations prior to treating hypoglycemia.

**2.** Do not wait for laboratory results before starting treatment; irreversible CNS damage may ensue from prolonged symptomatic hypoglycemia.

**Bibliography**

Aynsley-Green, A. Hypoglycemia in infants and children. *Clin. Endocrinol. Metab.* 11:159, 1982.
Cornblath, M., and Poth, M. Hypoglycemia. In S. A. Kaplan (ed.), *Clinical Pediatric and Adolescent Endocrinology.* Philadelphia: W. B. Saunders, 1982.
LaFranchi, S. Hypoglycemia in infancy and childhood. *Pediatr. Clin. North Am.* 34:961, 1987.

# Diabetic Ketoacidosis
Wah Jun Tze

Diabetic ketoacidosis (DKA) is defined as significant hyperglycemia (blood sugar > 17 mmol/liter or 300 mg/dl), ketonemia, ketonuria, and metabolic acidosis (pH < 7.3, $HCO_3$ < 15 mmol/liter) in the patient with diabetes mellitus. DKA is often the first presentation of diabetes mellitus in children. In known diabetics it may follow infection, trauma, or noncompliance with insulin therapy.

**I. Diagnosis and assessment**
   **A. History.** The clinical manifestations include a history of weight loss, vomiting, abdominal pain, polydipsia, urinary frequency, and polyuria. In all cases, events leading to the onset should be determined, a recent weight should be recorded for calculation purposes, and, in the known diabetic, the time and dose of the last insulin administration should be ascertained.
   **B. Examination.** Patients usually present with a distinctive clinical picture characterized by dehydration, Kussmaul's (deep, rapid) breathing, a fruity odor to the breath, and progressive cerebral obtundation. Other disorders that may resemble this presentation include uremia and salicylate intoxication. Look for signs of shock and establish the degree of dehydration by examining skin turgor, orthostatic changes in vital signs, capillary refill, and temperature of the extremities (see Chap. 23, sec. **II** and Chap. 4). Examine the child carefully for signs of infection or physical trauma. An accurate body weight must be determined before starting therapy.

**II. Principles of management.** There are no rigid guidelines for therapy. Management must be individualized, and the patient must be carefully monitored throughout treatment. The clinical response and biochemical status dictate ongoing management. The treatment principles are:
   **A.** Prompt correction of dehydration and electrolyte deficiencies.
   **B.** Insulin administration by continuous low-dose infusion regimen.
   **C.** Identification and treatment of precipitating factors.
   **D.** Prevention and control of complications such as shock,

oliguria, cardiac dysrhythmia, hypokalemia, and cerebral edema.

**E.** Gradual correction of metabolic disturbance, guided by frequent monitoring and assessment.

## III. Management

### A. Immediate

1. Assess and control breathing and circulation problems. Place the child on a cardiac monitor and give oxygen by mask. Dysrhythmias in the patient with DKA are usually due to hypokalemia.

2. Start two intravenous lines. Line 1 is for fluid and electrolyte replacement; line 2 is for continuous low-dose insulin infusion.

3. Obtain blood for measurements of blood gases, glucose, electrolytes, osmolality, blood urea nitrogen (BUN), creatinine, calcium, phosphorus, and complete blood count (CBC). Obtain a urinalysis in all patients and blood and urine cultures as indicated. Although the total body potassium level is decreased, serum potassium may be normal or increased secondary to cellular shift. Frequently, the child has a leukocytosis in the absence of infection.

### B. Fluid and electrolyte replacement—line 1. This is the most important aspect of therapy following initial clinical assessment. For treatment of patients in shock see Chap. 4.

1. **Requirements.** The fluid deficit in severe diabetic ketoacidosis is about 10–15% of ideal body weight (100–150 ml/kg); the sodium deficit is approximately 70–80 mEq/1000 ml of fluid loss. Half of the fluid and electrolyte deficit should be given during the first 8 hours; the remaining half is given over the subsequent 16 hours. Serum osmolality should decline gradually; a rapid decrease may contribute to cerebral edema.

2. **Fluid administration protocol**

   a. **Immediate.** Begin with a rapid infusion of intravenous normal saline as follows: for children less than 25 kg, give 250 ml; for children 25–50 kg, give 500 ml; for children greater than 50 kg, give 1000 ml.

   b. **First 2 hours.** After the initial normal saline infusion, change the solution to one-half normal saline given at a rate of 10 ml/kg/hour for 2 hours.

   c. **Third to eighth hours.** Administer the remainder of the first half of the estimated fluid deficit at 5 ml/kg/hour using one-half normal saline. Change to 5% or 10% dextrose with one-half normal saline when the blood glucose concentration approaches 14 mmol/liter (250 mg/dl).

   d. **Ninth to twenty-fourth hours.** Give the remaining half of the estimated fluid deficit as one-half normal saline, usually with dextrose added.

3. **Bicarbonate.** With fluid, electrolyte, and insulin administration, the metabolic acidosis usually corrects spontaneously. Bicarbonate used in the treat-

ment of DKA has been implicated in causing cerebral hypoxia, cerebral edema, and hypokalemia, and is therefore not recommended unless there is hypotension or shock associated with a pH of less than 7.00. In this case, give 1.0 mEq/kg of $NaHCO_3$ IV over 30–60 minutes.

**C. Insulin administration—line 2.** Continuous low-dose insulin infusion is an effective, reliable, and simple therapy for DKA. The rate of decline of blood glucose is predictable and linear for each patient, and the risk of hypokalemia is minimal.

   **1. Preparation.** Use regular insulin only, infused into a separate intravenous line (line 2). Make up a solution of *0.1* units/ml by adding 50 units of regular insulin to 500 ml of normal saline. In the child with evidence of normal renal function, add 15 mEq of KCl and 15 mEq of $KPO_4$ to each 500 ml of the insulin solution. $KPO_4$ is usually discontinued after the first 8 hours. Saturate the insulin-binding sites by allowing 50–100 ml of prepared solution to run through the tubing.

   **2. Initial dose.** Give a priming dose of regular insulin, 0.1 unit/kg body weight, by intravenous push.

   **3. Ongoing infusion.** Follow with an infusion of 0.1 unit/kg/hour—this equals a rate of 1 ml/kg/hour of solution as prepared in step 1 above. For example, the rate in a 30-kg child would be 30 ml/hour. Continue the insulin infusion until the blood pH is greater than 7.35.

   **4. Glucose infusion.** When the blood glucose level approaches 14 mmol/liter (250 mg/dl) change the solution in line 1 to 5% or 10% dextrose with one-half normal saline (see sec. **III.B.2.c** above).

**D. Monitoring.** Following initial therapy and blood work, regular monitoring of vital signs and neurologic status (including GCS scale—see Chap. 41) is indicated. Use a flow sheet to record blood work, intake and output, electrolyte infusion, dose of insulin, and vital signs. Determine ketones and glucose levels in urine specimens. Blood tests should be ordered as follows:

   **1.** Blood glucose levels hourly at bedside.

   **2.** Blood gas and electrolyte measurements every 2–3 hours during insulin infusion.

**E. Complications.** Complications of diabetic ketoacidosis include:

   **1.** Irreversible cerebral edema. Factors that may contribute to this often fatal complication include very rapid administration of a large volume of fluid and electrolytes, alteration of cerebral pH following a large dose of bicarbonate, and hypoxia.

   **2.** Hypokalemia.

   **3.** Cardiac dysrhythmia.

   **4.** Acute renal failure.

**IV. Disposition.** Children with shock, cerebral edema, or cardiac dysrhythmias should be admitted to an intensive care unit.

## V. Key points

1. The key to treatment of diabetic ketoacidosis is rehydration.
2. Use an insulin infusion to regain biochemical homeostasis.
3. Avoid bicarbonate therapy unless the child has hypotension or shock with a pH of less than 7.00.

### Bibliography

Brink, S. J. Diabetic Ketoacidosis. In *Pediatric and Adolescent Diabetes Mellitus*. Chicago: Year Book Medical Publishers, 1987.

Drash, A. K. The Complications of Diabetes Mellitus. In *Clinical Care of the Diabetic Child*. Chicago: Year Book Medical Publishers, 1987.

Sperling, M. A. Diabetic ketoacidosis. *Pediatr. Clin. North Am.* 31:591, 1984.

# 14

# Ear, Nose, and Throat Disorders

Keith H. Riding

I. **Otalgia.** Intrinsic otalgia can be caused by disease of the middle ear, external ear, or pinna. The majority of cases are due to otitis media or otitis externa. Many conditions can cause extrinsic pain that is referred to the ear (Table 14-1).

A. **Diagnosis and assessment**

1. **History.** Infants may have a history of tugging at a painful ear. Pain on mastication may be due to otitis externa, temporomandibular joint syndrome, or dental disorders. Pain on blowing the nose or swallowing suggests otitis media. Ear discharge and hearing loss is associated with acute otitis media and with otitis externa. In all cases, ask about trauma or previous surgery.

2. **Examination.** Note whether there is fever or signs of toxicity. Examine the pinna for signs of trauma or cellulitis. Pain on movement of the pinna suggests otitis externa or perichondritis. Examine the mastoid area for signs of erythema, swelling, or tenderness. On otoscopic examination look for maceration and inflammation of the canal (otitis externa) and examine the tympanic membrane noting its color, translucency, position, and mobility. Use a pneumatic otoscope to determine if there is decreased mobility—the most sensitive clinical indicator of an effusion. When ear pain is due to an extrinsic cause (see Table 14-1), the mischief is most likely to be found in the oral cavity; examine the throat, tonsils, teeth, and neck.

B. **Causes of otalgia**

1. **Acute otitis externa.** The prime symptom of otitis externa is pain that is made worse by chewing, talking, or moving the pinna. Other symptoms include pruritus of the ear, foul-smelling discharge, and loss of hearing. On examination erythema, discharge, and swelling of the canal are found.

   a. Most cases of **generalized** otitis externa are due to gram-negative bacteria such as *Pseudomonas aeruginosa* or *Proteus mirabilis*. There is usually a history of a foreign body, swimming, or trauma from attempts to clean the ear. Debris and cerumen accumulate and trap water, promoting infection.

   b. A furuncle is a **localized** staphylococcal infection that causes severe pain.

   c. Impetigo and *Herpes simplex* infection may also involve the external canal.

   d. **Management**

   (1) Clean the ear canal of debris by suction or by wiping with cotton pledgets. If pain is severe, provide analgesia with codeine, 0.5–1.0 mg/kg PO or IM prior to the procedure. Re-

**Table 14-1. Causes of otalgia in children**

| Type | Cause, path of referred pain | Examples, sites |
|---|---|---|
| Intrinsic | External ear | Otitis externa, foreign body, perichondritis, preauricular cyst/sinus, myringitis bullosa, trauma, tumor |
| | Middle ear, mastoid, and eustachian tube | Barotrauma, middle ear effusion, acute otitis media, mastoiditis, tumor, histiocytosis X |
| Extrinsic (referred) | Trigeminal nerve | Dental, jaw, TM joint, oral cavity |
| | Facial nerve | Bell's palsy, tumors, herpes zoster |
| | Glossopharyngeal nerve | Tonsil, oropharynx, nasopharynx |
| | Vagus nerve | Laryngopharynx, esophagus, thyroid |
| | Cervical nerves | Lymph nodes, cysts, cervical spine, neuralgia |
| | Miscellaneous | Migraine, aural neuralgia, salivary gland, sinuses, CNS |

Source: Adapted from W. D. Chasin. Causes of otalgia in children. In C. D. Bluestone, and S. E. Stool (eds.), *Pediatric Otolaryngology*, Vol. 1. Philadelphia: W.B. Saunders, 1983.

peat cleaning may be required on a daily basis if the inflammation is severe.

**(2)** Treat for 1 week with topical benzethonium chloride and hydrocortisone (Vosol HC) or an antibiotic-steroid medication such as framycetin-dexamethasone (Sofracort). One to two drops should be instilled q2–3h while the child is awake.

**(3)** If there is significant swelling of the canal, insert a preformed wick (Oto-wick by Xomed), or make one from ribbon gauze soaked in antibiotic ointment. Instruct parents to add the eardrops to the wick.

**(4)** A furuncle should be allowed to drain spontaneously. Incision may lead to perichondritis.

**(5)** Systemic antibiotics are indicated only when there is considerable surrounding cellulitis. In this case, treat with intravenous gentamicin and cloxacillin, oxacillin, or another suitable antistaphylococcal agent.

**(6)** Advise parents to keep the ear out of water and to avoid cleaning the ear canal in the future. Swabs of the canal for culture are misleading and unnecessary.

2. **Acute suppurative otitis media.** Otitis media usually follows an upper respiratory infection (URI). The common pathogens are *Streptococcus pneumoniae,* nontypable *Haemophilus influenzae, Branhamella catarrhalis, Streptococcus pyogenes,* and in the newborn, coliforms and *Staphylococcus aureus.* Pain, which may be intense, is always present in children who are old enough to localize (nearly all by age 3). The child may have a fever and look "toxic." Young infants often present with constitutional upset characterized by nausea, vomiting, and irritability. Never assume otitis media is the only cause of fever, toxicity, or irritability in a young child—there may be serious concurrent infections such as meningitis, pneumonia, or sepsis. The diagnosis can usually be confirmed by finding decreased drum mobility on pneumatic otoscopy or by finding a perforated drum and pus in the canal. Color and position of the drum can be misleading (e.g., if the child is crying, a normal drum may appear red).

   a. **Management.** Codeine, 0.5–1.0 mg IM or PO may be necessary for pain relief. The initial choices for antibiotic therapy include amoxicillin, 35–50 mg/kg/day PO divided q8h, or trimethoprim-sulfamethoxazole, 8 mg/kg/day as trimethoprim, PO divided q12h, given for 10 days. "Second line" drugs include amoxicillin trihydrate with potassium clavulanate (Clavulin), cefaclor (Ceclor), and erythromycin ethylsuccinate with sulfisoxazole (Pediazole). Decongestants or antihistamines are not indicated for the treatment of

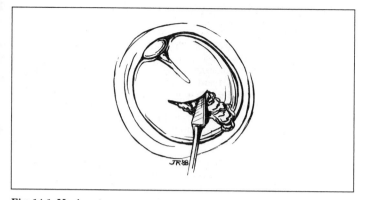

**Fig. 14-1. Myringotomy.**

children with otitis media. Arrange for follow-up in 2–3 weeks time.

  **b. Tympanocentesis**

    **(1) Indications.** Tympanocentesis is indicated in children with facial palsy, mastoiditis, CNS infection, or immune compromise, and in symptomatic babies under 8 weeks of age. It is often performed by an ENT surgeon.

    **(2) Equipment**

      **(a)** Otoscope with operating head or binocular operating microscope

      **(b)** 22-gauge lumbar puncture needle on a TB syringe or Senturia trap with wall suction

      **(c)** 70% alcohol solution

    **(3) Method**

      **(a)** Have an assistant restrain the child. Inspect the drum and clean any wax or debris from the canal.

      **(b)** To achieve antisepsis, fill the canal with 70% alcohol and drain.

      **(c)** Insert the needle into the canal and pierce the drum anteriorly and inferiorly, avoiding the posterior superior quadrant (Fig. 14-1).

      **(d)** Aspirate with the syringe or Senturia trap.

    **(4) Complications**

      **(a)** Bleeding

      **(b)** Infection

      **(c)** Ossicle damage

      **(d)** Laceration of membrane

**3. Acute serous otitis media.** Serous otitis media is present in all children with an upper respiratory tract infection. If bubbles are visible behind the drum, the diagnosis is certain. The drum often appears opaque, retracted, and immobile and is yellow, white, or red. Pain, if present, is rarely severe.

a. **Management.** Treatment is unnecessary in the child without pain who is old enough to localize. If there is pain or if the child is too young to localize it, treat as acute suppurative otitis media.

4. **Chronic perforation or tympanostomy tube that is discharging (chronic suppurative otitis media).** When water flows through an existing perforation or tympanostomy tube, the middle ear mucosa becomes irritated and inflamed. This condition is characterized by painless purulent discharge and in some cases by bleeding from inflamed mucosa or granulomatous tissue.

a. **Management.** Thoroughly clean the canal using a Q-tip with some of the cotton unwound from its end. Antibiotic drops should be instilled q2–3 hourly (i.e., framycetin) and worked into the middle ear by pumping the tragus 20–30 times. Systemic antibiotics are not required, and culture of the discharge is not indicated.

5. **Myringitis bullosa (hemorrhagica).** This very painful condition is characterized by blisters or blebs on the drum or skin of the deep ear canal that burst and release the blood within them. The middle ear is unaffected. The etiology is thought to be viral, although *Mycoplasma pneumoniae* has been demonstrated in one patient.

a. **Management.** Prescribe acetaminophen or codeine for analgesia. Although its effectiveness is unproved, oral erythromycin is often prescribed. Incision or rupture of the blebs is contraindicated; it will not help and may introduce infection.

6. **Acute mastoiditis with subperiosteal abscess**

a. **Mastoiditis.** Mastoiditis is due to an acute osteitis causing a breakdown of the bony trabeculae and abscess formation within the mastoid process. The organisms involved are identical to those that cause acute suppurative otitis media. Mastoiditis usually occurs 2–3 weeks after an untreated middle ear infection. The child presents with mastoid pain, discharge, and swelling over the mastoid and a characteristic sagging of the posterior ear canal. "Masked" mastoiditis occurs in the child who has been partially or ineffectively treated for otitis media.

b. **Postauricular periosteitis.** Periosteitis is a spread of inflammation from the mastoid mucosa to the periosteum that occurs during acute suppurative otitis media. It is seen in infants.

c. **Management.** All patients with mastoid infections should be admitted and referred to a surgeon. X rays are unnecessary; the diagnosis is clinical, and interpretation of the films is difficult. Obtain blood for complete blood count (CBC) and culture. The treatment of mastoiditis is usually surgical drainage, although early cases may respond to myringotomy and high-dose antibiotic therapy with cloxacillin or oxacillin, 150 mg/kg/day IV divided q6h or another suitable antistaphylococcal drug.

**7. Acute perichondritis of the pinna.** This infection usually occurs following a laceration, insect bite, or hematoma of the pinna. Erythema and swelling spread to involve the entire pinna, which is very painful and tender. Areas of fluctuation may occur with spontaneous rupture and drainage of pus. In severe cases, complete destruction of the cartilage may occur.

  **a. Management.** Consult an ENT surgeon for incision, irrigation, and admission for intravenous antibiotic therapy with gentamicin and cloxacillin, oxacillin, or another suitable antistaphylococcal agent.

**8. Infection of a pierced ear.** Pierced ear infection can result in mild infection or abscess formation. Mild infection should be distinguished from a metal allergy, which causes repeated mild inflammation of the lobule.

  **a. Management.** Mild infection often responds to aggressive cleansing with alcohol wipes, but removal of the stud or earring is usually required to allow drainage. To remove the earring with minimal discomfort use two pair of alligator forceps, one to grip the earring, the other to grip the stud. General anesthesia may be required for removal in the small child with an abscess. Give cephalexin or cloxacillin, 50 mg/kg/day PO divided q6h or another suitable antistaphylococcal drug for 10 days.

**C. Disposition.** Acute perichondritis and mastoiditis require semiurgent admission to hospital.

**D. Key points**

  **1.** The diagnosis of acute suppurative otitis media is unlikely in the child without ear pain who is able to localize.

  **2.** Do not incise or rupture blebs in children with myringitis bullosa.

**II. Trauma**

  **A. Laceration of the pinna** (see Chap. 35). These lacerations should be sutured under local or general anesthesia, depending on the age of the child and the extent of the laceration. Care should be taken to preserve as much of the cartilage as possible. Animal bites and tears must be carefully debrided prior to suturing. Treat with prophylactic phenoxymethyl penicillin, 50 mg/kg/day PO divided q6h for 10 days, and give a tetanus booster immunization to those at risk (see Appendix).

**B. Hematoma of the pinna.** This type of hematoma occurs after direct trauma and presents as a painful fluctuant swelling. Untreated, the clot organizes, and a "cauliflower ear" may develop.

  **1. Management.** A recent hematoma may be aspirated by large-bore needle. Older lesions should be incised, and the clot evacuated using meticulous sterile technique. A firm dressing, incorporating a mold (such as a dental stent) should be applied. Beware of perichondritis—arrange for follow-up within 24 hours with an ENT surgeon.

**C. Acute traumatic perforation of the tympanic membrane.** Perforation may be caused by a blow to the ear, a nearby explosion, or direct trauma. The latter is more common, often occurring when the child or parent is suddenly jostled while cleaning the ear. The canal is usually scratched and bleeding. Ossicular fracture or inner ear trauma should be suspected in the patient with vertigo or hearing loss.

  **1. Management.** In most cases, treatment with analgesics is all that is required. There is no indication for local cleaning or systemic or topical antibiotics. Instruct parents to keep water out of the ear and arrange follow-up in 6 weeks for examination and a hearing test. Patients with vertigo or severe hearing loss should be immediately referred to an ENT surgeon.

**D. Acute barotrauma.** A sudden increase in outside air pressure during aircraft descent or scuba diving can result in extreme negative pressure in the middle ear. This leads to hemorrhage into the middle ear with sudden onset of severe pain. On examination, the drum appears very retracted, opaque, red or purple, and immobile. There may be hemorrhage into the drum itself.

  **1. Management.** Treat with analgesics. Antibiotics are not required. Occasionally, myringotomy is indicated to provide pain relief.

**E. Nasal fracture.** Immediately following injury, there is usually swelling of the dorsum of the nose and minor bleeding. Periorbital bruising is almost pathognomonic of bony nasal fracture. When swelling is not marked, displacement can be diagnosed clinically. Check for associated facial bone fracture (see Chap. 35). Examine the inside of the nose for septal hematoma; it appears bilaterally as a soft, fluctuant, septal swelling, almost completely blocking the nasal passages. Septal hematoma can be complicated by infection, destruction of septal cartilage, and nasal collapse.

X rays to prove fracture should be ordered for medicolegal purposes only—they cannot be used to diagnose displacement. When injury is due to a motor vehicle accident, personal assault, or child abuse, legal evidence may be required, and careful documentation is important.

  **1. Management.** Lacerations and cartilaginous tears

should be repaired immediately. Through and through lacerations should be referred to a surgeon for layered closure and antibiotic therapy. If there is severe swelling, send the patient home for symptomatic treatment with ice packs and analgesics; arrange for follow-up in a few days after the swelling has lessened to determine if there is displacement. If there is displacement, consult a surgeon for repositioning. A fractured nasal bone becomes too fixed to be treated after 7–10 days. If septal hematoma is suspected, consult a surgeon for treatment with penicillin and evacuation under general anesthesia.

**F. Laceration of the tongue and soft palate.** This commonly occurs in the young child who falls with an object in the mouth. There may be laceration of the anterior tonsillar pillar, soft palate, or tongue. Occasionally, life-threatening injury occurs when a sharp object penetrates the cranial cavity or carotid artery.

  **1. Management.** Full-thickness lacerations and those with heavy bleeding should be sutured under general anesthesia. Superficial lacerations require no treatment and heal in a week. Analgesics and a soft diet help to reduce pain.

**G. Disposition.** Patients with septal hematomas and children with full-thickness or heavily bleeding tongue lacerations require semiurgent admission for surgery.

**H. Key points**

  **1.** X rays are indicated for medicolegal purposes only in children with nasal fracture.

  **2.** Traumatic perforation of the tympanic membrane usually requires symptomatic treatment only. Refer to a surgeon if there is vertigo or severe hearing loss.

**III. Epistaxis.** Bleeding from the anterior nose (Little's anterior septal area or Kiesselbach's plexus) accounts for the majority of cases of epistaxis. Bleeding is rarely severe, and patients can usually be managed on an outpatient basis. For a list of causes see Table 14-2.

**A. Diagnosis and assessment**

  **1. History.** Determine the amount of bleeding (size of towel or handkerchief used to stop the flow, and whether soaked or stained). Ask about risk factors such as forced air or dry heating, smoking, trauma (including nose picking), foreign body, infection, allergy, or high blood pressure. In children with recurrent or severe epistaxis consider the diagnosis of von Willebrand's disease or other bleeding diathesis.

  **2. Examination.** If bleeding has been severe, check for signs of hypovolemia and treat accordingly. Look for petechiae, purpura, and other areas of bleeding as evidence of a bleeding diathesis.

**B. Management**

  **1. Severe bleeding.** If blood loss is heavy or if there are signs of hypovolemia, start a large-bore intravenous line, give oxygen, and obtain a CBC, platelet count, prothrombin time (PT), partial thromboplas-

**Table 14-2. Causes of epistaxis**

| Class | Type | Examples |
|-------|------|----------|
| Common causes | Inflammation | Upper respiratory infection, childhood exanthems, allergic rhinitis/polyp |
| | Trauma | Dry air, nasal injury, nose picking |
| Uncommon causes | Bleeding diathesis | Dysfunctioning platelets, thrombocytopenia, coagulation defects |
| | Hypertension | |
| | Hereditary hemorrhagic telangiectasia (Osler-Rendu-Weber syndrome) | |
| | Neoplasm | Juvenile nasopharyngeal angiofibroma, rhabdomyosarcoma |

tin time (PTT), and cross-match. Suspect a bleeding diathesis in such cases. See Chaps. 4 and 19, Purpura and Bleeding Disorders, for specific treatment.

2. **Minor bleeding.** This group comprises the great majority of cases.

   a. **Identify the source.**
      Wear a gown and provide one for the child. Have the child sitting up in a chair, holding a kidney dish to catch any blood that spills. Gently lift the tip of the nose and examine each nasal cavity with a bright light. Severe posterior bleeding in a teenage boy may be due to juvenile nasopharygeal angiofibroma. These children may have a history of gradually increasing nasal obstruction.

   b. **Pressure.** If the source is anterior, squeeze the anterior nose between the thumb and index finger. If bleeding stops, have the parent or child squeeze for 20 minutes.

   c. **Cautery.** If pressure is ineffective, anesthetize the nose with a pledget of cotton dampened with 4% or 10% cocaine (preferred) or 4% lidocaine, with or without epinephrine. Place the pledget in the bleeding side and squeeze for 10–15 minutes. If bleeding stops hold a silver nitrate stick, firmly enough to bend the stick, on the offending blood vessel for 1 minute. Silver nitrate cautery is contraindicated in patients with bleeding diatheses.

   d. **Children with bleeding diathesis.** In these patients bleeding may be controlled by placing Gelfoam or Oxycel in the nasal cavity. Blood component therapy with FFP, factor concentrate, platelets, or cryoprecipitate may be required.

   e. **Packing.** If cautery is ineffective, the nose should be packed. Layer ¼- or ½-inch ribbon gauze soaked in antibiotic ointment from the bottom to the top of the nasal cavity, with the loose ends hanging from the nares. In children, posterior nasal packing should be performed only by an ENT surgeon. Following packing, inspect the pharynx to make sure that the bleeding has not been diverted. If bleeding has stopped, the child should be positioned in bed with the head elevated 20 degrees and the pack left in place for 48 hours. Improper packing may worsen the situation. If in doubt about the indications or method, consult an ENT surgeon.

   f. **Discharge.** If bleeding has been controlled and there is no suspicion of serious underlying disease, the child may be discharged. Instruct the parents to grease the nose with Vaseline, avoid hot air vents, and provide humidification with a cool mist vaporizer at the bedside. Caution against nose picking.

C. **Disposition.** Admit all children with hypovolemia and those who require posterior packing.

## D. Key points

1. Do not use silver nitrate cautery for the treatment of epistaxis in patients with bleeding disorders.
2. In children, posterior nasal packing should be performed by an ENT surgeon.

## IV. Infection

**A. Sinusitis.** The maxillary and ethmoid sinuses can be infected at any age. Frontal sinusitis does not occur in the young child (< 6 years) because the sinuses have not yet developed. In the classic case, there is a history of URI followed by sinus pain, fever, nasal obstruction, and rhinorrhea that is colorless to green in appearance. There may be erythema over the sinus and tenderness on palpation. The inferior turbinate often appears engorged, with pus visible in the middle meatus. Sinus x rays are unreliable for the diagnosis of sinusitis in children under 5 years of age.

1. **Management.** The treatment of sinusitis includes analgesics and 2–3 weeks of antibiotic therapy. The choice of antibiotics is similar to that described in sec. **I.B.2,** above. Local decongestants such as xylometazoline (Otrivin) or phenylephrine (Neosynephrine) drops or spray may be administered topically up to every 4 hours. Advise parents against the use of topical decongestants for more than 4 days because rebound swelling may occur. Systemic decongestants may also be used. Surgical drainage is indicated in refractory cases.

**B. Acute tonsillitis.** Symptoms and signs of acute tonsillitis include fever, dysphagia, tonsillar exudate, and cervical lymphadenopathy. Occasionally, severe tonsillar hypertrophy may lead to airway obstruction; this is most commonly seen in young children with Epstein-Barr virus (EBV) infection.

Over 85% of cases of tonsillitis are **viral** in etiology. Children with EBV infection may have additional findings of splenomegaly and generalized lymphadenopathy.

The commonest **bacterial** pathogen is group A beta-hemolytic streptococcus. Diphtheria, a rare cause of bacterial tonsillitis, is characterized by the presence of a membranous exudate extending from the tonsil onto the soft palate, tongue, anterior or posterior pillars, or posterior pharyngeal wall. Suspect gonococcal infection in sexually active teenagers or sexually abused children.

1. **Diagnosis.** When available, a positive result from a rapid streptococcal antigen test (Culturette, Directogen) of a throat swab can allow for immediate diagnosis and therapy. Always perform a culture in addition to antigen testing. If EBV is suspected, order a serum Monospot test. False-negative results for the Monospot test are nearly universal in children under the age of 3.

2. **Management**

   a. When rapid streptococcal antigen testing is not available, the treatment is symptomatic pending culture results. Children with documented group

A streptococcal infection should be given phenoxymethyl penicillin, 50 mg/kg/day PO divided q6h, or erythromycin, 30–50 mg/kg/day PO divided q6h.

  **b.** Children with airway obstruction require urgent ENT consultation. Steroids (dexamethasone, 1 mg/kg IV as a loading dose followed by 0.5 mg/kg/dose IV q6h) may be helpful to decrease swelling in EBV-induced airway compromise.

  **c.** Children with diphtheria should be admitted for monitoring and treatment with antitoxin and penicillin G, 150,000 units/kg/day IV divided q6h, or erythromycin, 50 mg/kg/day PO.

  **d.** For treatment of gonococcal infection, see Chap. 21, Sexually Transmitted Diseases.

**C. Peritonsillar abscess.** The organisms commonly found in peritonsillar abscess are group A streptococcus and *Staphylococcus aureus*. Patients typically have a history of progressive sore throat and the following three pathognomonic signs:

  **1.** Trismus—inability to open the mouth due to muscle spasm.

  **2.** Drooling—inability to swallow.

  **3.** Deviation of the uvula to the side opposite the infection, due to swelling on the affected side.

  **4.** In addition, there may be edema and erythema of the soft palate, toxicity, dysphagia, and a muffling of speech described as a "hot potato voice."

  **5. Management.** In the early stages, cellulitis that has not progressed to an abscess may be treated with intravenous penicillin, 100,000 units/kg/day divided q6h. Children with an abscess require incision and drainage under general anesthesia in addition to the following antibiotics:

   **a.** Clindamycin, 30 mg/kg/day IV divided q6h **or**

   **b.** Cloxacillin or oxacillin, 150 mg/kg/day IV divided q6h **and**

   **c.** Chloramphenicol, 50–75 mg/kg/day IV divided q6h.

**D. Retropharyngeal abscess.** Children under age 6 have retropharyngeal lymph nodes that can become infected (often following a URI) and form an abscess. The common isolates are group A streptococcus and *S. aureus*. The clinical picture may resemble acute epiglottitis, with dysphagia and difficulty in breathing—the child may drool and hold the neck rigidly extended if there is airway compromise. The diagnosis can be made by a lateral soft tissue neck x ray that demonstrates swelling and edema behind the pharynx (normally there is < 10 mm between the anterior pharynx and the body of C4).

  **1. Management.** When retropharyngeal abscess is suspected, consult a surgeon for treatment with incision and drainage. Obtain a blood culture, start an IV, and give intravenous antibiotics as in sec. **IV.C,** above.

**E. Cervical adenitis.** URIs often result in cervical lymphadenopathy. Occasionally, the lymph nodes are over-whelmed by bacterial infection and break down, forming an abscess. Bacterial lymphadenitis in the neck usually presents with a painful, enlarged (3–6 cm) swelling of a single node (submandibular, anterior cervical). There is usually erythema and warmth of the overlying skin, but fever is mild or absent. Nearly all cases are due to infection with *S. aureus* or group A streptococcus. Diagnosis can be confirmed by aspiration: anesthetize the skin over the node with 1% plain lidocaine, then carefully puncture the skin and aspirate the node with an 18-gauge needle. Send the aspirate for Gram's stain and culture. Take a throat culture when there are symptoms or signs of pharyngitis.

  **1. Management**
  - **a.** If lymphadenitis is suspected and the node is nonfluctuant, treat with PO cephalexin or cloxacillin, 50 mg/kg/day divided q6h and arrange for follow-up in 24–48 hours.
  - **b.** If the node is fluctuant, perform incision and drainage.
  - **c.** If the child is toxic or if the infection is unresponsive to oral therapy, obtain blood for CBC and culture and admit the patient for treatment with intravenous cloxacillin or oxacillin, 150 mg/kg/day divided q6h, or other suitable antistaphylococcal agent for 5–10 days.
  - **d.** In children with an atypical presentation or poor response to therapy, consider other causes of lymphadenopathy, including cat scratch fever, Kawasaki syndrome, EBV infection, and infiltrative neoplasm.

**F. Croup and epiglottitis.** See Chap. 6.

**G. Oral infections.** Oral infections may present as ulcers, gingivostomatitis, or thrush.

  **1. Ulcers**
  - **a.** Aphthous ulcers are painful grey lesions on a red base that can occur singly or in clusters anywhere on the oral mucosa. They usually heal in 1–2 weeks.
  - **b.** Herpangina is caused by Coxsackie A viruses and usually occurs in children under 4 years of age. The child has a sudden onset of fever and refuses to eat because of a sore throat. There is diffuse pharyngeal injection and ulcers on the fauces, tonsils, pillars, or soft palate.
  - **c.** Hand, foot, and mouth disease is also due to Coxsackie A viruses. Children often have fever, headache, malaise, and oropharyngeal vesicles that may occur anywhere on the oral mucosa and eventually change to shallow, painful ulcers. The diagnosis is confirmed by finding a vesicular eruption on the hands, feet, or buttocks.
  - **d.** Gingivostomatitis due to herpes simplex virus usually occurs in infants and toddlers, causing high fever and malaise. On examination, cervical

adenopathy, foul breath, gingivitis, and vesicles are found on the lips and oral mucosa; the vesicles eventually transform to painful ulcers. Resolution requires 10–14 days. Dehydration may occur owing to poor oral intake.

**e.** Vincent's angina is a very rare disease of young adults and adolescents that results in severe oral pain and is characterized by ulcerated interdental papillae covered by a pale pseudomembrane. There is a foul odor to the breath.

**f.** Other causes of mouth ulcers include varicella, EBV, and trauma (dental braces, retainer).

**g. Management.** In general, treatment is symptomatic. Fluid refusal secondary to pain may result in dehydration; advise parents to ensure adequate intake. Cold liquids or popsicles often decrease the pain and are better tolerated. A 1 : 1 mixture of lidocaine viscous 2% and diphenhydramine (Benadryl) elixir can be brushed onto the painful lesions with a Q-tip prior to meals. Do not allow the child to drink the solution, because toxicity with seizures may result. Admit children who are dehydrated or who refuse to drink for intravenous fluid administration. Refer cases of Vincent's angina to a dentist for debridement and treat with phenoxymethyl penicillin, 50 mg/kg/day PO divided q6h.

**2. Oral thrush.** Thrush is an infection due to *Candida* and is common in infants under 6 months, but it can also occur in children who have been treated with broad-spectrum antibiotics. When persistent in children over 1 year of age, it suggests immune compromise (T-cells). On examination, there are white patches that may occur throughout the mucosa. Treat with oral nystatin 1 ml (100,000 units) PO qid, continued until 2–3 days after visible evidence of infection has resolved. The drug must be well distributed in the mouth for maximal benefit, requiring deliberate rinsing or painting of all oral surfaces. Treat candidal skin infections with nystatin cream qid.

**H. Disposition.** Peritonsillar abscess, retropharyngeal abscess, severe cervical adenitis, and children with mouth ulcers who refuse to drink require admission.

**I. Key points**

**1.** Sinus x rays are unreliable in young children.

**2.** Airway obstruction due to EBV tonsillitis can be treated with intravenous steroids.

**V. Foreign bodies**

**A. Foreign bodies in the ear**

**1. Cerumen impaction.** This is not an emergent condition. Immediate removal is indicated when the tympanic membrane must be inspected. Otherwise, the parent is instructed to fill the ear canal with oil (any cooking oil will do) every night for 2 weeks and let the family physician remove the cerumen at his leisure. Advise against the use of Q-tips for ear cleaning, because this may worsen the impaction or injure the canal or tympanic membrane. Consult an ENT surgeon whenever there is difficulty in the treatment of foreign bodies in children.

**a. Management options**

(1) **Irrigation.** Use a syringe or a dental water pick—the latter is often better tolerated by the small child. Irrigate the ear canal with body temperature water, aiming the jet along the canal and behind the cerumen to push it out. Avoid irrigation in a child with a perforation or tympanostomy tube, as pain and infection may result.

(2) **Mechanical removal.** Use an otoscope with an operating head. Restrain the child and remove the cerumen with a wire loop or wax curette, taking care not to curette or scrape the ear canal.

(3) **Cerumenolytic agents.** Severe local reactions are common with these substances, especially if they are used incorrectly. They should be avoided in children with atopy because severe eczematous eruptions may result.

2. **Foreign bodies.** If the ear is bleeding, indicating a laceration of the canal wall or tympanic membrane, the foreign body must be extracted. Otherwise, if there is no complication, the object need not be removed immediately. Inexpert attempts at extraction can be harmful. Only one attempt should be made at removal; if this is unsuccessful, consult an ENT surgeon.

**a. Management**

(1) Use an otoscope with an operating head or binocular operating otoscope. The child should be lying down and should be restrained if necessary. Have an assistant steady the head.

(2) Look for barbs or hooks that may be stuck in the skin. Soft, unwedged objects are often best removed by syringing the ear with water (see sec. **V.A.1.a.(1)**). Do not syringe water-absorbing materials such as vegetable or wood fibers because swelling may result, making extraction more difficult.

(a) Tightly wedged objects may require endaural incision and removal under general anesthesia.

(b) Foreign bodies that have an edge should be removed with alligator or cup forceps under direct vision.

(c) Spherical foreign bodies are pulled out with a blunt hook or bent wire loop that is slid behind the object (Fig. 14-2).

(d) To remove a tick, fill the canal with 70%

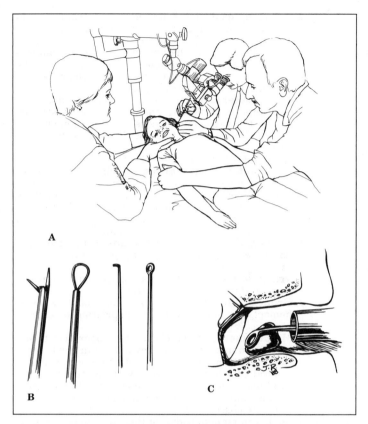

**Fig. 14-2. A. Removal of foreign bodies from the ear. B. Instruments for removal of foreign bodies from the ear. C. Removal of foreign bodies from the ear.**

alcohol. When the tick withdraws its head from the skin, remove it directly.

**B. Nasal Foreign Bodies.** These often become manifest with bleeding or unilateral nasal discharge.

   **1. Management.** Restrain the child and inspect the nose with a headlight. If swelling is severe, lidocaine 4% with epinephrine, or cocaine 4% or 10% can be dropped into the nose (beware of cocaine toxicity). Insert a hook or bent wire loop past the object, then pull it out. Make only one attempt; if this is unsuccessful, consult an ENT surgeon.

**C. Foreign bodies in the pharynx or nasopharynx.** Pharyngeal or nasopharyngeal foreign bodies may be present in the child who puts something into the mouth, has a choking spell, and then refuses food or appears uncomfortable with feeding. A nasopharyngeal foreign body causes the child to be "snuffly," with intermittent episodes of respiratory disturbance. A careful examination of the nose and throat does not always reveal the foreign body. A lateral soft tissue x ray of the neck may be helpful if the object is radiopaque.

   **1. Management.** A story suspicious of this diagnosis warrants examination under general anesthesia, even if the x rays and physical examination are normal. Refer the child to an ENT surgeon for treatment.

**D. Esophageal foreign bodies.** See Chap. 16.

**E. Foreign bodies in the larynx, trachea, or bronchi.** When a foreign body causes complete airway obstruction, the child rarely reaches the emergency room alive. For information on treatment of choking children, see Chap. 3, and for treatment and diagnosis of the child with a bronchial foreign body, see Chap. 7.

   **1. Laryngeal** foreign bodies can cause persistent pain, hoarseness, aphonia, cough, dyspnea, cyanosis, hemoptysis, or stridor.

   **2. Tracheal** foreign bodies may cause cough, wheeze, audible slap, or tracheal flutter.

   **3. Bronchial** foreign bodies may cause cough, wheeze, hemoptysis, and rhonchi on inspriation or expiration.

   **4. Management.** Order chest and upper soft tissue x rays; fluoroscopy can be invaluable in localizing a radiolucent object. Rigid endoscopic removal under general anesthesia is necessary. Do not tip the stable child upside down or try to remove the foreign body because this may convert a partial obstruction into a complete obstruction.

**F. Disposition.** Foreign bodies of the ear or nose that cannot be extracted in the emergency room should be scheduled for elective removal under general anesthesia. Pharyngeal or laryngeal foreign bodies require immediate removal in the operating room. Most esophageal and bronchial foreign bodies can be removed on an elective basis. Aspirated vegetable material should be treated immediately, before inflammation makes elective removal more difficult.

**G. Key points**

   **1.** Make only one attempt at foreign body removal—if unsuccessful, consult an ENT surgeon.

**Bibliography**

Bluestone, C. D., and Klein, J. D. *Pediatric Otolaryngology.* Vol. 1, p. 403. Philadelphia: W. B. Saunders, 1983.

Kaplan, E. I., Bell, F. H., Jr., Dudding, B. A., et al. Diagnosis of streptococcal pharyngitis: Differentiation of active infection from the carrier state in the symptomatic child. *J. Infect. Dis.* 123:490, 1973.

McCloskey, R. V., Eller, J. J., Green, M., et al. The 1970 epidemic of diphtheria in San Antonio. *Ann. Intern. Med.* 75:495, 1971.

Suen, J. Y., and Wetmore, S. J. (eds.). *Emergencies in Otolaryngology.* New York: Churchill Livingstone, 1986.

# 15

## Eye Disorders

Andrew Q. McCormick

I. **Examination of the young child's eye**
  A. **Setting.** Examine the patient in a quiet area with the parents present for assistance. A few attractive, small toys are helpful in gaining the young child's attention.
  B. **Ocular alignment.** Have the parent gently hold the child's head. Check the ocular alignment with a small light, looking for asymmetric positions of the corneal light reflexes.
  C. **Ocular movement.** Ocular movements can be assessed by having the child follow a moving toy. If one eye is kept closed due to discomfort, a drop of local anesthetic will bring quick relief from pain.
  D. **Visual acuity.** In infants and very young children, test visual acuity by ensuring that the affected eye can fixate and then follow an object while a parent gently covers the good eye.
  E. **Ophthalmoscopic examination.** Attract the child's attention to the circle of light projected by the ophthalmoscope. Dim the overhead lights and check both red reflexes simultaneously while standing a half meter from the child's face. Look for similarity in pupil size and the color of the red reflex. Move to within 5 or 6 inches of the child's face and refocus on the red reflex. Abnormality of color, clarity, or size of the red reflex indicates intraocular pathology. Pupil response to direct light can be assessed by moving the light from the brow to the pupil while viewing the pupil through the ophthalomoscope. Note the clarity of the cornea and the detail of the iris.
  F. **Slit-lamp examination.** Slit-lamp examination is often difficult in children under the age of 3. Having a child put his face up to such a daunting piece of equipment can be terrifying; if resistance is met, abandon the attempt and do what you can with the ophthalmoscope.
  G. **Fluorescein.** Fluorescein staining is indicated when corneal abrasion or herpes simplex keratitis is suspected. Wet the fluorescein strip with a drop of sterile local anesthetic and apply the strip to the margins of the slightly everted lower lid. Examine the cornea with a blue light or Wood's lamp.
II. **The red eye.** Most cases of red eye are due to conjunctival inflammation secondary to infection or allergy. Children with decreased visual acuity require urgent ophthalmologic consultation.
  A. **Diagnosis and assessment**
    1. **History.** Symptoms of conjunctival inflammation include light sensitivity, tearing, and itching. Ask about upper respiratory symptoms, pharyngitis, or fever. Foreign bodies, whether serious, as in penetrating injury, or benign, as with an eyelash in the eye, can also cause irritation and erythema. Iritis is rare in the child; it may be associated with trauma,

juvenile rheumatoid arthritis, sarcoidosis, or herpes simplex infection.

2. **Examination.** Begin by assessing visual acuity; if acuity is reduced, the child should be immediately referred to an ophthalmologist. Inspect the eye and conjunctivae; conjunctivitis is often accompanied by edema of the eyelid. Clouding of the cornea is associated with glaucoma, and a fixed or sluggish pupil response suggests glaucoma or iritis. If the child can be examined with the slit lamp, look for cells in the anterior chamber as evidence of iritis. When the diagnosis is unknown or when iritis, abrasion, or superficial foreign body is suspected, perform fluorescein staining to look for evidence of herpes simplex infection (dendritic branching pattern), or trauma.

B. **Causes of red eye**
   1. **Conjunctival infections**
      a. **Viral infection.** Viral infection is the most common cause of conjunctivitis. Upper respiratory signs or symptoms, preauricular adenopathy, and faint corneal opacities suggest the diagnosis. Severe inflammation may benefit from symptomatic treatment with an eye patch and acetaminophen. Topical antibiotics are indicated only when bacterial superinfection is suspected (see **b** below).

      b. **Bacterial infection.** Bacterial superinfection causes thick purulent discharge. Common pathogens are *Haemophilus influenzae* and *Streptococcus pneumoniae*. Obtain a swab of the discharge for Gram's stain and treat empirically with sulfacetamide 10% eye drops—1 drop q10min for the first 2 hours to sterilize the conjunctival sac, then q3–4h while awake—until culture and sensitivity results are available. Severe inflammation may benefit from symptomatic treatment with an eye patch and analgesics.

      c. **Gonococcal infection.** Gonococcal infection should be considered in any young child with a profuse purulent discharge. When gonococcal infection occurs in children beyond the neonatal period, suspect sexual abuse. The diagnosis is suggested by the presence of intracellular gram-negative diplococci on a Gram's stain of a conjunctival scraping (early) or discharge (late). Children with ophthalmic gonococcal infection should be admitted to hospital and treated with intravenous penicillin G, 50,000 units/kg/day divided q6h.

      d. **Chlamydia.** *Chlamydia trachomatis* causes conjunctivitis in infants up to 6 weeks of age. Classically, the baby has a mucopurulent or slightly blood-tinged eye discharge and may later develop pneumonitis. The diagnosis is made by immunofluorescence microscopy or culture of cells scraped from the lower lid conjunctiva with a cotton swab. Treat with erythromycin, 30–50 mg/kg/

day PO divided q6h for 4 weeks. When the diagnosis is confirmed, the mother should be treated with erythromycin or doxycycline PO (see Chap. 21, Sexually Transmitted Diseases).

   **e. Herpes simplex.** Herpes simplex keratitis may present with minimal redness and discomfort. The telltale dendritic ulcer with its branching pattern is often seen on fluorescein staining. Herpes zoster can also cause dendritic keratitis. Refer the child to a pediatric ophthalmologist for treatment.

2. **Acute iritis.** Acute iritis in the child usually results in mild symptoms. In most cases, visual acuity is reduced, and the pupil is decreased in size and reactivity. Pain is not always present. Slit-lamp examination of the anterior segment should be attempted in every child who presents with a nontraumatic red eye. Cellular deposits on the inner corneal surface or anterior lens surface appear as fine black dots in the red reflex, and the red reflex may be darker on the involved side. Refer all cases to an ophthalmologist for treatment with cycloplegics (atropine, homatropine) and steroids.

3. **Glaucoma.** Glaucoma is rare in children. It may be congenital or secondary to hyphema, surgery, or systemic disorders such as Sturge-Weber syndrome or neurofibromatosis. Children with glaucoma present with pain, tearing, and erythema. On examination, the eye is red, and the cornea may be cloudy. Visual acuity is decreased. When suspected, an ophthalmologist should be consulted immediately to verify the diagnosis and begin treatment.

C. **Disposition.** Admit all patients with gonococcal conjunctivitis. Children with acute angle closure glaucoma need admission; urgent surgery may be required.

III. **Eyelid inflammation**

A. A hordeolum or stye is a pyogenic infection of a lash follicle and may be secondary to blepharitis. Erythema, localized swelling, and tenderness at the base of the eyelash are present. Treat by plucking out the involved lash or by instructing parents to apply warm compresses for 10 minutes qid.

B. A chalazion results when a blocked meibomian gland leaks its contents into the subcutaneous tissue, resulting in a diffuse swelling of the lid. When onset is acute, it may produce discomfort. Treat with compresses made from teabags dipped in warm water, applied 10 minutes qid, to promote drainage. Refer to an ophthalmologist if symptoms are severe.

C. Blepharitis is an inflammation of the margins of the eyelid and may be associated with infection, seborrhea, or allergies. Patients with blepharitis have irritation and itching that is maximal at the lid margins. On examination there may be erythema, pustules, ulcers, and crusted lesions along the lid margin. Treat with warm compresses applied for 10 minutes qid and erythromycin ophthalmic ointment topically qid. Accompanying seborrhea of the face or scalp should be treated with 0.5% hydrocortisone ointment or selenium shampoo, respectively.

**IV. Periorbital and orbital cellulitis.** Diffuse erythema of the eyelids may be caused by allergy or cellulitis. **Allergic lid edema** is not painful but may be itchy—the child looks well and is afebrile.

**A. Diagnosis and assessment**

  **1. Periorbital cellulitis (preseptal cellulitis).** Periorbital cellulitis presents with edema and erythema around the eye without proptosis, ophthalmoplegia, or decreased visual acuity. Fever and pain are often present. When associated with skin trauma, the common pathogens are *Staphylococcus aureus* and group A streptococcus. In other cases, infection may be due to *H. influenzae* type b or pneumococcus.

  **2. Orbital cellulitis.** Orbital cellulitis presents with a painful, purple, or red swelling of the eyelids following an upper respiratory infection and is associated with ethmoid or maxillary sinusitis. There is variable proptosis with restriction of eye movement and decreased visual acuity. The patient is usually febrile and may have pain with eye movement or may complain of diplopia. When edema is severe, the lids become so tense that the globe cannot be examined. Most cases are due to *S. aureus,* streptococcus, pneumococcus, or *H. influenzae* type b. Complications of orbital cellulitis include abscess formation, blindness, and meningitis.

**B. Management**

  **1. Periorbital cellulitis.** Always obtain blood cultures and look for secondary foci of infection (meningitis, pneumonia). Treat with intravenous antibiotics for 7–10 days, beginning empirically with cefuroxime, 75–100 mg/kg/day divided q8h **or** cloxacillin or oxacillin, 150 mg/kg/day divided q6h, and chloramphenicol, 50–75 mg/kg/day divided q6h. In children who respond dramatically to treatment, with resolution of fever, erythema, and pain, oral antibiotics may be commenced and the child discharged after 3–5 days of IV therapy—assuming the bacteria is identified and sensitive to oral antibiotics.

  **2. Orbital cellulitis.** Start an intravenous line, obtain blood for CBC and culture, and take a swab of the eye for Gram's stain and culture. Rule out foci of secondary infection. In children who do not respond within 48 hours of commencing therapy, consult a surgeon and order a CT scan to rule out abscess formation. Treat with antibiotics for 2–3 weeks, beginning empirically with cloxacillin or oxacillin, 150 mg/kg/day IV divided q6h or another suitable antistaphylococcal agent and chloramphenicol, 75 mg/kg/day divided q6h **or** cefuroxime, 150 mg/kg/day IV divided q8h.

**C. Disposition.** Admit all patients with orbital cellulitis.

**D. Key points**

1. Most cases of conjunctivitis are viral in origin and do not require antibiotic therapy.
2. Gonococcal infection may present in children beyond the neonatal period. A Gram's stain should be performed on all children with profuse purulent eye discharge.
3. Children with decreased visual acuity associated with a red eye should be urgently referred to an ophthalmologist.

**V. The injured eye.** The corneoscleral wall of the eye is a protective envelope for the delicate structures within. Blunt or penetrating forces transmitted to the mostly fluid contents of the globe can have devastating effects on function. In patients with lacerations or perforating injury, give a tetanus booster immunization to those at risk (see Appendix).

**A. Diagnosis and assessment**

1. **History.** Inquire about the time and mode of trauma. In penetrating injuries, determine the type of material and its velocity. Ask if there has been pain, diplopia, or any other abnormality of vision since the injury.
2. **Examination.** When possible, begin with a measurement of visual acuity. Palpate the orbits and inspect the globe, lids, and orbital area for external evidence of trauma. Test ocular motility. Note pupil size, symmetry, and reactivity, corneal and anterior chamber clarity, and the quality of the red reflexes. Examine the fundi for evidence of papilledema and vitreous or retinal hemorrhage. Fluorescein staining and examination with a blue light source (Wood's lamp or slit lamp) may help to diagnose abrasion, burn, or a foreign body embedded in the cornea. Use of fluorescein is contraindicated when rupture of the globe is suspected.
3. **X rays.** Orbital x rays, including a Waters' view, are indicated in children with penetrating trauma, blow-out fracture, or metal-on-metal foreign body injuries. A CT scan may be useful in selected cases of eye trauma.

**B. Patterns of injury**

1. **Nonpenetrating injuries**

   a. **Subconjunctival hemorrhage.** Subconjunctival hemorrhage is relatively common after eye trauma—no therapy is required. Always rule out serious associated injury.

   b. **Traumatic iritis.** Following a blow to the eye, some degree of intraocular inflammation ensues. When the inflammation is out of proportion to the injury, the patient has traumatic iritis. Children with traumatic iritis usually complain of pain. On examination, the pupil is decreased in size, and protein and cells are visible in the anterior chamber on slit-lamp examination. Dilatation of the pupil with homatropine 5% usually brings rapid relief. Patch the eye and refer the child to an ophthalmologist for treatment. Steroids may be required if iritis is severe.

**c. Traumatic mydriasis.** Damage to the sphincter muscle of the iris following a blow to the eye may result in an oval, irregular, or dilated and fixed pupil. Traumatic mydriasis can be differentiated from the fixed, dilated pupil associated with brain herniation by the absence of associated neurologic signs and symptoms. There is no effective treatment. Patch the eye and refer to an ophthalmologist.

**d. Traumatic hyphema.** Blood in the anterior chamber results from indirect trauma to the iris. In most cases, the trauma is minor, and extensive ocular damage is absent. On examination, a hyphema initially presents with a diffuse decrease in anterior chamber clarity. Later, when the hyphema settles, it forms a clearly defined fluid level. The major complication of hyphema is glaucoma secondary to blood staining of the cornea; this may occur immediately or following a secondary hemorrhage 4 or 5 days after the injury. The management of hyphema includes sedation and rest in bed with the head of the bed elevated 20–30 degrees. Therapy with aspirin is contraindicated. Patch the eye and consult an ophthalmologist—consult immediately if raised intraocular pressure is suspected.

**e. Foreign bodies, superficial abrasions, and radiation burn**

**(1)** Conjunctival and corneal foreign bodies are usually very irritating and cause redness and profuse tearing. Most foreign bodies can be removed by brushing a cotton-tipped applicator over the conjunctival or corneal surface. Dental burrs or a 25-gauge needle tip may be used to remove the object when penetration is shallow. Although instillation of local anesthetic is usually necessary to gain the child's cooperation, it is toxic to corneal epithelium and should not be administered repeatedly. Following treatment, dress the eye with sulfacetamide eye ointment and an eye patch and prescribe regular acetaminophen for pain relief. Arrange for follow-up examination within 24 hours. Children with deeply embedded foreign bodies, particularly glass fragments, should be immediately referred to an ophthalmologist for removal of the object.

**(2)** Corneal abrasions result in pain, photophobia, and tearing. On examination there is conjunctival erythema, and fluorescein dye is taken up by the corneal defect. Treat with topical sulfacetamide ointment qid, an eye patch, and regular acetaminophen or codeine for pain. Advise the patient against wearing a contact lens for 4–5 days. Arrange for a follow-up examination within 24 hours.

(3) A radiation burn occurs secondary to prolonged ultraviolet light exposure. Diagnosis, assessment, and treatment are similar to those for corneal abrasion (see **(2)** above).

**f. Conjunctival lacerations.** The majority of conjunctival lacerations result from minor injuries such as finger or stick pokes and do not require suturing. If a large piece of subconjunctival connective tissue (Tenon's capsule) protrudes, refer the child to an ophthalmologist immediately.

**g. Small missile injuries.** Penetrating injury must always be considered when there is a history of the eye being struck by a rapidly moving small object (see sec. **V.B.2** below). Small missile injuries are commonly due to pellets fired from guns, small objects fired by sling shots, or fragments of metal or stone broken from a hammer or hammered object. Order an x ray before examining the eye. Small foreign objects may be seen in the conjunctival sac or globe, or posteriorly in the orbit. A rapidly traveling object can inflict serious damage if it strikes the eye; when in doubt about diagnosis or management, consult an ophthalmologist.

**h. Lid lacerations.** The child with a laceration involving the lid margin, the region of the lacrimal drainage system in the inner canthal region, or the lateral canthal area should be treated by an experienced surgeon, preferably a specialist in ophthalmic plastic surgery. Ocular penetrating injury should be considered in all children with lid lacerations.

**2. Penetrating injury.** Ocular penetration should be suspected if there is decreased visual acuity, pupil distortion, a shallow or absent anterior chamber (the iris is bowed forward and touches the inner corneal surface), or unexpectedly prominent swelling of the conjunctiva. Penetrating injuries of the eyelids may be associated with penetration of the globe, paranasal sinuses, or anterior cranial fossa.

When penetrating injury is suspected, urgent consultation with an ophthalmologist is required. Lay the child supine in a quiet dark room and keep NPO in anticipation of surgery. Place a rigid patch over the eye and provide sedation and pain relief with an analgesic such as codeine, 0.5–1 mg/kg IM.

**3. Orbital blow-out fracture.** Blow-out fractures usually occur when an object that is larger than the orbital opening strikes the orbit (i.e., tennis balls, baseballs). The resultant rise in orbital pressure may fracture the orbital floor, the roof of the maxillary sinus, or the nasal wall of the orbit into the ethmoid sinus. Serious damage to the globe is rare.

There may be mild enophthalmos and decreased sensation in the distribution of the infraorbital nerve over the ipsilateral maxillary prominence. Entrapment of soft tissues under the globe results in a restriction of vertical movement and diplopia that persists in the central position. Obtain an orbital x ray with a Waters' view. Children with uncomplicated fracture may be treated symptomatically with ice, elevation, and bed rest, arranging outpatient follow-up with an ophthalmologist. Elective surgery is delayed until the swelling subsides and globe position and ocular movements can be properly assessed.

4. **Chemical injury.** Alkali is more damaging than acid. In all cases, place a drop of topical anesthetic in the eye and irrigate for a minimum of 20 minutes with 1–2 liters of freely running, room temperature, normal saline. Give pain relief, patch the eye, and consult an ophthalmologist immediately.

C. **Disposition.** Children with gross traumatic hyphema, penetrating injury, rupture of the globe, or extensive lid lacerations require admission and urgent ophthalmologic consultation. Patients with lid laceration should be referred to an ophthalmic plastic surgeon for repair.

D. **Key points**
   1. Children with decreased visual acuity associated with trauma should be urgently referred to an ophthalmologist.

**Bibliography**

Aronoff, S. C. (ed.). *Advances in Pediatric Infectious Diseases,* Vol. 3. Chicago: Year Book Medical Publishers, 1988.

Duke-Elder, S. *System of Ophthalmology.* Vol. 14. *Injuries.* London: Henry Kimpton, 1972.

Israele, V., and Nelson, J. D. Periorbital and orbital cellulitis. *J. Pediatr. Infect. Dis.* 6:404, 1987.

# 16

# Gastrointestinal Disorders

## Abdominal Pain
Graham C. Fraser

In management of the child with abdominal pain, the first task is to determine whether assessment by a surgeon is required. The great majority of cases are nonsurgical. In general, disorders may be grouped according to age (see Table 16-1), although some diagnoses such as appendicitis can occur at any age, even in infancy.

**I. Abdominal disorders by age**

  **A. The infant** with abdominal pain is likely to have an organic cause. The common causes are gastroenteritis and urinary tract infection. Infantile colic is frequent between 3 and 13 weeks of age (see Chap. 20, Crying and Colic in Infants).

  **B.** The **preschool-aged child** also usually has an organic cause. Gastroenteritis, urinary tract infection, and constipation are common.

  **C. Extraintestinal causes of pain** include pneumonia (young child, toddler), urinary tract infection, and diabetic ketoacidosis.

  **D.** A large proportion of cases in the **school-aged and older child** are functional in etiology. Common organic causes are gastroenteritis, urinary tract infection, constipation, and appendicitis. In the adolescent female consider gynecologic disorders such as dysmenorrhea, mittelschmerz, and pelvic inflammatory disease (PID).

**II. Diagnosis and assessment.** Execution and interpretation of the abdominal exam is difficult in the fearful or anxious child; the approach should be quiet, orderly, and gentle.

  **A. History.** Every effort should be made to obtain the history from the child. The clinician should be seated at or below the level of the patient, in a room with as few distractions as possible. During the history taking, no attempt should be made to touch or examine the child. Always consider the possibility of nonaccidental injury; abdominal trauma is the second most common cause of death in victims of child abuse.

   **1. Past history.** In the past history, ask about previous abdominal surgery, sickle cell disease, ascites due to nephrotic syndrome or cirrhosis (primary peritonitis), and any recent contacts with infectious disease.

   **2. Characterization of pain.** Determine whether the pain is acute or chronic, steady or colicky, sharp or dull. Ask about severity and time course and whether it is relieved by such factors as change of posture (peritonism, abdominal wall injury), vomiting (obstruction), defecation (gastroenteritis), or medication. Pain that is truly colicky (regular waxing and waning quality) suggests obstruction of

**Table 16-1. Causes of abdominal pain in children**

Neonate
  Colic
  Constipation
  Acid reflux and regurgitation
  Malrotation
  Trauma/abuse
Infant
  Colic
  Gastroenteritis/constipation
  Intussusception
  Incarcerated inguinal hernia
  Trauma/abuse
Preschool-age
  HSP
  Gastroenteritis/viral illness
  Constipation
  Intussusception
  Neoplasm
  Meckel's diverticulum
  Malrotation
  Pancreatitis (traumatic, viral)
  Trauma/abuse
  Pneumonia
  Sickle cell crisis
  DKA
  UTI
School-age and older
  HSP
  Viral illness
  Appendicitis
  Ovarian cyst/torsion
  Neoplasm
  PID
  UTI
  Sickle cell crisis
  DKA
  Functional pain
  Trauma/abuse

Note: This is not an inclusive list.
Key: HSP = Henoch-Schönlein purpura, DKA = diabetic ketoacidosis, UTI = urinary tract infection, PID = pelvic inflammatory disease.

the gastrointestinal tract, genitourinary tract, or rarely, the hepatobiliary tract.

3. **Localize the pain.** When asked to "point to where it hurts," even very young children may localize pain accurately. In all cases, determine if the location of maximum pain has moved. Benign abdominal pain tends to be chronic or recurrent, periumbilical, and dull or crampy in nature. In general, the further from the umbilicus the pain is localized, the more likely it is to have a serious cause.

4. **Referred pain.** Peritoneal irritation tends to cause referred somatic pain that is worsened by movement. Children with peritoneal irritation often lie still with the hips flexed. Referred shoulder-tip pain occurs with diaphragmatic irritation and may be caused by pneumonia, peritonitis, or abscess. Referred testicular pain may be due to renal disease; back pain may be caused by pancreatitis or uterine disease.

5. **Accompanying symptoms**

   a. **Vomiting.** The child who is not vomiting is less likely to have an abdominal condition requiring surgery. Sustained or bilious vomiting suggests bowel obstruction. Hematemesis may be due to gastritis, peptic ulcer disease, esophagitis, or swallowed blood from any site (see Chap. 16, Gastrointestinal Bleeding).

   b. **Headache and high fever** tend to occur with viral illnesses rather than surgical conditions. An exception is the child with an appendiceal abscess, in which toxicity and high fever are common.

   c. **Appetite.** A child with a keen appetite is less likely to have a surgical cause of abdominal pain.

   d. **Bowel function.** Constipation is a common cause of abdominal pain and should always be considered, even when children and parents provide assurance to the contrary. Diarrhea usually has an infectious etiology but may also be due to inflammatory bowel disease or appendicitis. In all cases ask about blood or mucus in the bowel motions as evidence of colitis due to inflammatory bowel disease (IBD) or bacterial infection (see Chap. 16, Acute Diarrhea).

   e. **Urinary signs and symptoms,** including suprapubic pain, dysuria, frequency, and urgency, suggest urinary tract infection.

   f. **Gynecologic symptoms,** including vaginal discharge in a sexually active adolescent female, suggest PID. Vaginal bleeding is associated with PID, abortion, and ectopic pregnancy. Midcycle pain is usually due to mittelschmerz, whereas dysmenorrhea occurs at the onset of or just prior to the period.

   g. **Lower lobe pneumonia** can cause abdominal pain in the young child—ask about cough, fever, and a history of upper respiratory infection (URI).

B. **Examination**

   1. **General examination.** Observation is an important aspect of the examination. A child that is bright, happy, and interested in the surroundings is unlikely to be seriously ill. In contrast, the patient who lies quietly with flexed hips or knees may have serious pathology. In all cases, examine the chest and palpate or fist-percuss the costovertebral angles for tenderness. Consider a gynecologic examination in the adolescent female (see Chap. 18, sec. **I** and **II**).

**2. Activity tests.** Inability to perform the following activities suggests pain or irritation secondary to peritoneal irritation:

　**a.** Sit-ups. The child is asked to sit up straight from a lying position without the parent's assistance.

　**b.** Abdominal wall distention and indrawing. The child is requested to "push out your tummy" and then to "pull it in all the way."

　**c.** Straight leg raising. The right, left, and then both legs together should be raised, unassisted, without limitation.

　**d.** Heel jumps. The older child is asked to jump down from the bed, landing on the heels.

**3. Examination of the abdomen**

　**a. Inspection.** Look for scars as evidence of previous surgery. Swelling, distention, bruising, or external evidence of inflammation suggest serious intraabdominal pathology due to trauma or infection. Examine the inguinal and scrotal regions for hernias, and observe the movement of the abdominal wall during respiration for evidence of splinting due to pain.

　**b. Palpation.** This is the most important aspect of the examination. Feel gently in all quadrants for rigidity and masses, and watch the child's expression for guarding. Rebound tenderness is best determined by asking the child to cough or by percussing over the painful area.

　**c. Percussion.** Percussion is useful for diagnosing rebound tenderness (see sec. **b.** above) and for determining whether abdominal distention is due to fluid or gas. Children with intussusception may have absence of normal right lower quadrant resonance because the cecum has been displaced.

　**d. Auscultation.** Minor subtle variations in auscultation, such as "slightly increased" bowel sounds are seldom reliable. Complete absence of bowel sounds over a 2-minute period suggests ileus and peritonitis. With bowel obstruction, the bowel sounds may be increased.

　**e. Rectal examination.** A rectal examination is not required in all children with abdominal pain; small children who resist rectal examination are often wrongly determined to have rectal tenderness. It should be performed when it is likely to add useful information, as in cases of suspected intussusception or appendiceal abscess. Abdominal tenderness on rectal examination strongly suggests the diagnosis of peritonitis.

**C. Investigations.** When a surgical cause of pain is considered, order a complete blood count (CBC), differential count, measurements of electrolytes and glucose, and a urinalysis and urine culture. Include a cross-match if surgery is anticipated or if there is suspicion of trauma. Other blood tests, including measurements of blood gases, serum amylase, and liver function tests can be ordered as indicated. See Chap. 18 for appropriate gynecologic investigations. If infectious gastroenteritis is suspected, obtain a culture of the stool. When bowel obstruction or perforation is suspected, order plain supine and erect x rays of the abdomen. Other radiologic procedures to be considered include an upper GI series to rule out malrotation, a barium enema for diagnosis and treatment of intussusception, and a technetium scan for diagnosis of a Meckel's diverticulum.

**D. Principles of management**

  **1.** Evaluate the volume status. Hypovolemia or shock may be due to sepsis, third-space losses in the bowel or peritoneum, or trauma.

  **2.** Admit all patients with a suspicious abdominal mass, signs of peritoneal irritation, bowel obstruction, or other surgical lesion. When a surgical cause for abdominal pain is suspected, obtain blood work (see sec. **II.C** above) and start an intravenous line. Refer to a surgeon and keep the child NPO in anticipation of surgery. Do not give analgesics until instructed to do so by a surgeon.

  **3.** Blood cultures and antibiotic treatment are indicated for children suspected of peritonitis.

   **a.** When peritonitis is secondary to bowel perforation or appendicitis give ampicillin, 100 mg/kg/day IV divided q6h, gentamicin, 6 mg/kg/day IV divided q8h, and clindamycin, 30 mg/kg/day IV divided q6h for a minimum of 10 days.

   **b.** Primary peritonitis, usually due to *Streptococcus pneumoniae,* is associated with ascites in children with nephrotic syndrome or cirrhosis. Treat with penicillin G 150,000 units/kg/day IV divided q6h for 7–10 days.

  **4.** Children in whom there is no suspicion of surgical disease may be discharged. Instruct the parents to return if there is increasing pain or other suspicious symptoms. If there is doubt about the severity of the condition, observe the child for a few hours. In infants and toddlers, always check a urinalysis prior to discharge.

**III. Disposition.** Admit all children with suspected surgical causes for abdominal pain and children who are dehydrated or unable to tolerate oral fluid.

**IV. Key points**

  **1.** Rule out surgical causes (obstruction, peritoneal irritation, bleeding) in children with abdominal pain.

  **2.** An indirect examination by "activity tests" is often the best method of assessing the severity of abdominal pain in the young child.

  **3.** Rectal examination is not always indicated for the evaluation of the child with abdominal pain.

**Bibliography**

Jones, P. F. Active observation in management of acute abdominal pain in childhood. *Br. Med. J.* 2:551, 1976.

Jones, P. F. Acute abdominal pain in childhood, with special reference to cases not due to acute appendicitis. *Br. Med. J.* 1:284, 1969.

Winsey, H. S., and Jones, P. F. Acute abdominal pain in childhood: Analysis of a year's admissions. *Br. Med. J.* 1:653, 1967.

## Surgical Abdominal Disorders
### Graham C. Fraser and Gregory A. Baldwin

When children present with surgical disorders, close communication with the surgeon is of vital importance. Do not give pain medications prior to surgical assessment, and ensure that informed consent is obtained from parents or guardians before any procedure is performed.

I. **Acute appendicitis.** This is the most common cause of acute abdomen in children.
   A. **Diagnosis and assessment**
      1. **History.** Abdominal pain may be diffuse or localized to the right lower quadrant. In many cases pain lasts only a few hours. There is often repeated vomiting, diminished appetite, and headache. It is usually painful for the child to move, jump, or sit up. Young infants can present with vague, nonspecific symptoms such as anorexia, poor feeding, fever, and vomiting. Rupture can result in a temporary improvement in pain, followed by generalized peritonitis.
      2. **Examination.** The abdomen is tender, usually maximally in the right lower quadrant. Rigidity and guarding, while not always present, support the diagnosis of appendicitis. Abdominal wall movement is decreased (see Chap. 16, Abdominal Pain, sec. **II.B.2**), and rectal examination, if performed, may reveal localized tenderness on the right side. Patients are often moderately (5%) dehydrated.
      3. **Laboratory investigations.** The white blood count is usually mildly elevated (12,000–14,000, or 12–14 $\times$ 10$^9$/liter) with a left shift in the differential count. Pyuria may be seen in the absence of urinary tract infection and occurs secondary to bladder irritation.
   B. **Management.** When appendicitis is suspected, hospital admission and surgery are indicated. Consult a surgeon and keep the child NPO. Start an intravenous line and obtain blood specimens for CBC, differential count, measurement of electrolytes, and cross-match. Rehydrate with IV fluids (see Chap. 23, Fluid and Electrolyte Disorders). If peritonitis is suspected, take a blood sample for culture and treat with antibiotics as detailed in Chap. 16, Abdominal Pain, sec. **II.D.**

II. **Intussusception.** This form of acute intestinal obstruction is most common in the first year of life with a peak incidence at 10 months, although it can occur at any age. Most are ileocolic in type. In many cases the disease is preceded by an upper respiratory tract infection or diarrhea.

**A. Diagnosis and assessment**
   **1. History.** Onset of symptoms is rapid, with sudden, sharp abdominal pain and irritability or screaming, occurring regularly every 10–15 minutes. During these episodes the child may draw the legs up and turn pale. In most cases there is vomiting, which may be bilious and eventually becomes persistent. "Red currant jelly" stool, pathognomonic of intussusception, is common but does not occur in all patients.
   **2. Examination.** Children with intussusception may be lethargic with a decreased level of consciousness. On examination, the abdomen is soft. There is often a tender, sausage-shaped mass in the right upper quadrant and a "hollow" area with absence of percussion resonance in the right lower quadrant. Bowel sounds are increased. A rectal examination, which should always be performed, may detect a mass in the rectum, guaiac positive stool, or the characteristic bloody mucus on the glove.
   **3. X rays.** Plain abdominal films may appear normal in the presence of acute obstruction due to intussusception. Alternatively, signs of bowel obstruction (air-fluid levels in small bowel, no air distal to obstruction), decreased gas in the right colon, or a right-sided soft tissue mass may be seen.
**B. Management.** When intussusception is suspected, start an intravenous line and obtain blood samples for CBC, differential count, cross-match, and electrolytes and glucose. If there is evidence of peritonitis, obtain a blood culture and treat with antibiotics as described in Chap. 16, Abdominal Pain, sec. **II.D.3.** Consult a surgeon and a radiologist. If there is time, a flat plate x ray of the abdomen may be ordered. A barium enema will confirm the diagnosis and in most cases will reduce the intussusception. Reduction by barium enema should be attempted only when a surgeon is present. It is usually contraindicated if the duration of symptoms is more than 24 hours, if there is marked abdominal distention, evidence of peritonitis, heavy rectal bleeding, or shock. If the barium enema is unsuccessful or contraindicated, laparotomy and surgical reduction are required.

**III. Meckel's diverticulum.** This intestinal malformation is found in 2% of the population, usually 2 feet proximal to the ileocecal valve; it commonly presents in children under 2 years of age. Most children with a Meckel's diverticulum are asymptomatic; if ectopic gastric mucosa is present, ulceration can occur, resulting in painless rectal bleeding. Other complications include bowel obstruction and perforation. Diagnosis can often be made by technetium-99 scan.
   **A. Management.** Initial treatment is supportive, including resuscitation and transfusion. Once the diagnosis is confirmed, the diverticulum must be surgically excised.
**IV. Congenital hypertrophic pyloric stenosis.** This is a relatively common condition in babies (usually first-born males) in the first 2 months of life. Hypertrophy and hyperplasia of the pyloric musculature result in gastric outlet ob-

struction. Most cases present at 4–8 weeks with a history of increasing nonbilious vomiting after feeds, usually projectile in nature. Depending on the duration of vomiting, electrolyte and fluid depletion may be severe, often resulting in hypokalemic, hypochloremic alkalosis. Abdominal examination reveals a soft belly; a pyloric mass may be felt as a walnut-sized mass to the right of the midline in the epigastrium of most affected babies. Following clinical examination, abdominal ultrasound examination is the diagnostic method of choice; less often, an upper GI series is diagnostic, revealing a dilated stomach and a "string sign" due to narrowing of the pyloric canal.

A. **Management.** Treatment includes correction of fluid and electrolyte depletion followed by surgery. Consult a surgeon, start an intravenous line, and draw blood for CBC, BUN, type and screen, and electrolytes and glucose. If there is severe dehydration (see Chap. 23, Fluid and Electrolyte Disorders), give a bolus of normal saline, 10 ml/kg, and repeat until the patient is stable. Replace potassium losses with intravenous KCl, 30–40 mEq/liter of fluid infused (see Chap. 23, Fluid and Electrolyte Disorders). Place a nasogastric tube on low intermittent suction, and replace nasogastric losses with 5% dextrose one-half normal saline plus 20 mEq KCl/liter (add KCl only if renal function is normal).

V. **Volvulus.** Volvulus is a torsion of a loop of intestine that results in obstruction. Its incidence is highest in newborns and in children between 2 and 12 years of age. Factors predisposing to volvulus include an aberrant or abnormal mesentery, adhesions, Meckel's diverticulum, and malrotation. The diagnosis should be suspected in any child with acute onset of vomiting (which may be bile-stained), crampy abdominal pain, and obstruction. In some cases there may be a prolonged history of intermittent episodes of pain. Peritonitis can occur if there is necrotic bowel or perforation. Supine and erect abdominal x rays show evidence of obstruction with distended loops of bowel, air-fluid levels, and absence of gas distal to the level of obstruction (usually at the junction of the sigmoid and left colon).

A. **Management.** Start an IV, rehydrate, place a nasogastric tube, and obtain blood for measurement of electrolytes and cross-match. If there is peritonitis, take a sample of blood for culture and treat with IV ampicillin, gentamicin, and clindamycin (see Chap. 16, Abdominal pain, sec. **II.D.3**). Consult a surgeon. Treatment is accomplished by means of laparotomy and surgical detorsion.

VI. **Disposition.** Admit all patients with surgical abdominal disorders.

VII. **Key points**

1. Young infants with appendicitis usually present with vague signs and symptoms.
2. Most children with intussusception can be treated by hydrostatic reduction with barium enema. Exceptions include those patients with prolonged symptoms, peritonitis, and shock.

**Bibliography**

Hutchison, I. F., Olayiwola, B., and Young, D. G. Intussusception in infancy and childhood. *Br. J. Surg.* 67:209, 1980.

Ein, S. H., and Stephens, C. A. Intussusception: 354 cases in 10 years. *J. Pediatr. Surg.* 6:16, 1971.

Leope, L. L. *Patient Care in Pediatric Surgery.* Boston: Little, Brown, 1987.

Schwartz, S. I. (ed.). *Principles of Surgery* (4th ed.). New York: McGraw Hill, 1983.

## Constipation
Graham C. Fraser

Constipation is one of the most common causes of abdominal pain in childhood. The constipated child has hard stools that are difficult to pass and may cause considerable pain, although this may be denied by the child and family. The condition occurs commonly in infants on cow's milk formula and in children with anal fissure. Rarely, constipation may be due to serious disorders such as Hirschsprung's disease, hypothyroidism, or neurologic disorders (e.g., tethered spinal cord). **Spurious** constipation occurs when parents complain of infrequent bowel motions (up to q3 days), although the consistency of the stools is normal. This is more likely to occur in infants who are breast fed or underfed. Reassurance or instruction in feeding technique is generally all that is required.

I. **Diagnosis and assessment.** Abdominal pain due to constipation is often generalized and steady. The pain may be accompanied by nausea, but vomiting is unusual. Ask about stool frequency, consistency, and the presence of blood or mucus. On examination, the abdomen is often diffusely "uncomfortable" rather than tender, and the left colon is easily palpable and full of feces. Rectal examination and plain x ray are usually confirmatory; there may be evidence of anal fissure on rectal examination. In **Hirschsprung's disease** the rectum is usually empty of air, the rectal tone is increased, and there is an absence of stool in the ampulla.

II. **Management.** Most children with functional constipation benefit from a glycerin suppository. If this is ineffective, a Fleet enema can be gently administered; this should not be given to children in whom appendicitis or bowel obstruction is suspected. The infant with constipation or anal fissure should be treated with a mild osmotic agent such as corn (Karo) syrup, 15 ml or 1 tablespoon added to each 8 oz of formula. Ensure adequate volume of feeds. Outpatient management of chronic functional constipation in older children includes avoidance of constipating foods, oral administration of 15–75 ml of mineral oil twice daily, and follow-up with a family doctor.

III. **Disposition.** Patients with simple constipation can be managed as outpatients.

## IV. Key points

1. In infancy, constipation is commonly associated with cow's milk formula feeds and anal fissure.
2. Most cases can be treated with a mild osmotic agent (Karo syrup).

### Bibliography

Fitzgerald, J. F. Constipation in children. *Pediatr. Clin. North Am.* 8:299, 1987.

---

# Acute Diarrhea

Eric Hassall and Gregory A. Baldwin

Acute diarrhea is usually due to viral gastroenteritis. Extraintestinal infections (Table 16-2) often cause diarrhea in infants and toddlers. Serious abdominal pathology such as appendicitis, inflammatory bowel disease, and poisoning should always be considered. The complications of acute diarrhea include dehydration, electrolyte and acid-base disturbance, sepsis, protein-calorie malnutrition, and chronicity. Enteritis means small bowel inflammation; colitis refers to large bowel inflammation. Most infectious diarrhea is due to "gastroenteritis" or "enterocolitis."

## I. Diagnosis and assessment

A. **History.** Determine the duration of illness, diet, infectious contacts including pets and travel, and medications (antibiotics). Ask about vomiting and obtain a description of stool frequency, volume, consistency, urgency, and presence of blood or mucus. Ask about weight loss and inquire about urinary signs and symptoms such as frequency, urgency, and dysuria (see Chap. 23, Urinary Tract Infection). In most cases, infectious gastroenteritis presents with vomiting and diarrhea of rapid onset. Fever and headache are common, and abdominal pain is generally periumbilical or diffuse and crampy. Dysentery, the passage of blood and mucus in the stools, means that colitis is present. Infectious dysentery is usually bacterial, although infants and toddlers infected with rotavirus may also have blood and mucus in the stools.

---

**Table 16-2. Common causes of acute diarrhea**

Infectious enteritis (viral, bacterial, parasitic)

Extraintestinal diseases (otitis, pneumonia, urinary tract infection)

Antibiotic-related diarrhea

Inflammatory bowel disease

Hemolytic uremic syndrome/Henoch-Schönlein purpura

---

**B. Examination.** Examine the abdomen for masses, tenderness, and peritonism (see Chap. 16, Abdominal Pain, sec. **II.B.3**). Look for signs of acute dehydration and hypovolemia such as tachycardia, postural changes that cause changes in vital signs, dry mucous membranes, and sunken eyes (see Chap. 23, Fluid and Electrolyte Disorders). Document that diarrhea is in fact present—perform a rectal examination and obtain stool for investigation (see sec. **I.C** below). The presence of a purpuric skin rash suggests vasculitis due to Henoch-Schönlein purpura, hemolytic uremic syndrome, or rarely, sepsis. The diarrhea associated with these disorders is often bloody (see Chap. 19, Chap. 23, Hematuria, and Chap. 24, Limp). Consider the diagnosis of bacteremia in the ill patient (see sec. **III.C** below and Chap. 21, Bacteremia).

**C. Investigations**
   **1. Stool studies**
      **a.** In the majority of patients who are well with a brief history of uncomplicated, nonbloody diarrhea, dietary management without stool studies is acceptable. In all cases, gross examination of the stool for color, consistency, odor, blood, and purulent exudate is necessary. The presence of mucus and blood suggests colitis from any cause.
      **b.** In children with complicated, or bloody, or prolonged diarrhea (see sec. **III.A** below), the following stool studies are needed:
         **(1)** Perform cultures of fresh stool for bacterial enteropathogens including *Escherichia coli, Shigella, Salmonella, Yersinia enterocolitica, Campylobacter jejuni,* and *Clostridium difficile. Aeromonas hydrophila* and *Vibrio parahaemolyticus* are rarer bacterial pathogens. Send a specimen for determination of *C. difficile* toxin. Obtain a specimen to be used for microscopic examination for ova and parasites and for ELISA testing for rotavirus (Rotazyme). In *C. jejuni* infection a dark-field examination performed within 2 hours may show the typical "darting gull wing" appearance.
         **(2)** Test stool for pH and reducing substances. If the stool pH is less than 6.0 the child may have carbohydrate malabsorption. Mix 5 drops of stool water wrung out from the diaper or drawn up in a dropper with 10 drops of water and add a Clinitest tablet. In general, the presence of more than 1% reducing substance is abnormal (healthy breast-fed infants may have > 2% reducing substances). Carbohydrate malabsorption may be due to carbohydrate overload or disaccharidase deficiency.
         **(3)** Test for occult blood using Hemoccult strips.
         **(4)** Smear stool on a slide, apply methylene

blue, and look for polymorphonuclear leuko-cytes—their presence suggests colitis.
2. **Other studies.** Send a urine sample for urinalysis and culture. In children with high fever, toxicity, or other risk factors for bacteremia (see sec. **II.C** below), obtain a blood sample for culture. CBC, differential count, platelet count, BUN, and measurements of creatinine and electrolytes should be ordered in children who require admission.

## II. Specific disorders

A. **Food poisoning.** Exposure to toxins produced by *Staphylococcus aureus, Salmonella,* or *Clostridium perfringens* can result in acute onset of diarrhea, vomiting, and abdominal pain. Symptoms tend to occur within hours of ingestion and are usually of short duration ($<$ 24 hours).

B. **Viral causes of diarrhea.** In North America viruses account for 70–80% of cases of acute diarrhea. Common pathogens are rotavirus, Norwalk agent, and enteroviruses and adenoviruses. Viral infections decrease the absorptive surface of the small bowel; this type of lesion takes 3–6 days to heal. Rotavirus infection is especially common in infants, causing over 60% of cases of acute infectious diarrhea in this age group during the winter months. Infection with rotavirus presents with repeated vomiting and profuse, watery, foul-smelling stools for 5–7 days. Occasionally, rotavirus infection may result in enterocolitis with blood and mucus in the stool. Norwalk virus infection occurs in school-age children, typically causing "winter vomiting" illness. It usually lasts 1–2 days; myalgia and malaise are commonly associated.

C. **Bacterial causes of diarrhea.** In North America, the common bacterial enteropathogens are *C. jejuni, E. coli, Shigella, Salmonella,* and *Yersinia.* Bacterial enterocolitis often causes dysentery characterized by the passage of blood, mucus, and polymorphonuclear leukocytes in the stools. Vomiting is less common than in viral infection. The diagnosis is made by stool culture, although there are certain features particular to the various pathogens:
1. *C. jejuni* is often seen in children under 5 years of age.
2. *E. coli* is associated with travel and ingestion of undercooked hamburgers. It may precede the onset of hemolytic uremic syndrome (serotype 0157–H7).
3. *Vibrio* infection is more common in patients exposed to raw seafood or sea water.
4. *Shigella* infection can result in high fever and seizures, especially in children under 5 years of age.

**Risk factors for development of bacteremia** in children with bacterial diarrhea include age less than 1 year, immune deficiency or suppression, sickle cell disease (especially *Salmonella* infection), and preexisting malnutrition. Rarely, bacterial pathogens result in extraintestinal infection such as pneumonia and osteomyelitis.

## D. Antibiotic-associated diarrhea

1. Antibiotics may cause **transient diarrhea** that resolves after the antibiotic is stopped.

2. Rarely, *C. difficile* **colitis** can occur spontaneously in the absence of antibiotic administration, though it is usually seen during or after treatment with antimicrobials (all antibiotics other than rifampicin and parenteral aminoglycosides have been implicated). Onset may occur up to 6 weeks following antibiotic administration. The clinical presentation can vary from mild diarrhea to severe disease with bloody stools, fever, toxicity, abdominal pain, and distention. The diagnosis is made by the presence of *C. difficile* toxin and by a positive culture of *C. difficile* in fresh stool. Occasionally, the diagnosis must be made by colonoscopy, which reveals pseudomembranous colitis. Treatment is with oral vancomycin, 1 g/1.73 m$^2$/day (10–50 mg/kg/day) PO divided q6h for 14 days. Vancomycin is extremely expensive and may cost 200–400 dollars for a 10- to 14-day course. Metronidazole is also used, as it is much less expensive, although it may be less effective and associated with a higher relapse rate.

## E. Parasites

1. *Giardia lamblia.* This small bowel parasite is the most common parasitic cause of diarrhea in North America. Children may be asymptomatic or have diarrhea, flatulence, bloating, abdominal pain, or weight loss. Vomiting is infrequent, and there is no dysentery. Stools examined for ova and parasites are negative for trophozoites in up to 50% of cases. If *Giardia* is strongly suspected (patient is from an endemic area or has been exposed to inland lake water or a camping trip, if there is *Giardia* in the household, or if signs and symptoms are of recent onset), the child may be treated empirically with quinacrine, metronidazole, or furazolidone (for dosages see Table 16-3). Children with recurrent or persistent symptoms should be referred to a gastroenterologist.

2. *Entamoeba histolytica.* Although most cases are subacute, this parasite can cause severe dysentery with blood and mucus in stools. The most common extraintestinal manifestation is liver abscess. The diagnosis is made by serologic and stool examinations and by the presence of fecal monocytes on a stool smear (in contrast to polymorphonuclear leukocytes in bacterial colitis or inflammatory bowel disease [IBD]). All stages of amebiasis, including asymptomatic carriers, require treatment with diiodohydroxyquin or metronidazole (for dosages see Table 16-3).

3. *Dientamoeba coli* and *Blastocystis hominis.* These are parasites with an unclear correlation to symptoms: They are probably commensals rather than pathogens. If they are present in a concentration of

**Table 16-3. Treatment of infectious diarrhea**

| Infection | Indication for treatment | Medications |
|---|---|---|
| *Campylobacter jejuni* | Systemically ill, severe pain, duration > 3 days | (?)Erythromycin, 40 mg/kg/day PO divided q6h for 5–7 days |
| Enteropathogenic *E. coli* | Always treat if patient is symptomatic. If systemically ill or toxic use IV therapy | Neomycin, 100 mg/kg/day PO divided q6h. IV use: ampicillin, 100 mg/kg/day divided q6h, and gentamicin, 5 mg/kg/day divided q8h |
| *Shigella* | Always treat if patient is symptomatic | TMP-SMX, 10 mg/kg/day PO or IV divided q12h, or ampicillin, 100 mg/kg/day PO or IV divided q6h |
| *Salmonella* | Treat if patient is systemically ill, < 1 year age, has metastatic disease or sickle cell disease, or is immunocompromised. Do not treat chronic systemic carriers | Ampicillin, 100 mg/kg/day PO or IV divided q6h, or amoxycillin, 50 mg/kg/day PO divided q8h |
| *Clostridium difficile* | Watery/bloody diarrhea, pseudomembranes seen on colonoscopy | Vancomycin, 1 gm/1.73 m² (10–50) mg/kg/day PO divided qid for 14 days |
| *Aeromonas* | | (?) TMP-SMX, 10 mg/kg/day as TMP PO divided q12h for 5 days |
| *Giardia lamblia* | | Furazolidone, 8 mg/kg/day PO divided qid for 7–10 days, or quinacrine, 6 mg/kg/day PO divided tid for 7 days, or metronidazole 15 mg/kg/day PO divided tid for 5 days |

Key: TMP-SMX = trimethoprim-sulfamethoxazole.
Source: Adapted from R. L. Guerrant, J. A. Lohr, and E. K. Williams. Acute infectious diarrhea II: Treatment and prevention. *Pediatr Infect Dis* 5:353, 458, 1986.

tion of more than 5/high-power field in a child with recent onset of diarrhea, a course of treatment with metronidazole may be warranted (see Table 16-3).

   4. **Cryptosporidium.** This is a parasite of veterinary origin that primarily infests the small bowel but may also involve the colon. It causes acute, large-volume, watery diarrhea that is self-limited in hosts with normal immunity. Suspect immune compromise in the child with severe intractable disease; death may occur in these children due to fluid, electrolyte, and nutritional deficiency. There is no known effective treatment. Cryptosporidium is a leading cause of morbidity and mortality in AIDS patients.

III. **Management.** Most cases of acute diarrhea are self-limited. Symptomatic therapy and adequate hydration are often all that are required.

   A. **Intravenous fluids.** The first priority is assessment and treatment of dehydration (see Chap. 23, Fluid and Electrolyte Disorders). Admission and intravenous fluid therapy are usually indicated for patients who fulfill any of the following criteria:

      1. Under 3 months of age with bacterial diarrhea.
      2. Toxic or have underlying systemic illness.
      3. Severely dehydrated or cannot be rehydrated orally.
      4. Have large-volume, grossly bloody stools or significant abdominal pain.
      5. Compromised by chronic debilitating diseases, immune deficiency, or malnutrition.

   B. **Oral rehydration.** Most children can be successfully rehydrated via the oral route. In the child under 2 years of age, use commercially prepared oral rehydration solutions (ORS) such as Gastrolyte, Lytren, or Pedialyte RS. In the child over 2 years use an ORS if tolerated or clear fluids such as Gatorade or one-fourth strength apple juice.

      1. The breast-fed infant should continue to breast feed. ORS may be added as a supplement if there is significant dehydration.
      2. In formula-fed infants and older children, calculate the volume of fluid required for rehydration, maintenance, and replacement (see Chap. 23, Fluids and Electrolytes, sec. **II**) and divide into small aliquots given every 30–60 minutes. If this is tolerated and the hydration status is adequate, the child should be reweighed and may then be discharged home. Arrange for follow-up within 24 hours.
      3. Instruct the parents to continue administration of ORS or clear fluids for no longer than 24 hours. After 24 hours they should begin feeding with a diet high in starch and low in fat (BRAT diet, consisting of bananas, rice cereal, applesauce, and dry toast or crackers). In formula-fed children, formula should be reintroduced in reduced strength (one-half or one-fourth), increasing to full strength over 2 days. Diarrhea often continues or recurs. If the patient remains well hydrated and is gaining weight, advise the par-

**Table 16-4. Drugs that should be avoided in children with acute diarrhea**

Diphenoxylate (Lomotil)

Loperamide (Imodium)

Paregoric

Morphine

Codeine

Belladonna alkaloids (Donnagel, Donnatol, Diban)

Combinations of above (Pomalin)

Kaopectate

ents to persist with a gradual return to a regular diet.

4. Parents should be instructed to return with the child if oral intake is not tolerated or if symptoms become worse.

**C. Medications**

1. Antidiarrheal and antinauseant medications (Table 16-4) should not be used in children with diarrhea or vomiting—they may mask symptoms and promote bacteremia, fluid loss, and complications such as toxic megacolon.

2. In general, antibiotic therapy should be withheld until culture results are available, unless the child appears ill. For treatment guidelines see Table 16-3.

**IV. Disposition.** Admission should be considered in children who are:

1. Under 3 months of age with bacterial diarrhea.

2. Toxic or have underlying systemic illness.

3. Severely dehydrated or cannot be rehydrated orally.

4. Having large-volume, grossly bloody stools or significant abdominal pain.

5. Compromised by chronic debilitating diseases, immunodeficiency, or malnutrition.

**V. Key points**

1. In infants, consider extraintestinal causes of diarrhea such as urinary tract infection or otitis media.

2. Bacteremia is common in infants under 3 months of age with bacterial colitis.

3. Most children with acute infectious diarrhea can be orally rehydrated.

4. Do not use antidiarrheal medications in children with acute diarrhea.

**Bibliography**

Hyman, P. E., and Ament, M. E. Acute infectious gastroenteritis in children. *Pediatr. Ann.* 11:147, 1982.

Ament, M. E., and Barclay, G. N. Chronic diarrhea. *Pediatr. Ann.* 11:124, 1982.

Guerrant, R. L., Lohr, J. A., and Williams, E. K. Acute infectious diarrhea I and II. Epidemiology, pathogenesis, diagnosis, treatment and prevention. *Pediatr. Infect. Dis.* 5:353, 458, 1986.

# Gastrointestinal Bleeding
## Eric Hassall and Gregory A. Baldwin

There is a wide spectrum of disorders causing gastrointestinal bleeding in childhood. Hematemesis is usually due to esophageal varices or acid peptic disease (esophagitis, gastritis, peptic ulcer disease). Rectal bleeding is more common; the majority of cases are due to minor disorders such as anal fissure. Causes of heavy rectal bleeding include severe upper gastrointestinal bleeding, Meckel's diverticulum, or inflammatory bowel disease (IBD). See Table 16-5 for a list of age-related causes of rectal bleeding.

## I. Definitions
A. Hematemesis refers to the emesis of fresh (bright red) or old ("coffee grounds") blood. Fresh blood becomes chemically altered to a coffee-ground appearance within 5 minutes in the stomach.
B. Hematochezia is the passage of fresh (bright red) or dark maroon blood from the rectum. The source is usually the colon, although upper gastrointestinal bleeding that has a rapid transit can also result in hematochezia.
C. Melena is the passage of shiny, jet black stools of tarry consistency, which are strongly guaiac positive. The blood has been chemically altered during passage through the gut and usually originates from the upper gastrointestinal tract.

## II. Classification
A. **Apparent** gastrointestinal bleeding may be due to swallowed blood from the nasopharynx, as in epistaxis. In the newborn, swallowed maternal blood can be differentiated from the baby's own blood by an Apt test performed on the baby's stool. Hematemesis may be mimicked by red foods such as beets and red Jello or medications such as Tylenol elixir. Melenalike stools can occur in children who have ingested iron, bismuth, blackberries, or spinach.
B. **True upper gastrointestinal** bleeding occurs at a site proximal to the ligament of Treitz. Common disorders causing upper gastrointestinal bleeding include esophagitis, gastric erosions, peptic ulcer disease, Mallory-Weiss tear, or esophageal varices.
C. **True lower gastrointestinal** bleeding is due to a source distal to the ligament of Treitz. Minor bleeding presents as stool streaked with blood or the passage of a few drops of blood after stool is passed. It is commonly due to an anal fissure or polyp. Inflammatory disease such as IBD or infectious colitis results in diarrheal stool mixed with blood. Causes of heavy bleeding (hematochezia, clots) include IBD, Meckel's diverticulum, hemolytic uremic syndrome, Henoch-Schönlein purpura, and infectious colitis. Hemorrhoids are extremely rare in children

**Table 16-5. Causes of rectal bleeding by age of patient**

| Newborn | Infant to 2 years | 2 years to preschool | Preschool to adolescence |
|---|---|---|---|
| Viti K₁ deficiency | Anal fissure | Infectious diarrhea | IBD |
| Ingested maternal blood | Milk colitis | Polyp | Infectious diarrhea |
| | Infectious diarrhea | Anal fissure | Peptic ulcer |
| Infectious diarrhea | Intussusception | Meckel's diverticulum | Esophageal varices |
| Necrotizing enterocolitis | Polyp | Intussusception | Polyp |
| Hirschsprung's disease | Meckel's diverticulum | HUS | |
| | | HSP | |
| **Less frequent causes** | | | |
| Volvulus | Duplication | PUD | Anal fissure |
| Duplication | PUD | Esophageal varices | HUS |
| Vascular malformation | Vascular malformation | IBD | HSP |
| Stress ulcer | | | |

Key: HUS = hemolytic uremic syndrome, HSP = Henoch-Schönlein purpura, IBD = inflammatory bowel disease, PUD = peptic ulcer disease.
Source: Adapted from C. Hillemeier. Rectal bleeding in childhood. *Pediatr. Rev.* 5: 34, 1983.

under 16 years of age in the absence of portal hypertension or previous anorectal surgery.

## III. Diagnosis and assessment (Table 16-6)

### A. History

1. **Upper gastrointestinal bleeding.** In patients with upper gastrointestinal bleeding ask about forceful vomiting and use of ulcerogenic drugs (salicylates, nonsteroidal anti-inflammatory drugs, steroids). Inquire about previous episodes of bleeding, liver disease, and a family history of ulcers or gastrointestinal bleeding. Determine if there is pain and if so, its location, timing, and precipitating or relieving factors.

2. **Lower gastrointestinal bleeding.** Determine if there is blood only on the surface of the stool, mixed with the stool, true melena, or hematochezia, and if blood clots have been passed. Ask about diarrhea or constipation with large or hard stools and difficult or painful defecation. Inquire about infectious contacts, foreign travel, and antibiotic use.

### B. Examination

1. The immediate priority is to rule out hypovolemia (see Chaps. 4 and 23, Fluids and Electrolytes, sec. **II**).

2. Examine the nasopharynx for bleeding sites. Look for clubbing, pallor, and signs of malnutrition as evidence of chronic illness such as IBD. Purpura and petechiae suggest hemolytic uremic syndrome, Henoch-Schönlein purpura, acute coagulation disorder, or sepsis. Children with skin or mucous membrane telangiectasias or hemangiomas may have gut involvement, although these are very rare causes of gastrointestinal bleeding.

3. Examine the abdomen to rule out peritonism, masses (see Chap. 16, Abdominal Pain), hepatomegaly, and splenomegaly. Epigastric tenderness suggests acid peptic disease. Right lower quadrant tenderness may be due to IBD or infectious enterocolitis. A right lower quadrant mass suggests Crohn's disease or intussusception. Splenomegaly with distended abdominal veins with or without signs of chronic liver disease may be due to portal hypertension.

4. An anal fissure is best seen by spreading the buttocks and everting the anal canal. Most fissures are located at 6 or 12 o'clock, and there may be an accompanying skin tag.

5. Always perform a rectal examination to document the nature of the stool and whether there is diarrhea or blood. Even if the stool on the glove is red, always prove that it is strongly guaiac-positive by performing a Hemoccult test at the bedside. Feel for hard stool and a dilated rectum in children with chronic constipation and fissure.

## IV. Management

### A. The unstable child

1. In the child with heavy bleeding or hypovolemia, as-

**Table 16-6. Diagnosis of gastrointestinal bleeding**

| Site | Cause | Associated signs and symptoms |
|------|-------|-------------------------------|
| Upper | Medications | Ingestion of ASA, other NSAIDs |
| | Varices | Splenomegaly or evidence liver disease |
| | Esophagitis | Dysphagia, vomiting, dyspepsia, irritability in infants |
| | Peptic ulcer | Epigastric pain, meal-related, may be increased at night. Family history |
| Lower | Fissure | Bright red blood on surface of stool. Pain, constipation. Fissure often visible on anal eversion |
| | Polyp | Bright red blood on surface of stool. Painless. Very rarely palpable on rectal examination |
| | Milk colitis | Blood mixed with stool, diarrhea. Patient may have hypoproteinemia, edema |
| | Meckel's | Blood mixed with stool, hemochezia, clots. Usually a lot of blood |
| | IBD | Diarrhea, fever, abdominal pain, poor growth, associated signs and symptoms (joint pain, rash, iritis, etc.) |
| | Bacterial colitis | Abdominal pain, diarrhea, fever, antibiotics, infectious contact, ingestion of contaminated food, foreign travel |
| | HSP | Joint pain, purpura, abdominal pain, nephritis (casts, RBCs in urine) |
| | HUS | Diarrhea, renal failure, thrombocytopenia, microangiopathic hemolytic anemia |
| | Intussusception | Infant, young child. Intermittent abdominal pain, vomiting, pallor, red currant jelly stool, right-sided mass |
| | NEC | Neonate, perinatal hypoxemia, acidosis, sepsis. Onset of diarrhea, abdominal distension, DIC, shock, typical x-ray (see Chap. 16, Gastrointestinal Bleeding, sec. V). |

Key: HSP = Henoch-Schönlein purpura, HUS = hemolytic uremic syndrome, NEC = necrotizing enterocolitis, ASA = acetylsalicylic acid, NSAID = nonsteroidal anti-inflammatory drug, IBD = inflammatory bowel disease.

sess and control problems in the airway, breathing, and circulation. Give oxygen by mask, start two large-bore IV lines, and order a stat complete blood count (CBC), platelet count, cross-match, prothrombin time (PT), partial thromboplastin time (PTT), liver function tests, and measurements of electrolytes, BUN, and creatinine. A normal hemoglobin or hematocrit does not rule out severe acute bleeding. Give intravenous normal saline or Ringer's lactate in 10 ml/kg boluses until the patient is stable (see Chap. 4). Whole blood should be given if bleeding continues.

2. Insert a well-lubricated nasogastric (NG) tube of the largest bore possible after cutting side holes in the distal 5 cm of tubing. Perform lavage at least 3 times with 5 ml/kg of room temperature normal saline (see Chap. 27 for method). Do not use iced saline—it is of no benefit and may result in hypothermia. Failure to empty the stomach by lavage is usually due to NG tube blockage—remove and replace the tube. Esophageal varices are not a contraindication to the placement of a well-lubricated NG tube.

   a. **A clear return on lavage** makes the diagnosis of upper gastrointestinal bleeding unlikely, although occasionally duodenal ulcers may bleed only distally.

   b. Return of guaiac positive **fresh blood or coffee grounds** indicates upper bleeding. Begin treatment with an $H_2$ blocker (cimetidine or ranitidine) and antacids (Table 16-7).

   c. **Persistent return of fresh blood** indicates active bleeding and mandates aggressive intravenous fluid management.

3. When upper gastrointestinal bleeding is proved or suspected, begin treatment with ranitidine or cimetidine and antacids (see Table 16-7).

4. In children with evidence of liver disease, give vitamin K, 1 mg/year of age (maximum 10 mg) IV or SC, and fresh frozen plasma (FFP), 5 ml/kg IV over 15–30 minutes.

5. Vasopressin infusion may be used in children with massive or persistent upper gastrointestinal bleeding (see sec. **V.A.1** below); always consult with a gastroenterologist before commencing treatment.

6. Consult a gastroenterologist when possible.

**B. The stable child**

1. The stable child without heavy bleeding or signs of hypovolemia must be treated according to age and the suspected diagnosis. Always confirm the presence of blood in vomitus or gastric aspirate or stool using test cards (such as Gastroccult or Hemoccult) at the bedside. Trace positivity is of dubious significance.

2. Obtain a CBC to determine the significance of bleeding. Nasogastric lavage is usually unnecessary in

Table 16-7. Drugs used in the treatment of upper gastrointestinal bleeding

| Drug | Dosage | Interval | Route | Comments |
|------|--------|----------|-------|----------|
| Cimetidine | 20–40 mg/kg/day | q6–8h | IV, PO/NG | Give before meals and hs. Reduce dosage in renal failure |
| Ranitidine | 1.25–1.9 mg/kg/dose<br>2.5–3.8 mg/kg/dose | q6h bid | IV<br>PO/NG | Reduce dosage in renal failure |
| Antacid (Maalox TC, Amphogel) | 0.5 ml/kg/dose | Up to q2h | PO/NG | Can cause diarrhea. Aluminum or magnesium toxicity may occur in renal failure |
| Vasopressin | Per 1.73 m² the dose is as follows: Give 20 units in 5% D/W over 10 minutes; then continuous infusion of 0.2 units/min in 5% D/W. Double every 1–2 hr if active bleeding persists, to a maximum of 0.8 units/min | | IV | Adjust dose for child's size. Rapid IV push may cause bradycardia and hypotension. Vasopressin causes water retention and dilutional hyponatremia. Meticulous fluid balance is mandatory |

children with minor or nonacute gastrointestinal bleeding.

3. A thorough history and examination and consideration of age-related causes will usually lead to the diagnosis. However, the precise diagnosis is almost always made by flexible fiberoptic upper or lower endoscopic examination. Meckel's diverticulum can be diagnosed by Meckel's scan. Very rarely is angiography, a technetium-labeled red blood cell study, or surgery required for diagnosis. Barium contrast studies have little or no role in the actively bleeding patient.

## V. Specific disorders
### A. Upper gastrointestinal bleeding

1. **Esophageal varices.** Esophageal varices occur in children with portal hypertension secondary to an **extrahepatic cause** such as portal vein thrombosis, or an **intrahepatic cause** such as cirrhosis due to any of a number of disorders (e.g., biliary atresia, chronic hepatitis, Wilson's disease, alpha-1-antitrypsin deficiency). Varices are rare before 6 months of age. Onset of bleeding is often sudden and severe and may be spontaneous or precipitated by ulcerogenic drug ingestion (salicylates, nonsteroidal anti-inflammatory drugs) or an upper respiratory tract infection.

   a. **Management.** Following resuscitation, these children should be immediately referred to a gastroenterologist for consideration of treatment with vasopressin, Sengstaken Blakemore tube tamponade, or endoscopic sclerotherapy. Insert an NG tube in all cases. Obtain blood for CBC, liver function tests, ammonia, cross-match, PT, PTT, and measurement of AST (SGOT), ALT (SGPT), alkaline phosphatase, bilirubin, total protein, and albumin, and give vitamin K and FFP (see sec. **IV.A** above).

2. **Peptic ulcer.** Acute **stress ulcers** occur in the stomach and are associated with sepsis, head injury, multiple trauma, burn, hypoxemia, or acidosis. Chronic **peptic ulcer** disease can occur in children of all ages but is unusual under 5 years. Duodenal ulcer is much more common than gastric ulcer in children. There is often a strong familial history of peptic ulcer disease in these patients. Typical symptoms of meal-provoked or meal-relieved pain may be absent in young children, in whom the pain may be poorly localized. Children over 10 years of age are more likely to have symptoms typical of "adult" peptic ulcer disease. *Campylobacter pylori* antral gastritis is present in most children with primary chronic duodenal ulcer disease.

   a. **Management.** In the child with significant bleeding, insert an NG tube and give antacids and IV ranitidine or cimetidine to keep the gastric pH $\geq$ 5 (beware of magnesium or aluminum toxicity from antacids in patients with renal failure). Early consultation with a gastroenterologist is advised. Upper gastrointestinal endoscopic examination is mandatory for diagnosis: It should be performed after the patient is volume repleted and stable and after lavage has rendered the stomach clear of blood and antacids. Barium studies are of little use in the actively bleeding patient. Therapy and treatment of refractory bleeding may include intravenous vasopressin, prostaglandins, somatostatin, angiographic arterial embolization, and surgery. Fortunately, these are rarely needed.

3. **Esophagitis.** Peptic esophagitis due to gastroesophageal reflux is the most common form of esophagitis in children. Other causes include esophageal dysmotility with poor acid clearance (usually secondary to CNS disorders), ingestion of caustic substances, infections (cytomegalovirus, herpes, *Candida*), chemotherapy, and radiotherapy. Esophagitis may present with hematemesis or iron deficiency anemia; heavy bleeding is rare. The older child may describe dysphagia with burning epigastric or substernal pain. Children less than 3 years of age may present with vomiting, irritability, or abnormal posturing. Symptoms are often worse during or after feeds or when the child is lying flat. Associated problems include failure to thrive, anemia, pulmonary disease, and stricture. The diagnosis of esophagitis is made by endoscopy with biopsy and esophageal brushings.

   a. **Management.** These children should be treated with an antacid or an $H_2$ blocker for symptomatic relief. Refer the child to a gastroenterologist for outpatient assessment.

4. **Gastritis.** Acute "stress" gastritis is associated with sepsis, head injury, burns, hypoxemia, and acidosis. Drugs such as salicylates and nonsteroidal anti-inflammatory drugs (NSAIDs) may cause gastritis, as may ingestion of iron or alcohol, enteroviruses, *Campylobacter pylori,* eosinophilic gastroenteropathy, Crohn's disease, and Henoch-Schönlein disease. Endoscopy with biopsy is usually diagnostic.

   a. **Management.** Initial management includes therapy with antacids and $H_2$ blockers until a specific diagnosis is made at endoscopy.

5. **Mechanical causes.** Gastric erosions and Mallory-Weiss tears due to forceful vomiting are common causes of upper gastrointestinal bleeding in children. Endoscopy may be required to make the diagnosis.

B. **Lower gastrointestinal bleeding**
   1. **Meckel's diverticulum.** See Chap. 16, Surgical Abdominal Disorders.
   2. **Intussusception.** See Chap. 16, Surgical Abdominal Disorders.
   3. **Inflammatory bowel disease.** Inflammatory bowel disease, although common in children aged 8–18 years, may also occur in younger children. It is rare in those

under 2 years of age. The typical presentation includes growth delay, abdominal pain, weight loss, fever, and diarrhea with or without blood. Rectal bleeding may vary from microscopic loss to severe hemorrhage causing shock. Other complications include toxic megacolon (decreased bowel sounds, hypovolemia, dilated colon), abscess (Crohn's disease), obstruction, perforation, and sepsis.

    **a. Management.** When IBD is suspected, obtain blood for CBC, erythrocyte sedimentation rate, and serum albumin measurement. Ensure that stool cultures are negative, and refer the child to a gastroenterologist. **Narcotic analgesics, antidiarrheal agents, or barium enema may cause toxic megacolon in the ill patient and should be avoided.**

**4. Polyps.** Most polyps in children are juvenile in type and are benign, although multiple polyposis syndromes do occur and may be premalignant. Polyps generally present with painless blood streaking in stools or passage of bright red blood clots. Heavy blood loss is rare. Polyps are rarely palpable on rectal examination. Diagnosis is made by flexible fiberoptic colonoscopy with polypectomy. Barium studies are not indicated except in rare syndromes involving small bowel polyps.

    **a. Management.** Refer the patient to a gastroenterologist for endoscopy and polypectomy.

**5. Anal fissure.** Anal fissure is the most common cause of blood streaking on the surface of the stool in the infant and young child. Constipation is often diagnosed by the history and abdominal and rectal examinations. Fissures are best seen by spreading the rectal mucosa with the fingers to evert the anal canal; most are located posteriorly at the 6 o'clock position. Fissures are often seen only in the well-sedated child because anal sphincter spasm may prevent adequate examination. Chronic anal fissures may also occur in Crohn's disease.

    **a. Management.** If treatment is not undertaken, constipation persists owing to fearful stool withholding, and a cycle ensues, resulting in chronic fissure. Sitz baths provide symptomatic relief, and stool softeners such as mineral oil or docusate (Colace) may also help (see Chap. 16, Constipation). Patients refractory to these measures after 6 weeks of treatment should have the diagnosis verified by examination under sedation. Anal stretch, performed under sedation, is often curative. Surgical treatment is hardly ever required and should be avoided for fissures due to Crohn's disease.

**6. Cow/soy milk colitis.** Cow's milk protein may cause enteritis and colitis. About 50% of these patients also have soy protein intolerance. They may present with a history of diarrhea and bloody stools or, when blood loss is microscopic, iron deficiency anemia. Protein-losing enteropathy may lead to hypoproteinemia.

   **a. Management.** Always exclude other causes of enterocolitis, especially infection. The child should be switched to a formula that does not contain the offending antigen and treated with iron replacement therapy if he is anemic (see Chap. 19).

**7. Necrotizing enterocolitis (NEC).** Necrotizing enterocolitis is usually seen in preterm newborns, although it may occur in the term infant with a history of sepsis, acidosis, and hypoxemia. In general, babies present in the first 4 weeks of life. Presenting signs include irritability, poor feeding, bloody diarrhea, and abdominal distention with adynamic ileus. Severe disease may result in apnea, shock, thrombocytopenia, and disseminated intravascular coagulation (DIC). Order supine and erect abdominal x rays to look for pneumatosis intestinalis and free air in the peritoneum or portal system. Obtain blood for CBC, differential count, platelet count, PT, PTT, culture, and measurement of electrolytes, arterial blood gases, BUN, and glucose. Electrolytes, CBC, and the platelet count should be monitored every 6 hours.

   **a. Management.** Control problems in the airway, breathing, and circulation. The child may be in shock from sepsis or hypovolemia; if so, resuscitate with FFP, 5–10 ml/kg/dose, until he or she is stable. Place the child on continuous or low intermittent NG suction, keep NPO, and give intravenous alimentation. Following a septic workup (cerebrospinal fluid, blood, urine, and stool cultures), treat with intravenous vancomycin, 45 mg/kg/day divided q8h (30 mg/kg/day divided q12h if the patient is under 7 days old) and cefotaxime, 150 mg/kg/day divided q8h (100 mg/kg/day divided q12h if under 7 days). Consult a surgeon and transfer the child to an intensive care unit.

**VI. Disposition.** Admit all children with more than trivial hematemesis or rectal bleeding. A patient with severe gastrointestinal bleeding should be admitted to the intensive care unit.

**VII. Key points**

1. The earliest sign of significant gastrointestinal bleeding is often a raised resting heart rate.

2. The most common error in management of the child with severe gastrointestinal bleeding is inadequate volume replacement. Start two large-bore IV lines and infuse fluid boluses of a crystalloid or colloid substance until stable.

3. Determine that gastrointestinal bleeding has in fact occurred. Test all suspicious stools with guaiac (Hemoccult) at the bedside. If no stool is available for testing or inspection, perform a rectal examination to obtain stool.

**4.** Cow/soy milk enterocolitis almost always occurs in patients under 1 year of age and is almost never seen in patients over 2 years of age.

**5.** Giardiasis does not cause gastrointestinal bleeding.

**6.** Barium studies are of little value in the diagnosis of the actively bleeding patient. Upper or lower flexible fiberoptic endoscopic examination is usually diagnostic and may be therapeutic.

**7.** Narcotic analgesics, antidiarrheal agents, or barium enema may precipitate toxic megacolon and should be avoided in patients with acute diarrhea.

### Bibliography

Ament, M. E., Berquist, W. E., Vargas, J., et al. Fiberoptic upper endoscopy in infants and children. *Pediatr. Clin. North Am.* 35:141, 1988.

Hassall, E., Barclay, G., and Ament, M. E. Colonoscopy in children. *Pediatrics* 73:594, 1985.

Hyams, J. S., Leichtner, A. M., and Schwartz, A. N. Diagnosis and management of gastro-intestinal hemorrhage. *J. Pediatr.* 106:1, 1985.

## Liver Failure
### Eric Hassall

Liver failure occurs when the synthetic and excretory functions of the liver decline, compromising the clinical status of the child. Failure of **synthetic function** is reflected by a prolonged prothrombin time and decreased serum albumin; failure of **excretory function** is manifest by increased serum bilirubin and ammonia levels. The clinical and biochemical manifestations of liver failure are listed in Table 16-8 and the causes according to age in Table 16-9.

**Table 16-8. Clinical and biochemical manifestations of liver failure**

Jaundice

Gastrointestinal bleeding due to portal hypertension

Ascites

Hepatic encephalopathy

Palmar erythema or spider angiomas

Hypoalbuminemia

Coagulopathy

Raised transaminases (AST, ALT) and alkaline phosphatase

Hyperammonemia

Note: Not all of these features are required to diagnose liver failure. Abnormal liver function tests (raised AST, ALT) may reflect liver damage but do not indicate liver failure per se. Similarly, portal hypertension may be seen in the absence of liver disease.

**Table 16-9. Causes of liver failure**

| Type | All ages | Onset more common in newborn |
| --- | --- | --- |
| Idiopathic | **Cryptogenic cirrhosis** | **Idiopathic neonatal hepatitis** |
| Infectious | **Hepatitis B, non-A, non-B (NANB)**, delta, cytomegalovirus, Epstein-Barr virus, adenovirus, Coxsackie virus, disseminated herpes, rubella, bacterial sepsis, leptospirosis | Hepatitis B, TORCH, syphilis |
| Vascular | Shock, hypoxemia, ischemia, venoocclusive disease, acute Budd-Chiari syndrome | |
| Toxic | **Drugs** (acetaminophen, salicylates, ketoconazole, phenytoin, valproic acid, iron, antineoplastic drugs) Ethanol, CCl₄, halothane, penthrane, mushrooms (*Amanita phalloides*) | **Parenteral nutrition** |
| Metabolic | **Alpha-1-antitrypsin deficiency**, Reye's syndrome, Wilson's disease, hemochromatosis | **Alpha-1-antitrypsin deficiency**, tyrosinemia, galactosemia, GSD, Wolman's disease, HFI |
| Other | | **Biliary atresia**, polycystic disease, congenital hepatic fibrosis |

Note: Disorders causing hyperammonemia without liver failure (urea cycle, amino acidemia, organic acidemia) are excluded from this list.
Key: Common causes denoted by bold lettering. HFI = hereditary fructose intolerance, GSD = glycogen storage disease.
*Uncommon under 2 years of age.

## I. Diagnosis and assessment

**A. History.** In children with **acute onset of liver failure** inquire about exposure to infectious agents or persons, blood products including gamma globulin, tattoos, ear piercing, drugs, and toxins, including anesthetic agents. Ask about travel and a family history of jaundice or liver disease. In the **infant** ask about the pregnancy, birth weight, feeding history (inborn errors of metabolism, galactosemia, hereditary fructose intolerance [HFI]), hemolysis, anemia, or maternal history of hepatitis. In **children with known liver disease** determine if there are precipitating factors such as intercurrent infection (urinary tract infection, sepsis, primary bacterial peritonitis), dehydration, hypokalemic alkalosis (often due to overdiuresis), gastrointestinal bleeding, high dietary protein intake, or recent high-volume paracentesis of ascitic fluid.

**B. Examination.** Look for signs of liver failure as listed in Table 16-8. Examine the abdomen and determine liver size, consistency, and tenderness. Perform a full neurologic examination. Measure vital signs and look for orthostatic changes that may indicate acute or chronic blood loss (see Chap. 23, Fluids and Electrolytes, sec. **II**). Perform a rectal examination to identify the presence of melena or fresh blood in the stool, and test the stool specimen for occult blood (using a Hemoccult card). (See Gastrointestinal Bleeding.) Children requiring emergency treatment for liver failure are invariably jaundiced, with the exception of patients with Reye's syndrome. There may be evidence of coagulopathy including purpura, or bleeding or oozing from areas subjected to trauma (gums, venipuncture sites). The initial signs of hepatic encephalopathy are confusion and vomiting, with progression to irritability, stupor, hyperreflexia, and asterixis (liver flap). Obtundation, coma, areflexia, apnea, and seizures are signs of end-stage encephalopathy.

**C. Investigations**

1. **To assess severity of liver failure.** Obtain blood for complete blood count (CBC), differential and platelet counts, prothrombin time (PT), partial thromboplastin time (PTT), reticulocyte count, and measurements of AST (SGOT), ALT (SGPT), alkaline phosphatase, bilirubin, total protein, albumin, ammonia, electrolytes, serum osmolality, BUN, creatinine, blood gases, and glucose. Send a urine specimen for measurement of sodium, specific gravity, and osmolality.

2. **To determine etiology of liver failure.** When the cause is unknown, send specimens of blood for hepatitis serologic examination (A IgM, B-surface antigen, B-surface antibody, and B-core antibody), and blood culture. Send urine samples for urinalysis and culture in all cases. Other investigations that may be ordered as indicated include toxic screen, measurements of serum iron, ferritin, copper, ceruloplasmin,

and alpha-1-antitrypsin, syphilis serologic examination, TORCH titers, and acute viral titers for Coxsackie virus, adenovirus, and reovirus. Measurements of urine reducing substances, organic acids, amino acids, and a 24-hour urine specimen for copper measurement may also be ordered as indicated. Obtain a specimen of ascitic fluid for culture when peritonitis is suspected, and perform an eye examination (including slit-lamp examination) to look for Kayser-Fleischer rings as evidence of Wilson's disease.

## II. Management

### A. Principles of emergency management

1. Reverse hepatic encephalopathy by treating the metabolic disturbances and any precipitating factors.
2. Stop gastrointestinal bleeding.
3. Prevent onset of hepatorenal syndrome by careful fluid management and early recognition of decreased renal function (as shown by oliguria or increased serum creatinine level).
4. Rule out and treat sepsis and hypoglycemia.
5. Institute careful nutritional management.

### B. The unstable child. The following steps are recommended for the acutely ill child with encephalopathy or bleeding. Consult a gastroenterologist when possible.

1. Assess and maintain airway, breathing, and circulation. Give oxygen by mask. Start a large-bore intravenous line, check blood sugar level by Dextrostix, and send blood specimens for investigations (see sec. **I.C,** above). Infuse 10% dextrose in water at a rate according to the patient's fluid status.
2. If there is suspicion of sepsis, begin therapy with intravenous ampicillin, 200 mg/kg/day IV divided q6h, and gentamicin, 5.0 mg/kg/day IV divided q8h, after cultures have been obtained.
3. Insert the largest nasogastric (NG) tube the child will tolerate and perform lavage with 5 ml/kg of room temperature normal saline. If there is bleeding, treat aggressively with antacids, $H_2$ blockers (cimetidine, ranitidine) or vasopressin (see Chap. 16, Gastrointestinal Bleeding). If the PT is prolonged for more than 3 seconds over control values, give vitamin K, 1–5 mg IV or SC daily, whether the patient is bleeding or not. Fresh frozen plasma (FFP), 5–10 ml/kg given intravenously over 30–60 minutes, may be required if there is bleeding or if PT and PTT are markedly prolonged.
4. Treat encephalopathy by decreasing ammonia production as follows:
   a. Give lactulose through an NG tube, 1–2 ml/kg q4h, until profuse, watery diarrhea occurs. When stools are watery and clear, decrease the amount and frequency of lactulose. Lactulose may cause abdominal distention or discomfort.
   b. If lactulose is not tolerated, give neomycin, 50

**Table 16-10. Diagnosis of hepatorenal syndrome**

Chronic liver disease with ascites

Slow onset azotemia

Good renal tubular function:
  Urine osmolality greater than that of serum
  Urine sodium concentration very low (<10 mmol/liter or 10 mEq/liter)
  Urine to serum creatinine ratio greater than 30

No sustained benefit from intravascular volume infusion

Source: Adapted from S. Sherlock. *Diseases of the Liver and Biliary System* (6th ed.). London: Blackwell Scientific Publications, 1981.

mg/kg/day through NG tube divided q6h. Lactulose and neomycin do not need to be given concurrently.

**c.** If the child is constipated and is not receiving lactulose, treat with an enema or magnesium citrate, 4 ml/kg via NG tube.

**5.** Carefully monitor fluid status with strict intake and output measurements. Children with hepatic failure may have oliguria due to the hepatorenal syndrome or established acute tubular necrosis (Table 16-10).

**a.** Intravenous albumin is indicated in children with **oliguria due to poor renal perfusion** (prerenal failure—see Chap. 23) or respiratory embarrassment secondary to ascites. The dose is 1 gm/kg (4 ml/kg of 25% solution) infused over 1–2 hours intravenously and repeated PRN or q12h.

**b.** Diuretics may be indicated for the treatment of the child with ascites or oliguria. Frequently monitor and maintain serum electrolyte levels as near to normal as possible. The total body sodium level is high and potassium is low; use low-sodium or sodium-free IV fluids (10% dextrose in water with or without one-fourth normal saline), and if potassium-losing diuretics are used, add potassium to the IV fluid and give spironolactone.

**6.** Nutrition must be maintained; branched-chain amino acid solutions given intravenously (Hepatamine) or PO (Hepatic Aid), or special enteral formulas (Portagen or Pregestemil) are often required.

**7.** Monitor the following laboratory values:

**a.** Every 12 hours initially: CBC, platelet count, PT, PTT, ammonia, glucose, serum osmolality, electrolytes, BUN, creatinine, and urine electrolytes and osmolality.

**b.** Daily: bilirubin, AST, ALT, alkaline phosphatase, and albumin levels, and blood and urine cultures.

**c.** Many children with acute liver failure require Foley catheter and central venous pressure (CVP) line placement to monitor fluid status accurately.

**C. The stable child.** The child with mild chronic enceph-

**Table 16-11. Drugs used in liver failure**

| Drug | Dose |
| --- | --- |
| Lactulose | 1–2 ml/kg/dose via NG tube q4–6h in patients in hepatic coma. Decrease dose and frequency if stools are watery or encephalopathy resolves |
| Neomycin | 50 mg/kg/day PO/NG divided q6–8h |
| Albumin | 1 gm/kg/dose IV over 15–30 minutes |
| Furosemide | 1.0 mg/kg IV/PO |
| Chlorothiazide | 20–40 mg/kg/day PO divided q12h |
| Hydrochlorothiazide | 2–5 mg/kg/day PO divided q12h |
| Spironolactone | 1–3 mg/kg/day PO divided q12h |
| Ranitidine | see Chap. 16, Gastrointestinal Bleeding and Table 16-7 |
| Cimetidine | see Chap. 16, Gastrointestinal Bleeding and Table 16-7 |
| Vasopressin | see Chap. 16, Gastrointestinal Bleeding and Table 16-7 |

alopathy from liver failure can be managed as follows (Table 16-11):

1. Admit the patient and place him or her on a high-carbohydrate diet with a largely vegetable protein intake, the quantity of which will vary with the degree of encephalopathy and the serum ammonia level. Do not routinely give a low-protein diet because malnutrition may result.
2. Prescribe lactulose to give 1–2 soft stools daily (10–30 ml/day in the older child and 2.5 ml bid in children under 1 year of age).
3. Diuretics may be given to the patient with ascites. Always include a potassium-sparing diuretic such as spironolactone.

**III. Disposition.** Admit all children with acute liver failure. Patients with encephalopathy or gastrointestinal bleeding should be managed in the intensive care unit.

**IV. Key points**

1. The initial management of the child with liver failure includes diagnosis and treatment of sepsis, hypoglycemia, encephalopathy, and gastrointestinal bleeding.
2. Decreased urine output in the patient with liver failure may be due to acute tubular necrosis or hepatorenal syndrome.

**Bibliography**

Epstein, M. Hepatorenal syndrome. In J. E. Berk et al. (eds.). *Bockus Gastroenterology* (4th ed.). Philadelphia: Saunders, 1985.

Hoyumpa, A. M., et al. Hepatic encephalopathy. *Gastroenterology* 76:184, 1979.

Westaby, D., and Williams, R. Portal hypertension. In J. E. Berk et al. (eds.). *Bockus Gastroenterology* (4th ed.). Philadelphia: Saunders, 1985.

---

# Vomiting
Eric Hassall

Vomiting is a common presenting complaint in pediatrics, since it has both systemic (see Table 16-10) and gastrointestinal causes. Extraintestinal causes such as urinary tract infection and otitis media are frequent in the infant and toddler. See also Chap. 16, Acute Diarrhea.

I. **Diagnosis and assessment**
   A. **History.** Determine the frequency and quantity of the vomitus and whether it contains blood, bile, or undigested food. Ask if it is effortless or forceful, and determine its relationship to meals and posture. Ask about toxic ingestion, previous medical disease, head injury, and CNS signs and symptoms such as irritability, lethargy, neck stiffness, and headache. Vomiting due to increased intracranial pressure often occurs in the early morning, is effortless, and is not associated with nausea. A history of diarrhea or fever suggests gastroenteritis. Bowel obstruction is suggested by a history of previous surgery, colicky pain, vomiting after meals, or continuous bile-stained or feculent vomiting.
   B. **Examination.** Determine the degree of dehydration in all children who have been vomiting (see Chap. 23, Fluids and Electrolytes, sec. **II**). Feel the fontanel, test for neck stiffness, and examine the CNS including the level of consciousness, coordination, reflexes, and cranial nerves. In infants and children who are unable to complain of earache, rule out otitis media. Carefully examine the abdomen for masses, distention, tenderness, guarding, and rebound. Rectal examination may demonstrate tenderness (appendicitis, pelvic inflammatory disease [PID], peritonitis), mass (intussusception), or a narrow distal anorectal segment (Hirschsprung's disease), or it may provide stool for examination (see Chap. 16, Abdominal Pain; Acute Diarrhea).
II. **Causes of vomiting**
   A. **Systemic disease.** See Table 16-12.
   B. **Gastrointestinal disease**
      1. **Infant** (under 2 years). **Gastroesophageal reflux** accounts for most cases of recurrent vomiting in infancy. It may be due to an incompetent lower esophageal sphincter, hiatal hernia, or delayed gastric emptying. Esophagitis, per se, from any cause may

**Table 16-12. Systemic causes of vomiting**

| Type | Example |
| --- | --- |
| Infectious | Fever, sepsis, tonsillitis, otitis media, pneumonia, hepatitis, bacterial enterocolitis with sepsis |
| Genitourinary | UTI, pyelonephritis, UPJ obstruction, testicular, ovarian torsion |
| CNS | Meningitis, encephalitis, increased ICP, labyrinthitis, tumor, migraine, Reye's syndrome, seizure, congenital anomalies of brain |
| Metabolic | DKA, adrenal crisis, inborn errors of metabolism, renal or hepatic failure |
| Other | Raised intraabdominal pressure, cyclic vomiting, psychogenic vomiting, high blood pressure, pregnancy, heat excess, cancer causing nausea and anorexia |
| Toxic ingestion | Salicylates, theophylline, caustics, caustic agents, lead, digoxin, food poisoning (*S. aureus* preformed toxin, *Clostridium perfringens*). |

Key: UTI = Urinary tract infection, UPJ = ureteropelvic junction, ICP = intracranial pressure, DKA = diabetic ketoacidosis.

**Table 16-13. Causes of bowel obstruction**

| Age | Examples |
| --- | --- |
| Infant | Duodenal atresia, duodenal bands, duplication cyst, malrotation, volvulus, incarcerated hernia, intussusception, Meckel's diverticulum with torsion. Hirschsprung's disease, gastric web. |
| Child | Malrotation, volvulus, intussusception, Meckel's diverticulum with torsion, incarcerated hernia, posttraumatic obstruction (duodenal hematoma, ruptured viscus), SMA syndrome, adhesions |

Key: SMA = Superior mesenteric artery.

cause vomiting. Other common causes of vomiting are overfeeding or underfeeding, pyloric stenosis, cow or soy milk protein intolerance, and gastroenteritis. Severe vomiting may be due to partial or complete bowel obstruction (Table 16-13).

2. **Child** (2–12 years). Common gastrointestinal disorders causing vomiting in children include gastroenteritis, gastroesophageal reflux (see sec. **II.B.1,** above), food poisoning, acid peptic disease, hepatitis, and pancreatitis. Maintain a high index of suspicion

for surgical disorders such as appendicitis or bowel obstruction (see Table 16-13).

**3. Adolescent.** Common causes in the adolescent include gastroenteritis, food poisoning, acid peptic disease, Crohn's disease, appendicitis, psychogenic vomiting, cholecystitis, pregnancy, and PID.

III. **Management of the vomiting child.** Complications of vomiting include aspiration in obtunded or mentally handicapped children, dehydration, and electrolyte imbalance with hypochloremic, hypokalemic alkalosis. Forceful vomiting may result in a Mallory-Weiss tear or erosion of the gastric cardia. Recurrent vomiting may cause esophagitis.

A. **Fluid status**

1. Some children with nonsurgical causes of vomiting will tolerate oral rehydration (see Chap. 16, Acute Diarrhea).

2. Start an intravenous line and administer IV rehydration in children who are unable to tolerate oral fluids, who are > 5% dehydrated, or who have serious underlying disease (see Chap. 23, Fluids and Electrolytes, sec. **II**). Obtain blood for measurement of glucose, electrolytes, and BUN, and a urine specimen for urinalysis, urine culture, and measurement of specific gravity. Additional investigations, including x rays, ultrasound examination, and blood samples for measurement of ammonia, blood gases, and amylase, toxic screen, culture, and other tests may be ordered as indicated.

3. Do not use antiemetic drugs such as phenothiazines or antihistamines because they may mask or delay diagnosis of serious causes of vomiting.

B. **Bowel obstruction.** When bowel obstruction is suspected start an intravenous line, draw blood for CBC, electrolytes, and cross-match, and consult a surgeon. Place a nasogastric (NG) tube, and order supine and erect or cross-table lateral films—the presence of multiple air-fluid levels and air in the small bowel is highly suggestive of obstruction.

C. **Gastroesophageal reflux.** In general, a happy thriving baby under 18 months of age with small amounts of vomiting requires no treatment or investigation. Complications of gastroesophageal reflux include failure to thrive, pulmonary disease, choking or apneic episodes, hematemesis, anemia, irritability, and abnormal posturing with feeds. Children who present with any of these complications should be referred to a gastroenterologist for investigation with 24-hour intraesophageal pH monitoring, endoscopy, manometry, and gastric emptying studies. Barium studies alone are unreliable.

IV. **Disposition.** Admit all patients with significant dehydration, bowel obstruction, serious underlying systemic disease, and those who are unable to tolerate maintenance oral fluid therapy.

V. **Key points**

A. The majority of cases of vomiting are due to gastroesophageal reflux and its causes, acute gastroenteritis, or systemic disorders such as tonsillitis, otitis media, or urinary tract infection.

**B.** Many children with vomiting will tolerate oral rehydration and maintenance fluid therapy.

**C.** Ensure that a surgical cause for vomiting is not present.

**D.** Do not use antiemetic drugs in children with vomiting.

### Bibliography

Silverberg, M., and Daum, F. *Textbook of Pediatric Gastroenterology* (2nd ed.). Chicago: Yearbook, 1988.

Silverman, A., and Roy, C. C. (eds.). *Pediatric Clinical Gastroenterology*. St. Louis: Mosby, 1983.

## Upper Gastrointestinal Foreign Bodies
Eric Hassall

Children may swallow a variety of items including coins, button batteries, marbles, pins, and pieces of toys. In most cases the child is under 5 years of age or is mentally handicapped. Occasionally the child has an initial brief gagging or choking spell. Subsequent symptoms depend on the location and nature of the foreign body: An object in the esophagus may cause discomfort, drooling, and partial upper airway obstruction; an object in the stomach is usually asymptomatic unless the ingested object is corrosive or sharp.

**I. Coins and marbles.** On a posteroanterior x ray of the neck and chest, a coin in the esophagus is seen flat side on, whereas a coin in the trachea is seen edge on. A coin in the stomach that is smaller than a quarter (24 mm in diameter) will usually pass without difficulty in children over 2 years of age. Coins lodged in the esophagus should be immediately removed endoscopically before pressure necrosis leads to fistula formation.

**A. Management.** Indications for endoscopic removal of coins and marbles beyond the esophagus include:

**1.** Presence of the object for more than 3–4 weeks in the gastrointestinal tract.

**2.** Known gastric outlet anomaly or intestinal stricture downstream.

**II. Button batteries.** Most button batteries pass through the gastrointestinal tract without problem. Batteries that become lodged in the gastrointestinal tract can cause damage secondary to mechanical pressure necrosis, alkaline burn, or low-voltage electrical burn.

**A.** A button battery that is lodged in the **esophagus** is a true emergency and urgent removal is required. It is important to distinguish between a coin and a battery on x ray; on the posteroanterior view, the battery has concentric double densities, whereas on a lateral view the edges are rounded and a stepoff is visible at the junction of the cathode and anode. A coin appears flatter and has a sharper edge on the lateral view.

**B.** A button battery in the **stomach** is usually passed without difficulty. Indications for immediate removal include large battery size in a small child, presence in the stomach for more than 24 hours, or symptoms of pain, vomiting, or bleeding.

**C.** An **intestinal** button battery rarely causes problems. Once past the third part of the duodenum, endoscopic removal from above is impossible. Most are passed within 72 hours, although it may take up to 14 days. Purgation may be performed to hasten transit time.

**III. Principles in treatment of gastrointestinal foreign bodies**

**A.** If there is a history of foreign body ingestion, instruct the parents or nursing staff to keep the child NPO until x rays have been obtained.

**B.** Obtain x rays of the neck, base of the skull, chest, and abdomen. Always order at least two perpendicular views to locate the object accurately. Radiolucent objects such as glass, bone fragments, aluminum ring pull-tabs on drink cans, plastic, or wood may be seen on fluoroscopy or on an upper GI series using barium.

**C.** A child who has a food bolus obstruction of the esophagus almost always has an underlying abnormality, such as a web, motility disorder, or stricture. Therefore, even if the obstruction has passed, the patient should be referred for flexible fiberoptic evaluation of the gastrointestinal tract, an upper GI series, and possible esophageal manometry and pH study.

**D.** Consult a gastroenterologist or other endoscopist for management. In general, flexible fiberoptic endoscopy is the procedure of choice. Sharp, pointed foreign bodies in the esophagus such as fishbones, nails, pins, needles, and blades are best removed by rigid endoscope or flexible endoscopy using an overtube. Children with foreign bodies at the level of the pharynx or cricopharyngeus muscle should be referred to an ear, nose, and throat (ENT) surgeon. Some advocate removal of upper gastrointestinal foreign bodies in an unanesthetized child with a Foley balloon in the esophagus or a magnet attached to an orogastric catheter. Young children usually struggle during such procedures, and the foreign body may be dropped, resulting in airway obstruction and death. **The procedure of choice is endoscopy with removal of the foreign body under direct vision, under general anesthesia with an endotracheal tube in situ.**

**IV. Disposition.** In most cases, foreign body removal can be accomplished as an outpatient surgical case, with discharge 3–6 hours after the procedure.

**V. Key points**

**A.** Always obtain x rays in children in whom foreign body ingestion is suspected. Keep NPO until the course of action is decided.

**B.** Consult with a specialist skilled in the management of ingested foreign bodies in children.

**C.** The method of choice for removal is by endoscopy under general anesthesia with a protected airway.

## Bibliography

Webb, W. A. Management of foreign bodies of the upper gastrointestinal tract. *Gastroenterology* 94:204, 1988.

# 17

# Genitourinary Disorders

Gerald U. Coleman

I. **Renal trauma.** Most renal trauma results from blunt injury, such as a motor vehicle accident or a fall from a swing onto a bar or a bicycle onto a curb. Underlying renal anomalies are believed to be more common in children who are investigated for renal injury.

  A. **Diagnosis and assessment**

    1. **Examination.** Direct signs of renal injury include a mass in the flank, tenderness in the costovertebral angle (CVA), and gross or microscopic hematuria. Flank ecchymoses is an indirect sign of injury. The degree of hematuria is not a reliable indicator of severity of injury. For diagnosis and assessment of other causes of hematuria, see Chap. 23, Hematuria.

    2. **Investigation**

      a. **Intravenous pyelogram (IVP).** An IVP is indicated whenever renal injury is suspected, including all multiple trauma victims with hematuria, flank mass, CVA tenderness, or undiagnosed shock or when there is penetrating injury to the flank, back, or abdomen. After giving the radiocontrast medium, take films at 1, 5, 10, and 20 minutes.

        (1) Look for **fractures of the twelfth rib or lumbar transverse processes** as indirect signs of renal injury.

        (2) Hematuria with a normal IVP suggests **contusion,** the most common type of injury.

        (3) When there is no renal appearance of contrast media, suspect a **vascular pedicle injury;** urgent angiography and surgery must be considered in these children.

        (4) Extravasation of contrast from the collecting system indicates possible **laceration or collecting system injury.** Distortion of the collecting system or failure of calyces to fill also suggests collecting system injury.

      b. **Renal ultrasound.** Ultrasound examination may be used in nonurgent cases to look for disruption, segmental areas of increased echogenicity, or perirenal fluid collection.

      c. **Renogram.** A radioisotope renogram may help to determine blood flow when the kidney is poorly seen on IVP or when there are underlying obstructive renal anomalies.

  B. **Management.** Most renal injuries are treated nonoperatively with intravenous fluid and blood replacement and follow-up ultrasound examinations.

    1. **Resuscitation.** Assess and control any problems in the airway, breathing, and circulation. Up to 25% of renal trauma is associated with other injuries, especially liver trauma. Start an intravenous line and draw blood for a complete blood count (CBC) and

cross-matching, liver function tests, and measurements of amylase, BUN, creatinine, and serum electrolytes.

   **2. Monitoring.** Closely follow the patient's vital signs. Obtain each voided specimen or 2-hourly catheter specimens for gross and microscopic analyses.

   **3. Investigation.** Arrange an IVP. Nonvisualization of a kidney or extravasation of dye should prompt urgent arteriography or renogram. Keep these children NPO until they are seen by a urologist (see sec. **I.A.2.a.(3)**).

   **4. Stabilization.** Children who are stable should have serial renal ultrasound examinations to follow development of renal hematomas and repeated hemoglobin measurements to rule out occult injury causing hemorrhage.

**C. Disposition.** Admission to an intensive care unit is indicated if the child is in shock or has sustained multiple injuries. If an isolated renal injury is present, admit the child to a surgical ward for monitoring. Immediate surgery is necessary when there is renal pedicle injury or uncontrolled bleeding.

**II. Bladder trauma.** These rare injuries usually result from a fall or a blow to a full bladder. Pelvic fracture is frequently associated.

**A. Diagnosis and assessment.** Bladder rupture causes urine leakage into the peritoneum, causing an initial presentation of suprapubic tenderness, inability to void, hematuria, pallor, and hypotension. These signs are followed 24–48 hours later by peritoneal irritation with fever, vomiting, guarding, rigidity, and rebound tenderness. The diagnosis is made by performing a static cystogram with anteroposterior and oblique or lateral x rays; in most cases there is obvious peritoneal extravasation of dye. Always consider the possibility of concomitant urethral injury (see sec. **III** and **IV** below).

**B. Management.** Start an intravenous line, keep the child NPO, and obtain blood specimens (see sec. **I** above). Children with pelvic fracture may be hypovolemic from blood loss and require fluid resuscitation. Pass a Foley catheter (for correct size see Table 17–1), and immediately consult a urologist for operative repair.

**C. Disposition.** Children with significant isolated bladder and urethral injury require emergency surgery and postoperative care on a surgical ward.

**III. Rupture of the prostatomembranous urethra.** This usually occurs in boys who are run over by a motor vehicle. Pelvic crush fracture occurs in all cases and commonly involves the pubic rami. Suspect prostatomembranous urethral rupture in the trauma victim with a suprapubic mass, inability to void, blood at the urethral meatus, or a boggy anterior mass on rectal examination.

**A. Management.** Obtain a retrograde urethrogram, which can be performed when pelvic x rays are taken. To obtain a urethrogram, pass an 8F Foley catheter just inside the distal glandular urethra and inflate the balloon to oc-

**Table 17-1. Foley catheter size for age**

| Age (years) | Size (F) |
| --- | --- |
| Girls | |
| 0–12 | 10–12 |
| 12–adult | 16 |
| Boys | |
| 0–5 | 8 |
| 6–10 | 10 |
| 11–15 | 12 |
| Over 15 | 16 |

clude it. Allow a water-soluble contrast medium (10% Renografin) to flow by gravity through the catheter into the urethra, and obtain oblique films. Extravasation of contrast into pelvic soft tissue indicates urethral rupture. Consult a urologist immediately for suprapubic cystotomy and catheter realignment of the urethra. **Do not attempt to pass a catheter into the bladder.**

**IV. Rupture of the bulbous urethra.** Typically, this injury occurs in boys who sustain a straddle injury after falling astride a fence, monkey bar, or manhole cover. Patients with bulbous urethral rupture present with severe pain on voiding and blood at the meatus. There may be a tender mass, hematoma, or extravasation of urine into the perineum. A retrograde urethrogram reveals extravasation into the soft tissue of the perineum.

**A. Management.** Make a gentle attempt to pass a small Foley catheter (see Table 17-1 for correct size). If the catheter does not pass, the urethral injury is complete, and immediate surgical consultation for cystotomy and primary repair is required.

**V. Penile and scrotal trauma.** Traumatic injuries include penile amputation, zipper injury, and scrotal skin amputation.

**A. Management.** The amputated portion of the penis or scrotal skin should be immediately cleaned, wrapped in sterile gauze that has been soaked in Ringer's solution, and put in a sterile plastic bag that is placed on ice. Urgent surgery is indicated. Zipper injury may require general anesthesia in a young uncooperative child. If the child is cooperative, inject 1% plain Xylocaine (lidocaine) around the area that is caught, close the zipper, cut it through at the base, then open it to release the skin.

**B. Disposition.** Admit all patients with significant genitourinary trauma.

**C. Key points**

1. Order an IVP in all children suspected of renal trauma. Nonappearance of a kidney on IVP may be due to severe injury—consult a urologist immediately.

2. Blood at the meatus in a boy with a fractured pelvis

indicates disruption of the urethra. Urinary diversion and repair are necessary.

**VI. Acute scrotal swelling.** Boys with a history of pain and swelling of the scrotal contents require immediate assessment to determine if there is torsion of the testis: Uncorrected, there is a 50% chance of loss of the testis from infarction within 8–12 hours. Other causes of scrotal swelling include incarcerated inguinal hernia, torsion of the appendix testis, acute epididymitis, orchitis, and idiopathic scrotal edema.

**A. Diagnosis and assessment**

   **1. History.** Determine the onset, duration, severity, and character of the pain. Inquire about abdominal or inguinal swelling (incarcerated hernia), underlying urinary tract anomaly, or passage of purulent urine (epididymoorchitis).

   **2. Examination.** Examine the abdomen as well as the testis. Feel the testis, noting position, size, and presence of tenderness on palpation or elevation.

**B. Management.** All patients with acute painful testicular swelling should be suspected to have testicular torsion and referred to a surgeon. Keep the child NPO pending surgical assessment and obtain a urine specimen for urinalysis and culture.

**C. Causes of testicular swelling**

   **1. Nonpainful swelling.** Nonpainful causes of acute scrotal swelling include varicocele, hydrocele (transilluminates), uncomplicated inguinal hernia, Henoch-Schönlein purpura, and tumor (the testis often feels hard and irregular).

   **2. Painful swelling**

      **a. Testicular torsion.** The typical patient presents with sudden onset of pain and swelling after vigorous exercise. Some children complain of nausea and vomiting. On examination, there may be dark discoloration of the overlying scrotum. The testis is exquisitely tender and rides high in the scrotum—pain is increased when the scrotum is elevated. When scrotal edema is present for more than 24 hours, diagnosis by palpation can be difficult. The diagnosis may be confirmed using Doppler sonography and radioisotope flow studies, but these should never delay surgery. Management includes exploration and detorsion with orchidopexy on the nontorsed side.

      **b. Incarcerated inguinal hernia.** There is usually an inguinal component to the swelling of an incarcerated hernia, frequently with bruising of the overlying skin. Occasionally, the testis is infarcted when strangulation occurs. Immediate exploration is indicated when strangulation is suspected.

      **c. Torsion of the appendix testis.** The onset of pain is more gradual than it is in testicular torsion. A "blue dot sign" may be seen through the skin at the superior pole of the testes in the early stages, but severe edema can make the diagnosis difficult and necessitates surgical exploration.

  **d. Acute epididymoorchitis.** This is a rare condition in prepubertal boys. The urine is almost always purulent, and there is usually an underlying urinary tract anomaly such as an ectopic ureter or posterior urethral valves. Children with this disorder should be treated with trimethoprim-cotrimoxazole, 8 mg/kg/day as trimethoprim PO divided q12h, or amoxicillin, 50 mg/kg/day PO divided q6h for 10 days, after a urine sample has been obtained for culture. For treatment of patients in whom sexually transmitted disease is suspected, see Chap. 21, Sexually Transmitted Disease.

  **e. Mumps orchitis.** In these patients the symptoms of testicular inflammation are overshadowed by the systemic symptoms of mumps. Treatment is symptomatic, with analgesia and bed rest if the pain is severe.

  **f. Idiopathic scrotal edema.** Idiopathic scrotal edema is a form of urticaria that starts in the scrotum and may extend posteriorly in the perineum toward the anus and sometimes onto the shaft of the penis. A slightly violaceous color is noted. There may be hyperesthesia, but the testis within feels normal and is not tender. The condition usually resolves within 2 days.

**D. Disposition.** All suspected cases of testicular torsion require emergency exploration and repair with an overnight postoperative stay on a surgical ward.

**E. Key points**

  **1.** Consider the diagnosis of torsion in all children with acute onset of testicular pain and swelling.

  **2.** Surgical exploration is indicated when testicular torsion is suspected.

**VII. Inflammatory disease of the penis**

**A. True phimosis.** Phimosis, the inability to retract the foreskin over the glans, is a rare condition that is seen in prepubertal boys. It is due to chronic inflammation (balanitis xerotica obliterans) that causes scarring and thickening of the preputial opening. True phimosis must be differentiated from nonretractability of the foreskin, which occurs physiologically in boys up to the age of 4.

  **1. Diagnosis and assessment.** Phimosis presents with pain and ballooning of the prepuce during voiding. A glistening pale scar is present at the preputial opening with variable amounts of edema and erythema. There may be concurrent balanitis or meatitis.

  **2. Management.** The child should be referred to a urologist for elective circumcision.

**B. Paraphimosis.** Paraphimosis occurs when the preputial ring is retracted past the corona of the glans penis and is not immediately reduced. The resultant bacterial

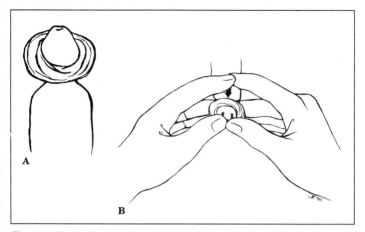

Fig. 17-1. Reduction of paraphimosis. (From Klauber GT and Grannum R. In Kilalis, King and Belman. Disorders of the male external genitalia. *Clin. Pediatr. Urol.* 2:825–863, 1985.)

infection and lymphedema of the entrapped prepuce and glans cause progressive pain and swelling. Urethral obstruction can occur if swelling is marked. If vascular compromise is severe, the glans looks pale—a precursor to gangrene.

  **1. Management.** Reduction should be attempted immediately. Prior to reduction, the child should be sedated with codeine (1 mg/kg) or Demerol (1 mg/kg) by injection.

    **a.** Apply Xylocaine (lidocaine) jelly topically to the area.

    **b.** Remove the edema by applying gentle pressure on the glans with the index and middle fingers until the fluid has all been expressed.

    **c.** Place the thumbs on the glans and fingers on the prepuce. Push with the thumbs and pull with the fingers to move the foreskin over the glans (Fig. 17-1).

    **d.** Following reduction, treat with systemic antibiotics (trimethoprim-cotrimoxazole or amoxicillin—for doses see sec. **VI.C.2.d,** above). Refer the child to a urologist for interval circumcision.

    **e.** If reduction fails, consult a urologist because a dorsal slit is required.

**C. Acute balanitis.** Balanitis is an acute inflammation of the prepuce and glans penis. It may be caused by *Staphylococcus epidermidis,* hemolytic streptococcus, or enteric gram-negative bacilli. It occurs most commonly in the toddler, when preputial separation creates a relatively raw surface that is ideal for invasion of bacteria.

  **1. Diagnosis and assessment.** Most cases present

with dysuria and purulent discharge through the preputial opening. On examination there is marked swelling, redness, and edema of the prepuce, which is often not retractable. In severe cases, inflammation may extend onto the penile shaft.

2. **Management.** Obtain a swab of the prepuce for Gram's stain and culture, and treat the child with sitz baths and oral broad-spectrum antibiotics: ampicillin, amoxicillin, or trimethoprim-sulfamethoxazole (see sec. **VI.C.2.d,** above, for dosage). Resolution of swelling and pain can be expected within 24–48 hours. A history of repeated episodes of balanitis is a relative indication for circumcision.

**D. Hair tourniquet of penis.** In infants, penile edema may be the result of a loose hair that encircles the base of the penis, causing strangulation. There is usually a deep circular groove at the base, but the hair may be difficult to see. Use cool compresses to decrease swelling, then gently wash with warm water. If the hair does not come free, it must be carefully cut. Following removal, observe the child until the swelling has resolved.

**E. Disposition.** Most patients with phimosis, paraphimosis, and balanitis do not require emergency admission or surgery but can be managed as outpatients. Irreducible paraphimosis may require an emergency dorsal slit.

**F. Key points**
1. Paraphimosis can usually be reduced manually.
2. True phimosis must be differentiated from nonretractable foreskin, which is normal in boys under 4 years of age.

**VIII. Dysuria.** Painful voiding is a common presenting symptom in children in the emergency department. In all cases, consider the diagnosis of urinary tract infection or sexually transmitted disease.

**A. Diagnosis and assessment**
1. **History.** Ask about recent trauma and the onset, character, and location of the pain. Determine if there has been any hematuria and its timing in relation to voiding (see Chap. 23, Hematuria).
2. **Examination.** Examine the abdomen to determine if the bladder is distended and look at the genitalia and the urethral opening for evidence of trauma, irritation, or discharge.
3. **Investigation.** A urinalysis and urine culture are essential. Renal ultrasound examination and a catheter-voiding cystourethrogram should be obtained following urinary tract infections, usually 2–3 weeks after completion of antibiotic treatment (see Chap. 23, Urinary Tract Infection).

**B. Dysuria in boys.** In boys, painful voiding may be due to true phimosis, paraphimosis, or acute balanitis (see sec. **VII, A, B,** and **C** above). In addition, dysuria may be the result of any of the following:
1. **Meatal ulceration.** This type of ulceration is usually due to the child's diaper rubbing on the glans penis in patients with an ammoniacal diaper rash.

Treat with sitz baths, and, if the condition is purulent, 1% hydrocortisone ointment topically, tid.

2. **Lower urinary tract inflammatory disease**
   a. **Ascending bacterial urethral contamination.** Bacterial infections in infants and toddlers are more common in uncircumcised males (see Chap. 23, Urinary Tract Infection).
   b. **Acute viral hemorrhagic cystitis** is usually due to an adenovirus infection, which causes burning urination and terminal hematuria with urinary frequency (see Chap. 23, Hematuria).
   c. **Chemical cystitis** may be due to antineoplastic agents such as cyclophosphamide.

3. **Obstruction**
   a. **Anterior or posterior urethral valves** and other uncommon urethral obstructive anomalies can cause dysuria. If this is suspected, refer the child to a urologist.
   b. **Dysfunctional voiding.** This may be due to detrusor-sphincter dysnergia, in which high intravesical pressure is opposed by an unrelaxed external sphincter. The patient has episodic suprapubic pain and daytime urinary incontinence (damp pants syndrome). If this is suspected, refer the patient to a urologist.
   c. **Rare malignancies of the prostate and bladder** base (sarcomas) result in obstructive voiding.

4. **Trauma.** Zipper trauma results in frenular lacerations. Masturbation may also cause urethral irritation and dysuria.

5. **Sexually transmitted disease.** In the sexually active male perform Gram's stain and culture on a sample of urethral discharge for examination for gonorrhea and *Chlamydia* (see Table 21-5).

C. **Dysuria in girls.** In adolescent females, vulvovaginitis may be the cause of dysuria (see Chap. 18).
   1. **Chemical vulvovaginitis** can be caused by bubble baths, detergents used to wash underpants, disinfecting agents, or synthetic materials in the underwear. Treatment is by avoidance of offending agent(s). See Chap. 18, sec. **III.**
   2. **Ammoniacal vulvovaginitis (diaper rash).** This rash may be complicated by a monilial infection. Treatment is by air exposure or an emollient such as hydrophilic petrolatum. Treat suspected monilial infection with nystatin cream qid.
   3. **Labial adhesions** may occur in children with thin hypoplastic vulvar skin and may result in bacterial infection. Treat bacterial infection with cloxacillin, given PO 50 mg/kg/day divided q6h; cephalexin, 35–50 mg/kg/day divided q6h; or erythromycin, 40 mg/kg/day divided q6h. Do not attempt to force apart the labia. Topical application of Premarin cream twice daily will facilitate separation.
   4. **Sexual abuse** can result in dysuria secondary to labial tears, lacerations, bruising, or gonococcoal infec-

tion. See Chaps. 18 and 21 for assessment and management.

5. **Vaginal foreign bodies** can cause an intensely purulent and bloody vaginal discharge. See Chap. 18.

6. **Sexually transmitted disease.** In sexually active females urethritis is most often caused by *Chlamydia* infection and is associated with suprapubic tenderness, pyuria without hematuria, dysuria, urgency, and negative urine bacterial culture. Obtain a urinalysis and a urine culture. If there has been a discharge but none is available for culture, perform a urethral swab (insert the swab 2.5 cm into the urethra) for *Chlamydia* and *Gonococcus*. For treatment, see Table 21-5.

**D. Disposition.** In general, children with dysuria do not require admission to hospital.

**E. Key points**

1. Consider the diagnosis of sexually transmitted disease in children with dysuria.

2. Chemical vulvovaginitis is a common cause of dysuria in females.

**Bibliography**

Gonzalez, E. T., Jr., and Guerriero, W. G. Genitourinary Trauma in Children. In Kelalis, King, and Belman (eds.). *Clinical Pediatric Urology.* Vol. 2. Philadelphia: Saunders, 1985. Pp. 1125–1156.

Johnston, J. H. Acquired Lesions of the Penis, the Scrotum and the Testes. In D. I. Williams and J. H. Johnston (eds.). *Pediatric Urology* (2nd ed.). London: Butterworth, 1982. Pp. 467–475.

Klauber, G. T., and Sant Grannum, R. Disorders of the Male External Genitalia. In Kelalis, King, and Belman (eds.). *Clinical Pediatric Urology.* Vol. 2. Philadelphia: Saunders, 1985. Pp. 825–863.

McConnell, J. D., Wilkinson, M. D., and Peters, P. C. Rupture of the bladder. *Urol. Clin. North Am.* 9:293, 1982.

Morehouse, D. D. Emergency management of urethral trauma. *Urol. Clin. North Am.* 9:251, 1982.

Peters, P. C., and Bright, T. C., III. Blunt renal injuries. *Urol. Clin. North Am.* 4:17, 1977.

# 18

# Gynecology

Shirley A. Reimer and Karen Wardill

I. **Gynecologic examination.** The gynecologic examination performed in the emergency department is often the child's first—a gentle, empathetic approach is important. Describe the procedure and give warning when pain or discomfort is expected. Young girls usually prefer to have the mother present.

A. **Premenarchal female.** Always begin with a general examination. Look for adenopathy, pharyngitis, skin disease, and evidence of puberty (Tanner stage). Inspect the external genitalia, and identify the vaginal orifice by spreading the labia. In the young child, insertion of a lubricated feeding tube may help to locate the vagina; if this is unsuccessful, suspect imperforate hymen or vaginal agenesis. Premenarchal females rarely require a standard pelvic examination unless there is trauma with bleeding or suspicion of a foreign body; examination is then usually done under general anesthesia. There are several positions to consider for examination: (1) the supine lithotomy position on the mother (see sec. **I.A.1.a** below), (2) the knee-chest position (see sec. **I.A.1.b** below), (3) sitting in a semireclining position, (4) the left lateral position.

1. **Vaginal examination**

a. **Supine examination.** With the mother seated, place the infant on her lap in the "frog leg" position. In the older child, have the mother lie flat on the table, and lay the child supine on the mother's abdomen, using her legs as stirrups. **Labial adhesions** may be seen in the young child and are due to irritation or inflammation. Do not attempt to force apart the labia. Topical application of estrogen cream twice daily will facilitate separation.

b. **Knee-chest examination.** This position permits visualization of the vagina and cervix without using instruments. The child rests her head on one side on folded arms and supports her weight on bended knees positioned 6–8 inches apart. Encourage her to take deep breaths and let her "tummy sag"—have an assistant hold the buttocks laterally and upward to open the hymenal ring. When the vagina opens, perform the examination with magnification and a light source such as an otoscope without a speculum—see Fig. 18-1. When a more detailed examination is required, consult a gynecologist.

2. **Rectoabdominal examination.** Rectoabdominal examination is indicated when a foreign body or pelvic mass is suspected and is not visible on vaginal examination. With the patient lying on her back, the examiner's index or fifth finger is inserted into the

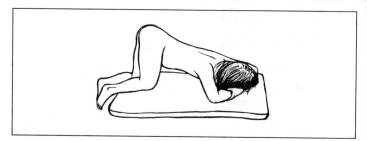

**Fig. 18-1. Gynecologic examination. Knee-chest position.**

rectum while the other hand is placed on the abdomen for bimanual palpation. The cervix can usually be palpated in the midline.

**B. Adolescent female.** If the patient desires it, the parents should be asked to leave the room. Females may perform the examination alone; a male should be accompanied by a female assistant. The patient should be undressed and gowned with the bladder emptied prior to examination. Examination may be carried out with the patient in the supine or semireclining position; the latter is often preferred because it facilitates eye-to-eye contact.

  **1. Inspection of genitalia.** In the frog-leg position, note the hygiene, Tanner stage, and clitoral size and inspect the pubic hair, labia, and introitus. For the normal diameter of the hymenal opening according to age, see Table 39-1.

  **2. Vaginoscopy.** Indications for a speculum examination in the emergency room include bleeding, pain, suspicion of sexually transmitted disease, trauma, sexual abuse, or failed knee-chest examination. The preferred instruments in the young or virginal patient are a 0-degree endoscope (female urethroscope, hysteroscope) or a Huffman pediatric speculum. If neither is available, a nasal speculum or otoscope may be used. For appropriate specula for hymenal size, see Table 18-1. Note the appearance of the cervix and vaginal mucosa and any discharge, bleeding, or lesions. Take cultures and smears as indicated by the history and examination.

  **3. Bimanual examination.** Bimanual examination is appropriate in the patient with a large hymenal opening and gynecologic complaints, abdominal pain, or a history of trauma or sexual abuse. Feel the cervix and determine if the os is open. Lateral movement of the cervix may cause pain in patients with pelvic inflammatory disease (PID) or ectopic pregnancy. Palpate the uterus and adnexae (including the ovaries) for size, tenderness, and masses. The uterus and ovaries are often impalpable in the infant or young child.

**Table 18-1. Speculum sizes**

| Type | Situation |
| --- | --- |
| Nasal speculum | Very small hymenal opening |
| Huffman ($\frac{1}{2}$ × $4\frac{1}{2}$ in.) | Small opening |
| Pederson (1 × $4\frac{1}{2}$ in.) | Sexually active adolescent |
| Graves ($\frac{5}{8}$ × 3 in.) | Sexually active adolescent |

Source: Grace, E. M. Prepubertal and Adolescent Gynecology. In J. W. Graef, and T. E. Cone (eds.), *Manual of Pediatric Therapeutics*. Boston: Little, Brown, 1985.

   **4. Rectal examination.** When a vaginal examination cannot be performed, usually because the parents have refused, an experienced clinician can often assess the situation with a rectal examination, confirming any suspicion of underlying disease with a pelvic ultrasound examination.
 **C. Investigations**
   **1. Papanicolaou smear.** This should be performed whenever a speculum examination is done on a sexually active female. Use a wooden spatula to scrape the squamocolumnar junction by rotating it 360 degrees around the external os. Smear and spread the specimen on a glass slide. Rotate a cotton swab or cytobrush 360 degrees in the endocervical canal, smear, and spread the specimen on a second slide. Label the slides, fix, dry, and send to the cytology laboratory.
   **2. Wet preparations.** These are useful for the microscopic diagnosis of vaginal discharge. In the prepubertal child, collect vaginal specimens with a saline-dipped Q-tip or an eye dropper. In the adolescent take the sample from the vaginal pool with a swab. Mix 1 drop of the specimen with 1 drop of warm saline, place on a slide with a cover slip, and view under a microscope for motile trichomonads. On another slide mix 1 drop of the specimen with 1 drop of 10% KOH, add the cover slip, and look for fungal mycelia. When indicated, perform a Gram's stain.
   **3. Cultures**
      **a. Gonorrhea.** Take samples with a Q-tip from the urethra, endocervix, rectum, and pharynx. Use Transgrow or Thayer-Martin culture medium.
      **b. Chlamydia.** Clean the endocervix with a swab, then take a second swab and rotate it for 20 seconds in the endocervix. Roll the swab on Microtrak or place in a Chlamydiazyme tube or culture medium and send it to the laboratory.
      **c. Yeast, *Trichomonas, Gardnerella*.** Take a swab from the vagina or vaginal pool and send it in the transport medium to the laboratory.
   **4. Human chorionic gonadotropin pregnancy test-**

**Table 18-2. HCG pregnancy tests**

| Test | Number of days after conception that test becomes positive |
| --- | --- |
| Serum radioimmunoassay | 9 |
| Serum radioreceptor assay | 9 |
| Urine hemagglutination inhibition | 28 |
| Urine latex fixation | 32 |

**ing.** Human chorionic gonadotropin (HCG) is secreted by the syncytiotrophoblast cells beginning 8 days after fertilization. Several types of HCG are available (Table 18-2). Urine pregnancy tests are less sensitive than blood HCG measurements. False-positive urine HCG results may occur in the presence of significant proteinuria and following use of drugs such as methadone, phenothiazines, and progestational agents.

  5. **Pelvic ultrasound.** Ultrasound examination is useful in cases of suspected PID with hydrosalpinx, pyosalpinx, or pelvic abscess. Ultrasound can also detect ovarian cysts, tumors, foreign bodies, pregnancy, and some congenital anomalies.

**D. Key points**
   1. A standard pelvic examination is rarely required in the prepubertal female.
   2. Pelvic ultrasound examination is invaluable in the diagnosis of gynecologic disorders in the young child.

**II. Abdominopelvic pain in the adolescent.** The differential diagnosis of lower abdominal pain in pubertal females includes gastrointestinal, genitourinary, and psychogenic disorders (Table 18-3). When pain is severe, rule out serious organic disease such as PID, ectopic pregnancy, appendicitis, and threatened abortion.

**A. Diagnosis and assessment**
   1. **History**
      a. **General history.** Take a thorough history, including a description of the pain, bowel function, urinary symptoms, and constitutional symptoms. A past history of bowel problems, abdominal surgery, or recurrent urinary tract infections may suggest the diagnosis.
      b. **Gynecologic history.** Enquire about the age of menarche, regularity of periods, dates of the last two menstrual periods, and contraceptive methods. Establish whether the patient is sexually active. The pattern of any abnormal bleeding or pain should also be sought. A history of pain with bleeding should prompt suspicion of ectopic pregnancy or abortion. Midcycle pain may be due to mittelschmerz, whereas dysmenorrhea classically begins at or just prior to the beginning of the

**Table 18-3. Causes of pelvic or lower abdominal pain in the adolescent female**

| Type | Example |
| --- | --- |
| Gastrointestinal | Irritable bowel<br>Lactose intolerance<br>Inflammatory bowel disease<br>Gastroenteritis<br>Appendicitis |
| Urinary tract | Pyelonephritis<br>Urinary tract infection |
| Gynecologic | Dysmenorrhea<br>Pregnancy (ectopic, abortion)<br>Pelvic inflammatory disease<br>Ovarian cyst |
| Psychogenic | Reaction anxiety<br>Secondary gain<br>Depression<br>Conversion hysteria<br>School phobia |

Source: Adapted from Barr, R. G. Abdominal pain in the adolescent female. *Pediatr. Rev.* 4:281, 1983.

period. Fever and vaginal discharge suggest PID. If PID is suspected, request that the parents leave the room and take a complete sexual history, including number of partners, type of intercourse (oral, anal, genital), previous history of sexually transmitted disease (STD), and any use of an intrauterine contraceptive device (IUD).

**2. Examination**

   **a. General examination.** Determine the vital signs. Palpate the inguinal regions for adenopathy or hernias. Examine the abdomen for tenderness (including costovertebral tenderness), peritonism, and masses. Perform a rectal examination in patients with acute severe pain to determine if tenderness, masses, or fluid are present in the cul-de-sac.

   **b. Gynecologic examination.** Perform a complete examination (see sec. **I** above). Rule out the presence of imperforate hymen in the virginal patient. Examine the cervix for discharge (PID), bleeding, and signs of pregnancy (see sec. **VI** below) and assess the size of the uterus. Adnexal masses or tenderness suggests PID, ectopic pregnancy, or ovarian cyst, whereas increased pain on cervical motion may be due to ectopic pregnancy or PID.

**3. Investigations.** Collect samples for Gram's stain, gonorrhea culture, *Chlamydia* Microtrak or culture, and Pap smear. Examine a midstream urine specimen to screen for urinary tract infection and pregnancy if indicated. If serious pathology is suspected, obtain blood for complete blood count (CBC), erythrocytic sedimentation rate (ESR), and culture. Order a stat serum beta HCG test and a type and crossmatch if ectopic pregnancy is suspected.

**B. Principles of management. In any sexually active female with pelvic or lower abdominal pain, the first priority is to rule out ectopic pregnancy and abortion.**

1. Carefully assess the patient for signs of sepsis or hypovolemia. If hypovolemic, give oxygen, start a large-bore intravenous line, and administer fluids (see Chap. 4).

2. Avoid vigorous pelvic examination when serious pathology such as ectopic pregnancy is suspected.

3. If there is any doubt about the diagnosis or management consult a gynecologist.

**C. Gynecologic causes of pain**

1. **Pelvic inflammatory disease.** Pelvic inflammatory disease should be suspected in the nonvirginal female with pelvic or lower abdominal pain. Fever, cervical discharge, and pain on cervical motion are commonly associated signs. There is often irregular vaginal bleeding, and there may be signs of peritonism. **Always consider the diagnosis of ectopic pregnancy.** See Chap. 21, Sexually Transmitted Diseases for specific diagnosis and management.

2. **Pregnancy.** Normal pregnancy may present with symptoms of vague abdominal or pelvic pain. Complicated pregnancy (ectopic, abortion) should be suspected when pain is accompanied by vaginal bleeding or shock; initial management of complicated pregnancy includes assessment and treatment of hypovolemia or sepsis and referral to a gynecologist (see sec. **VI**).

3. **Dysmenorrhea.** Dysmenorrhea is crampy lower abdominal pain with menses, beginning within 24 hours of the flow and lasting for up to 24 hours. In some patients, dysmenorrhea starts 2–4 days before the onset of menstrual flow. Associated symptoms include nausea and vomiting, diarrhea, lower backache, thigh pain, headache, fatigue, and dizziness.

   **a. Diagnosis.** In the virginal patient, examine the vulva to rule out imperforate hymen. When dysmenorrhea is severe, perform a bimanual examination to exclude PID and other gynecologic causes of pain.

   **b. Management.** Give analgesia: Nonsteroidal anti-inflammatory medications such as naproxen, 125 mg PO bid, flurbiprofen, 50 mg PO tid, or ibuprofen, 400 mg PO q6h are usually effective. Bed rest and local heat may also help. For nausea and vomiting prochlorperazine or promethazine may be prescribed. If these measures fail or if the pain is severe, refer the patient for outpatient gynecologic assessment, oral contraceptive therapy or laparoscopic examination as required.

4. **Mittelschmerz.** Mittelschmerz is ovulatory discomfort secondary to peritoneal irritation. Pain may be severe and occurs in one or both lower abdominal quadrants at midcycle, lasting minutes to several hours. Rarely, mittelschmerz may mimic serious disorders such as appendicitis, torsion of an ovarian cyst, or ectopic pregnancy. The diagnosis is suggested by the midcycle timing and an absence of identifiable pathology.

a. **Management.** Treatment is usually not required owing to the transient nature of the pain. Local heat and analgesia with nonsteroidal antiinflammatory agents may be helpful (see sec. **II.C.3,** above).

5. **Ovarian cysts**

a. **Diagnosis.** Cysts with secondary bleeding, torsion, or rupture may cause acute onset of severe lower abdominal pain. Signs of peritonism are usually present. A tender adnexal mass is often felt on bimanual palpation.

b. **Treatment.** Keep the patient NPO, start an IV, obtain blood for CBC and cross-match, and order an ultrasound examination. Consult a gynecologist for further evaluation, laparoscopy, and possible laparotomy.

D. **Disposition.** Admit all patients suspected of abortion, ectopic pregnancy, severe PID, or rupture, bleeding, or torsion of an ovarian cyst. Suspected cases of ectopic pregnancy or incomplete or septic abortion require immediate evaluation and stabilization.

E. **Key points**

1. In the sexually active female with abdominopelvic pain rule out abortion, ectopic pregnancy, and PID.

2. Dysmenorrhea can usually be treated with nonsteroidal antiinflammatory agents, local heat, and bed rest.

III. **Vaginitis. Apparent** vaginitis is usually due to physiologic leukorrhea. There is a white discharge without any associated symptoms. Most female newborn babies have a physiologic excess of vaginal fluid that may become blood-stained; it usually disappears within 7–10 days and requires no treatment. Similarly, in females approaching menarche, there may be an excess of vaginal fluid. Normal vaginal flora may include nonhemolytic streptococci, diphtheroids, and *Escherichia coli.*

**True** inflammation of the vagina may be nonspecific (polymicrobial and due to disturbed homeostasis) or due to a particular pathogen. In sexually active or sexually abused children, condylomas are common, as are gonococcal, *Chlamydia,* candidal, *Gardnerella,* and *Trichomonas* infections. Vaginal colonization with *Chlamydia* acquired at birth may persist up to 12–24 months of age.

A. **Diagnosis and assessment**

1. **History.** Vaginal discharge is the hallmark of vaginitis—note its color, odor, consistency, duration, and quantity. The presence of associated symptoms such

as pruritus, pain, bleeding, or dysuria should be sought. Pubertal girls often have dysuria in addition to discharge. Inquire about previous episodes of discharge, menstruation, recent medications, and the relationship of symptoms to sexual activity. Always consider the diagnosis of sexual abuse. Bacterial vaginosis due to *Gardnerella vaginalis* is the most common type of vaginitis in sexually active females. Suspect foreign body when there is blood or very foul purulent discharge in the young child.

2. **Examination.** Examine the abdomen for masses and tenderness, the inguinal areas for adenopathy, and the skin for signs of dermatitis or other disorder. Perform a careful vulvar and vaginal examination (see sec. **I**), noting erythema, vesicles, warts, or signs of trauma. A foreign body is often best felt on rectal examination, although retained toilet tissue paper is usually impalpable.

3. **Investigations.** Obtain specimens with saline-moistened swabs or an eye dropper (see sec. **I.C**). Perform a wet preparation, test the pH, and send a specimen to the laboratory for Gram's stain and culture for gonorrhea, other bacteria, *Chlamydia,* and *Candida.* Send a urine sample for urinalysis and culture.

B. **Management**

1. **Perineal hygiene.** Hygiene is an important aspect in the care of children with vaginitis. Educate the child or parent about general measures that may be causing or aggravating the vaginitis. Daily cleaning, wiping the perineum from front to back, and the wearing of white cotton underpants may help to resolve the problem. Advise against the use of tight underclothing, bubble baths, irritant soaps, or deodorants. Laundry detergents used to clean the underwear may also be aggravating. In general, the adolescent should be advised against douching. Tampons, especially deodorized tampons, should be avoided until the vaginitis has resolved.

2. **Prepubertal girls.** In prepubertal girls (Table 18-4), vulvovaginitis is usually due to poor hygiene (for management, see sec. **III.B.1** above). Suspect sexual abuse, especially when there is infection with a sexually transmitted agent. Most foreign bodies can be gently removed with a forceps or flushed with saline using a small catheter; general anesthesia may be required for the very young or uncooperative patient. Rarely, severe pruritus requires treatment with antihistamines (hydroxyzine, Benadryl). Consider the diagnosis of pinworm infestation if itching is severe and becomes worse at night. In general, do not treat simple vulvovaginitis with antimicrobials until the diagnosis is confirmed.

3. **Pubertal girls.** Perform a speculum examination in the sexually active female with vaginitis and either abdominal or pelvic pain or a purulent, foul, or

**Table 18-4. Etiology of vulvovaginitis in the prepubertal child**

| Type | Examples |
|------|----------|
| Nonspecific vulvovaginitis (most common) | Pinworms, foreign body, poor hygiene |
| Specific infections | Group A streptococcus, *Strep. pneumoniae, N. meningitides, Candida, Shigella, Staph. aureus, H. influenzae, N. gonorrhoeae,* condyloma accuminatum, *G. vaginalis,* herpes, *Chlamydia trachomatis* |
| Polyps, tumors | |
| Systemic illness | Measles, chickenpox, scarlet fever, Steven-Johnson syndrome, Crohn's disease |
| Vulvar skin disease | Seborrhea, psoriasis, dermatitis, scabies |
| Trauma | |
| Psychosomatic vaginal complaints | |
| Miscellaneous | Draining pelvic abscess, prolapsed urethra, ectopic ureter |

bloody discharge. Use local palliative measures such as oatmeal colloidal bath, medicated soaps, sitz baths in warm water, air drying, and regular hygiene until culture results are available.

IV. **Key points**

A. In the prepubertal girl, vaginal discharge is usually due to poor hygiene. Infection with a sexually transmitted organism implies sexual abuse.

B. Gardnerella is the most common cause of vaginitis in sexually active females.

V. **Dysfunctional uterine bleeding.** Dysfunctional uterine bleeding (DUB) is defined as a variety of bleeding manifestations of anovulatory cycles. It is a diagnosis of exclusion; serious pathology as listed in Table 18-6 must always be ruled out. When vaginal bleeding occurs in the premenarchal child, be alert to the possibility of foreign body, trauma, or tumor. Consult a gynecologist when in doubt.

A. **Diagnosis and assessment**

1. **History.** Take a full menstrual history, noting menarche, frequency and regularity of menses, length of flow, and number of pads or tampons used. Often gushes of blood and clots are passed. Determine the sexual and medication history and whether there has been trauma, endocrine disease, psychosocial stress, weight change, or chronic illness.

2. **Examination**

a. **General examination.** Examine the patient for

**Table 18-5. Vulvovaginitis**

| Etiology | Symptoms | Diagnosis | Management |
|---|---|---|---|
| Bacterial vaginosis or *Gardnerella vaginalis* (nonspecific vaginitis) | Fishlike odor, grey or clear discharge | pH 5 to 5.5; clue cells on wet mount. "Whiff test" add 10% KOH - emits fishy odor | Metronidazole[a], or ampicillin[b] PO for 1 week |
| *Trichomonas vaginalis* | Frothy, purulent, foul-smelling discharge; occurs with or just after menses | Motile flagellates and PMNs on wet mount; pH 6 to 7 | Metronidazole for both partners PO, 2 gm once in adolescent |
| *Candida albicans* | Pruritus; white, cheesy, thick discharge and inflammation | Budding filaments on 10% KOH prep, pH 4–5; Nickerson's medium | Nystatin or imidazoles or gentian violet 1% topical |
| *Candida glabrata* | Burning, thick white, cheesy discharge and inflammation | pH 4 to 5. Spores only on KOH preparation | Imidazoles, gentian violet topically for 1 application |
| *Chlamydia trachomatis* | Mucopurulent cervicitis, urethral syndrome, PID; may be asymptomatic | Swab cervix and take culture or monoclonal preparation (Microtrak) or ELISA assay (Chlamydiazyme); Leave swab in cervical canal 20–30 seconds | See Chap. 21, Sexually Transmitted Disease |
| *Neisseria gonorrhoeae* | Purulent discharge or asymptomatic | Positive culture, Gram's stain | See Chap. 21, STD |

| | | | |
|---|---|---|---|
| Herpes simplex | Pain and burning dysuria, erythema, dysuria | Tzanck smear to detect giant cells; immunofluorescence; culture | First episode, use acyclovir; See Chap. 21, STD |
| Condyloma accuminata (human papilloma virus) | Warts, itching. Often with other STD | Obvious lesions on perineum, anus, vagina, or cervix | Podophyllin 10% to 20% topically or trichloroacetic acid. Refer to gynecologist |
| Leukorrhea (estrogen effect) | Creamy grey-white nonpruritic discharge | Epithelial cells on microscopy | Perineal hygiene |
| Foreign body | Very foul smelling; occasionally bloody discharge | Pelvic or rectal examination | Visualize and remove with forceps or flush. May need general anesthesia |
| Nonspecific vulvitis and intertrigo | Local pain, erythema | By exclusion—tight clothing, obesity, poor hygiene | Steroid cream, hygiene, or antifungal agents |
| Syphilis (Treponema pallidum) | Chancre, adenopathy, secondary skin lesions, condylomata lata, mucous patches, systemic symptoms | VDRL, FTA-ABS tests; dark-field microscopy | See Chap. 21, Sexually Transmitted Disease |

[a] Metronidazole dose in adolescent and older child 500 mg q6h
[b] Ampicillin dose in adolescent and older child, 500 mg q6h

**Table 18-6. Causes of irregular vaginal bleeding**

| Type | Examples |
|---|---|
| Pregnancy | |
|   Normal | |
|   Complicated | Abortion |
| Vulval/vagina | |
|   Inflammation | Vulvovaginitis |
|   Foreign body | Retained toilet tissue |
|   Tumors | Consider diethylstilbestrol exposure |
|   Trauma | Rape, coitus |
|   Physiologic | Newborn 5–10 days |
| Cervix | |
|   Erosion | |
|   Tumor | Polyps, carcinoma |
| Uterus | |
|   Inflammation | Endometritis, IUD use |
|   Hormonal medication | Birth control pill |
| Uterine tubes | |
|   Inflammation | Salpingitis |
|   Ectopic pregnancy | |
| Extragenital causes | |
|   Endocrine | Thyroid, adrenal, medication |
|   Anovulation | Stress, weight change, exercise |
|   Blood dyscrasias | Thrombocytopenia, bleeding diathesis |

signs of anemia or hypovolemia, including pallor and orthostatic changes in vital signs (see Chap. 23, Fluids and Electrolytes, sec. **II**). Look for ecchymoses, petechiae, or bleeding from gums as evidence of blood dyscrasia. Examine the breasts for signs of pregnancy and the abdomen for masses, enlarged uterus, or tenderness (PID).

**b. Pelvic examination.** Inspect the vulva for bleeding sources or signs of trauma. Insert a speculum and look for local lesions and evidence of injury, pregnancy, or infection. Perform a bimanual examination in the older child (see sec. **I**).

**c. Investigations.** Take vaginal and cervical swabs when indicated by the history or examination. Draw blood for CBC, platelet count, serum HCG, prothrombin time (PT), and partial thromboplastin time (PTT). An ultrasound examination may be necessary.

**B. Management.** Menstruation in the young adolescent is frequently anovulatory and irregular; reassurance is all that is required in such cases. For management of systemic disorders that lead to vaginal bleeding, see sec. **VII** below and Chap. 19.

1. **Patient is stable without anemia or hypovolemia.** In these patients the hemoglobin and hematocrit are normal, and there is usually a history of prolonged menstrual flow, persistent spotting, or frequent menses. Treat with Provera 10 mg PO daily for 10 days (day 18–28) every month for 3 consecutive cycles, *and* ferrous gluconate, 300 mg/day PO.

2. **Patient has persistent bleeding or heavy flow with anemia**

   a. **Hypovolemia.** If there is a very low hematocrit (< 28%), postural changes in vital signs (see Chap. 23, Fluids and Electrolytes, sec. **II**), or other evidence of hypovolemia, give oxygen, start a large-bore intravenous line, draw blood for cross-match, and urgently consult a gynecologist. Ectopic pregnancy and abortion must be ruled out.

   b. **Normovolemia.** Numerous regimes using hormonal medication may be used. The following is one management option:

      (1) Start treatment with Ortho-Novum, 1/50 21s, 1 PO q16h for 5–7 days, then bid for the next 5–7 days. The patient should then be cycled with low-dose oral contraceptives for 3 months. Arrange for follow-up in 24–36 hours.

      (2) Consult a gynecologist; intervention may be necessary if the flow does not stop in 24–36 hours.

**C. Disposition.** Admit all patients with signs of hypovolemia or persistent heavy flow.

**D. Key points**

1. Vaginal bleeding in the prepubertal child may be due to foreign body, trauma, or tumor.

2. Rule out ectopic pregnancy or abortion when vaginal bleeding occurs in a nonvirginal patient.

## VI. Trauma

**A. Vulvar and vaginal hematoma.** These injuries are usually secondary to blunt trauma or laceration. There is often intense pain, which is referred to the ipsilateral leg and abdomen. Perform a careful examination to try to delineate the lesion, and beware of signs of severe occult hemorrhage. Ascertain if the patient is able to void.

1. **Management**

   a. **Vulvar hematomas.** Hematomas are usually treated conservatively with a tight pressure dressing. Ice, analgesia, and stool softeners may also be helpful. If the hematoma is increasing in size, incision and drainage, ligation of the bleeding point, and packing may be required. The pack is removed in 24 hours. Start broad-spectrum antibiotics (ampicillin) if the lesion is drained. Urethral or suprapubic catheterization may be required if urinary retention occurs secondary to pain or pressure from the hematoma. X ray of the pelvis may be necessary to rule out a fracture.

Give a tetanus booster immunization to those at risk.

b. **Vaginal hematomas.** Small lateral wall hematomas often stop bleeding without intervention. Larger hematomas require evacuation and ligation of bleeding vessels. See sec. **VI.A.1.a** above for management. If a vessel is torn above the pelvic floor, a retroperitoneal hematoma may form, and laparotomy is required. In all cases consult a gynecologist for assessment and examination under anesthesia to exclude deep pelvic, genitourinary, and rectal injury. Give a tetanus booster immunization to those at risk (see Appendix).

B. **Perineal and vulvar lacerations.** These injuries are usually caused by a fall on a sharp stick, bicycle handle, or toy. The most common area of injury is the outer labium majorum. Blood loss is usually minor but may be heavy when injury is deep or if the corpora cavernosum beneath the labium majorum are involved. The patient may present with a lacerated hymen and little bleeding or pain; a detailed intravaginal examination is mandatory to rule out upper vaginal or deep pelvic injury. In all cases, rule out laceration of the vagina or rectum.

   1. **Management.** Control bleeding with a pressure dressing, Gelfoam, or Oxycel and consult a gynecologist immediately. General anesthesia may be required to repair the wound and rule out penetration causing deep pelvic or abdominal injury. An ultrasound study should be ordered if deep injury is suspected. Give a tetanus booster immunization to those at risk (see Appendix).

C. **Vaginal lacerations.** Vaginal lacerations are usually associated with vulvar injury and involve the lateral vaginal walls. Blood loss and pain are usually minimal. If the laceration extends to the vaginal vault, exploration of the pelvic cavity is necessary to rule out deep pelvic injury.

   1. **Management.** Bladder and bowel integrity must be confirmed by catheterization and rectal examination. The extent of the laceration and the presence or absence of deep pelvic injury must be determined. Consult a gynecologist for intravaginal examination and repair under anesthesia. Tetanus booster immunization should be given to those at risk (see Appendix).

D. **Disposition.** Patients with large vulvar or vaginal hematomas can often be managed with local measures but may require treatment with incision and drainage. Patients with suspected retroperitoneal hematomas or lacerations of the perineum, vulva, or vagina require examination and repair under anesthesia.

E. **Key points**

   1. Vulvar and vaginal hematomas are usually treated conservatively but may require exploration to rule out deep pelvic injury.

   2. If there is any evidence that an object has entered

the vagina, (including a hymenal tear), perform an intravaginal examination to rule out deep pelvic injury.

VII. **Pregnancy.** More than 1 million adolescents become pregnant each year in the United States. Consider the diagnosis of pregnancy in all pubertal females seen in the emergency department.

A. **Diagnosis and assessment**

1. **History.** Conduct the interview privately. Take a full sexual history, noting the type of contraception used, if any. Ask about the last menstrual period (timing and normalcy) and weight gain. Inquire about symptoms such as fatigue, nausea and vomiting, urinary frequency, and enlargement, tenderness, or tingling of the breasts.

2. **Examination.** Perform a full examination. Breast examination during pregnancy reveals enlargement, deep pigmentation of the nipples, and protrusion of Montgomery follicles in the areolae. Cutaneous signs of pregnancy include striae gravidarum, linea nigra, and vascular spiders. If the uterus is palpable, measure the symphysis-to-fundal height. Amplified (Doppler) auscultation of the fetal heart sounds may be heard at 10–12 weeks. Unamplified heart sounds are heard at 20 weeks. Perform a full pelvic examination. Determine the uterine size and note if there is softening of the cervix on palpation (Hegar's sign—seen at 6 weeks), violet discoloration of the vagina (Chadwick's sign—seen at 8 weeks), or cervical dilatation.

3. **Determination of gestational age.** There are a number of methods of determining gestational age. The most reliable is a calculation based on the last menstrual period when it is known with certainty. Other methods include the HCG pregnancy test (see sec. **I.C.4**), ultrasound examination, and uterine examination. The uterus is the size of an orange at 8 weeks, grapefruit size at the symphysis pubis at 12 weeks, midway between the umbilicus and symphysis pubis at 16 weeks, and is usually palpable at the umbilicus at 20 weeks.

B. **Complicated pregnancy.** First-trimester bleeding may be caused by cervical lesions, spontaneous abortion, ectopic pregnancy, or trophoblastic disease. It occurs in 25% of all pregnant patients.

1. **Spontaneous abortion.** Abortion is the termination of pregnancy before the fetus is viable. Most cases occur between 2 and 4 weeks postimplantation. The diagnosis should be considered in any adolescent female with pain and vaginal bleeding.

a. **Diagnosis**

(1) **History.** Determine the sexual history, menstrual history, use of contraception, and the date contraception was discontinued. Ask the patient about any symptoms of pregnancy (see sec. **VII.A.** above). The presence

of abdominal pain, passage of clots or tissue, and quantity and pattern of bleeding should also be determined (see sec. **V** above).

(2) **Examination.** Look for signs of hypovolemia or shock (see Chap. 4). Perform an abdominal and pelvic evaluation—determine uterine size and tenderness, whether the cervical os is open or closed, and if tissue is visible in the os or vagina. If the os is open, a ring forceps will be admitted beyond the internal os without resistance.

b. **Initial management.** Initial management involves assessment and treatment of hypovolemia and sepsis. Obtain blood for cross-match and Rh status in all cases. When possible, order a serum HCG measurement and pelvic ultrasound study. Specific management depends on the type of abortion and the hemodynamic status of the patient; always refer the patient to a gynecologist. Rh-negative women with an aborted fetus and Rh incompatibility should receive $Rh_o$(D antigen) immune globulin.

c. **Type of abortion**

(1) **Threatened abortion.** In threatened abortion vaginal bleeding occurs after a period of amenorrhea. The internal os is closed, and uterine size is appropriate for dates. There may be uterine cramping, but the bleeding is often painless.

(a) **Management.** Perform a speculum examination to exclude extraplacental causes of bleeding. The management of threatened abortion includes bed rest and avoidance of coitus. Advise the patient to return if bleeding is heavy or prolonged or if tissue is passed.

(2) **Inevitable abortion.** In inevitable abortion the internal os is open, and there is usually heavy bleeding and uterine cramping. Tissue may be visible in the cervical os but has not been passed. There may be progression to complete or incomplete abortion.

(a) **Management**

(i) Admit the patient to hospital, start an intravenous line, and order a CBC and cross-match.

(ii) Tissue caught in the cervical os may result in shock—gently remove it with a ring forceps.

(iii) Place 20 units of oxytocin in 1000 ml of 5% dextrose in water and infuse this solution over 1–2 hours. Ergonovine IM or oxytocin IV may be required if bleeding is severe.

(3) **Complete abortion.** In complete abortion the total gestational sac and placenta are ex-

pelled in the first trimester and may not be noticed by the patient. The diagnosis must be made by ultrasound examination. Many gynecologists are now deferring dilatation and curettage (D and C) in early cases.

**(4) Incomplete abortion.** When abortion is incomplete, vaginal bleeding occurs and may be profuse. The patient complains of cramping lower abdominal pain, and fragments of tissue are passed. On examination the internal os is open, and products of conception may be visible within. Order an ultrasound examination to determine whether products remain in the uterus. Management is the same as that described for inevitable abortion (sec. **VII.B.1.c.(2)** above).

**(5) Septic abortion.** Usually there is a history of interference in cases of septic abortion. Patients present with vaginal bleeding, abdominal pain, and signs of local sepsis (metritis, parametritis) or generalized sepsis (peritonitis, fever). Other causes of an acute abdominal condition and sepsis must be excluded.

    **(a) Management**

        **(i)** Place two large-bore intravenous lines and resuscitate the patient with IV fluid (see Chap. 4). Give tetanus booster immunization to those at risk (see Appendix).

        **(ii)** In the critically ill patient start treatment with triple antibiotics: penicillin, 12–18 M units/day IV divided q6h *and* gentamicin or tobramycin, 1.5–1.7 mg/kg/dose IV q8h *and* clindamycin, 600 mg IV q6h.

        **(iii)** Obtain an urgent CBC, cross-match, cervicovaginal cultures, and blood culture prior to giving antibiotics.

        **(iv)** Immediately consult a gynecologist for examination and evacuation of the uterine contents.

**(6) Missed abortion.** This occurs when there is intrauterine retention of dead products of conception. It often occurs in patients who have had prior symptoms of threatened or incomplete abortion. The uterus is small for dates, and the os is usually closed. The diagnosis is confirmed by ultrasound examination. A missed abortion must be differentiated from a tumor or an incorrectly dated pregnancy.

    **(a) Management.** Obtain a CBC, blood type and antibody screen and Rh determination. Consult a gynecologist for treatment. Specific treatment depends on gestational age:

    **(i)** If the abortus is less than 12 weeks old, a D and C is usually required.

    **(ii)** If it is over 12 weeks, an oxytocin drip may be administered. The patient should be monitored for hypofibrinogenemia and disseminated intravascular coagulation (DIC), which can develop up to a month or more after fetal death.

**2. Ectopic pregnancy.** Ectopic pregnancy occurs when the fertilized ovum implants in a location other than the lining of the uterus. The most common site is the fallopian tube. The incidence is increased in females with a history of salpingitis, appendicitis, endometriosis, tubal surgery, or IUD use.

  **a. Diagnosis.** There is a wide spectrum of clinical presentation, from mild pain and discomfort to hemorrhage and shock. Pain may occur in the lower abdomen or upper abdomen, or it may be generalized. Symptoms of pregnancy may or may not be present. In the classic case of **ruptured** ectopic tubal pregnancy, normal menses are replaced by slight vaginal bleeding and sudden onset of severe, sharp, lower abdominal pain. Abdominal examination reveals peritonism. On pelvic examination there is pain on motion of the cervix (cervical excitation), and the posterior fornix may bulge with blood in the cul-de-sac. An adnexal mass may be present. Fifty percent of patients have diaphragmatic irritation with shoulder tip pain. A high index of suspicion combined with timely use of procedures and laboratory investigations is vital to successful management. Complications include infertility, DIC, and death due to shock.

  **b. Management**

    **(1)** When ectopic pregnancy is suspected, immediately consult with a gynecologist and arrange for possible culdocentesis or laparotomy.

    **(2)** Keep the patient NPO, start two large-bore intravenous lines, and obtain blood for beta HCG, CBC, and cross-match. Up to 50% of patients with ectopic pregnancies have a negative pregnancy test result.

    **(3)** If the patient is stable, perform a **gentle** pelvic examination and obtain a pelvic ultrasound study; have a physician in attendance at all times and frequently monitor vital signs and hematocrit.

**3. Pregnancy prevention.** Offer the "morning after pill" to adolescent females at risk for pregnancy who deny consensual intercourse since their last normal period.

  a. Give an oral contraceptive such as Ovral, two tablets PO immediately, followed by two tablets in 12 hours. Treatment must be started as soon as possible, never more than 72 hours after coitus.

  b. Nausea is a common side effect, and dimenhydrate may be prescribed concurrently.

  c. Because of the association with fetal anomalies, the patient must be warned of the risks if pregnancy results. Advise her that withdrawal bleeding is likely to occur within a week and that she is not protected against pregnancy **after** taking the medication.

  d. Arrange for a follow-up pregnancy test and contraceptive counseling advice with a family doctor or family planning clinic.

**C. Disposition.** Admit patients with incomplete, inevitable, or septic abortion and patients with ectopic pregnancy for emergency surgery. The pregnant teenager who is well should be seen for follow-up with her partner by an adolescent gynecologist, family planning counselor, or other appropriate specialist.

**D. Key points**

  1. Suspect ectopic pregnancy in all females who present with symptoms of pregnancy, vaginal bleeding, and lower abdominal pain.

  2. A negative pregnancy test does not rule out ectopic pregnancy.

  3. Do not carry out a vigorous pelvic examination in cases of suspected ectopic pregnancy. Order a serum beta HCG test, cross-matching, and ultrasound examination, and consult a gynecologist immediately.

  4. In cases of suspected abortion, order a pelvic ultrasound examination and serum beta HCG and determine if the cervical os is open and whether tissue has been passed.

  5. Placental tissue that is seen in the cervical os should be gently removed or shock may result.

  6. In the treatment of patients with septic abortion, early fluid resuscitation and antibiotic therapy are vital.

**Bibliography**

Barr, R. G. Abdominal pain in the adolescent female. *Pediatr. Rev.* 4(9):281–289, 1983.

Emans, S. J. H., and Goldstein, D. P. *Pediatric and Adolescent Gynecology.* Boston: Little, Brown, 1982.

Huffman, J. W., Dewhurst, C. J., and Capraro, V. J. *The Gynecology of Childhood and Adolescence.* Philadelphia: Saunders, 1981.

Reese, R. E., and Douglas, R. G. D. *A Practical Approach to Infectious Diseases* (2nd ed.). Boston: Little, Brown, 1983.

Speroff, L., Glass, R. H., and Kase, N. G. (eds.). *Clinical Gynecologic Endocrinology and Infertility.* Baltimore: Williams & Wilkins, 1983.

Sweet, R. Importance of differential diagnosis in acute vaginitis. *Am. J. Obstet. Gynecol.* 152:247, 1985.

# Hematology and Oncology

Paul C. Rogers

**I. Anemia.** Anemia is caused by decreased production or decreased survival of red blood cells. Normal hematologic values, and therefore the definition of anemia, vary with age (see Appendix IV). Iron deficiency due to faulty nutrition is the most common cause. In most cases, clinical evaluation and a few simple laboratory tests can differentiate benign causes of anemia from serious disease.

**A. Diagnosis and assessment** (Table 19-1).

**1. History.** Determine the onset, duration, and past history of anemia, including any previous transfusions (Table 19-1). In general, children who appear well and are asymptomatic or have only mild symptoms such as lethargy and fatigue probably have **chronic onset anemia.** Children with **acute onset anemia** are more likely to have dramatic symptoms such as postural dizziness or exertional dyspnea.

**2. Examination.** Pallor is often visible. Examine the vital signs and look for orthostatic changes as evidence of hypovolemia due to acute blood loss. Tachycardia, gallop rhythm, and hepatomegaly are evidence of high-output heart failure. Petechiae, purpura, or mucosal bleeding suggests coincidental thrombocytopenia due to marrow failure, infiltration, or coagulopathy. The child with jaundice probably has hemolytic anemia, whereas the finding of hepatosplenomegaly or lymphadenopathy should arouse suspicion of malignancy.

**3. Investigation**

**a.** In the **unstable child,** obtain blood for urgent cross-match and investigations as listed in sec. **I.A.3.b.** and **c.** below.

**b.** In the **stable child** without evidence of abnormal bleeding, obtain a complete blood count (CBC) with red blood cell (RBC) indices, a white blood cell (WBC) and differential count, platelet count, reticulocyte count, and peripheral smear.

**c.** If the child is **jaundiced,** include a direct antibody test (Coombs') with the initial investigations. Observe the color of the urine and test it for blood, hemoglobin, bilirubin, and urobilinogen.

**d.** Other investigations that may be ordered include coagulation studies in cases of abnormal bleeding and bone marrow aspiration when marrow infiltration or replacement is suspected.

**4. Interpretation of investigations** (Fig. 19-1)

**a.** The CBC will indicate whether there is a pure anemia or a decrease in other cell lines due to aplastic anemia or marrow infiltration (lymphoma, leukemia, neuroblastoma).

**b.** Anemia with a **raised reticulocyte count** may

**Table 19-1. Clinical clues to the diagnosis of anemia**

| Cause of anemia | Diagnostic clues |
| --- | --- |
| Acute blood loss | Hypovolemia, shock |
| Chronic blood loss | Diarrhea, vomiting, epistaxis, hematuria or heavy or frequent menstrual periods |
| Infiltrative malignancy (neuroblastoma/leukemia) | Bone pain, abdominal pain, purpura, weight loss |
| Acute hemolysis | Acute onset, bright orange urine, jaundice |
| Congenital red cell abnormalities (Sickle cell, G6PD, thalassemia) | Neonatal jaundice, family history of jaundice, anemia, cholecystectomy or splenectomy |
| Dietary/nutritional (iron deficiency) | Otherwise healthy toddler, high intake of milk |
| Marrow failure | Medications (chloramphenicol, chemotherapy), recent infection, chronic inflammatory disorder (JRA, IBD) |

Key: JRA = juvenile rheumatoid arthritis, IBD = inflammatory bowel disease

be due to hemolysis or blood loss. **If the reticulocyte count is decreased,** the cause may be marrow failure or replacement.

   c. In most cases, detailed investigation of chronic anemia should be performed on an outpatient basis. The most common cause of microcytic, hypochromic anemia is iron deficiency.
**B. Principles in management of anemia**
   **1. General.** Admit all children with acute onset anemia who are symptomatic or when there is suspicion of severe disease such as marrow infiltration or aplasia. For management of iron deficiency, see sec. **I.B.3** below. Stable children in whom a cause other than iron deficiency is suspected should be seen for follow-up within 48 hours; further investigations can be arranged at that time.
   **2. Transfusion**
      **a.** Order transfusion for children with blood loss or marrow failure who have symptomatic hypovolemia.
      **b.** In the child with high-output heart failure, give blood transfusion slowly with 5–10 ml/kg of packed red blood cells at 2 ml/kg/hour, and give furosemide (Lasix), 1 mg/kg intravenously at the midpoint of transfusion.
      **c.** Transfusion should be delayed in clinically stable

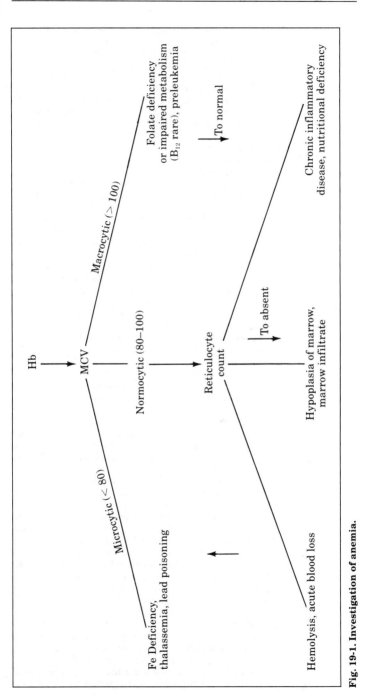

**Fig. 19-1. Investigation of anemia.**

children with hemolytic anemia until the diagnosis is established. Early liaison with the blood bank is essential. In antibody-mediated hemolysis, utilize blood that is as antigenically equivalent to the patient's own blood as possible.

3. **Iron deficiency anemia.** If iron deficiency is suspected, treat the child empirically with ferrous sulfate, 6 mg/kg/day of elemental iron PO divided tid. Arrange for a follow-up CBC and reticulocyte count in 1 week, at which time there should be a high reticulocyte count.

C. **Hemolytic anemia**

1. **Specific disorders**

a. **Hemolytic uremic syndrome (HUS).** HUS occurs predominantly in young children with a history of gastroenteritis—often with bloody diarrhea—and decreased urine output followed by pallor, petechiae, and purpura. The blood smear reveals a microangiopathic hemolytic anemia with distorted red blood cells. In addition, there is evidence of renal failure (BUN and creatinine are increased) and thrombocytopenia. Consult a nephrologist for management of renal failure (see Chap. 23). In general, these children should not be transfused unless the hemoglobin falls to less than 70 gm/liter (7.0 gm/dl).

b. **Thrombotic thrombocytopenic purpura (TTP).** The presentation of TTP is similar to that of HUS, but it usually occurs in older children. Manifestations include fever, purpura, neurologic signs, and renal failure. The peripheral smear is identical to that of HUS. Consult a nephrologist when this diagnosis is suspected.

c. **Toxic causes** (nonimmune). Toxic causes include drugs, venoms (snakes, spiders), and infections such as malaria. The peripheral smear often shows changes typical of intravascular hemolysis and occasionally spherocytes.

d. **Autoimmune hemolytic anemia** (direct Coombs' positive). Direct Coombs'-positive hemolysis with warm (IgG, complement) antibody may be seen following viral illness, medication use (antibiotics, antimalarials), or autoimmune disorders (systemic lupus erythematosus [SLE]). Hemolysis can progress rapidly and may result in heart failure. The etiology makes cross-match difficult; consult with the blood bank and try to use blood that is as antigenically equivalent to the patient's blood as possible. Treat with prednisone, 2.0 mg/kg/day PO divided q12h, and consult a hematologist.

D. **Sickle cell anemia.** Sickle cell anemia is an autosomal recessive disorder of hemoglobin synthesis that is seen commonly in black children. Heterozygotes (sickle trait) are usually asymptomatic. Homozygotes (SS) produce sickle hemoglobin and develop clinical complications of sickle cell disease. Diagnosis is suggested by the sickle shape of the red cells seen on peripheral smear and sickle screen test, and is confirmed by hemoglobin electrophoresis.

1. **Complications of sickle cell disease (SS).** Children with sickle cell disease are prone to crises that may be precipitated by hypoxia, acidosis, dehydration, or infection. The normal range for hemoglobin in these children tends to be 55–95 gm/liter (5.5–9.5 gm/dl).

   a. **Anemic crises**

      (1) Splenic sequestration. This is a potentially fatal complication, common between 6 months and 6 years of age, before autoinfarction of the spleen occurs. Due to pooling of a large volume of blood in the spleen, hypovolemia occurs, often with shock and massive splenomegaly.

      (2) Aplastic crisis. Aplastic crises frequently follow a viral (often parvovirus) infection that results in impaired production of red cells. Due to ongoing hemolysis and decreased red cell production, patients become severely anemic. On laboratory examination, the normally high reticulocyte count is very low.

      (3) Megaloblastic crisis. In sickle cell disease folate utilization is increased owing to a high cell turnover. Folate deficiency may result in pancytopenia with hypersegmentation of the neutrophils and megaloblastic changes in red cells.

      (4) Hyperhemolysis. Hyperhemolysis occurs in the child who also has glucose 6-phosphate dehydrogenase (G6PD) deficiency; there is rapid destruction of red blood cells precipitated by viral illness or oxidant ingestion (see sec. **I.E** below).

   b. **Vasoocclusive crisis.** This is the most common type of crisis in the child with sickle cell disease. Decreased deformability of the red cells results in occlusion of the microvasculature, causing tissue infarction. The child presents with pain: frequently bone (often the femoral or humeral head), abdominal, or chest pain. Severe crises can lead to aseptic necrosis of bone. Dactylitis, with swollen and sore hands and feet (hand-foot syndrome), is often seen in toddlers. Autosplenectomy is universal by age 6 years. Other severe complications include pulmonary infarction, retinopathy, and cerebrovascular accident with hemiplegia.

   c. **Other complications**

      (1) Infection. Children with sickle cell disease have an increased risk of pneumococcal, meningococcal, *Hemophilus influenzae type b,* staphylococcal, and *Salmonella* infections. These infections may manifest as sepsis, meningitis, pneumonia, or osteomyelitis.

**(2)** Cholelithiasis. Cholelithiasis causes right upper quadrant pain and jaundice. The incidence of cholelithiasis increases with age.

**(3)** Genitourinary system problems. Papillary necrosis causes renal colic and hematuria. An acquired tubular absorption defect may result in an inability to concentrate urine, with polyuria, enuresis, and nocturia. Obstruction of the corpus cavernosum can result in priapism.

**(4)** Hepatic sequestration.

**2. Management**

**a. Resuscitation.** Resuscitation may be needed in children with splenic sequestration, stroke, pulmonary infarction, or sepsis. Assess and control airway, breathing, and circulation and give oxygen by mask. Start an intravenous line and draw blood for CBC, differential and reticulocyte counts, platelet count, cross-match, culture, and measurement of blood gases, glucose, and electrolytes.

**b. Transfusion.** Transfusion is indicated in patients with extensive pulmonary infarction, cerebrovascular accident, sequestration or severe anemia (hemoglobin < 40 gm/liter or 4.0 gm/dl) from aplastic crisis or hyperhemolysis. Give packed red blood cells (saline-washed if possible), 5 ml/kg at a rate no faster than 2 ml/kg/hour. When rapid transfusion is necessary in the child with high-output heart failure, stroke, or severe pulmonary involvement, consider partial exchange transfusion through a peripheral vein with 50–100 ml aliquots of equal parts of the patient's blood exchanged for whole blood. Monitor closely for signs of fluid overload.

**c. Infection**

**(1)** Fever. Suspect and treat bacterial infection in any child who is toxic or who has no focus of infection with an oral temperature of ≥38.0°C if under 2 years of age or ≥38.5°C if over 2 years. Obtain blood and other appropriate cultures and start treatment with intravenous cefuroxime, 150 mg/kg/day divided q8h. When there is concurrent diarrhea, consider treatment with cefotaxime as an alternative.

**(2)** Mild fever. In the child over 2 years of age with a temperature of less than 38.5°C and no signs of toxicity or sepsis, obtain a urinalysis and blood for culture and a CBC. If the child is under the age of 12 years, treat with amoxicillin, 50 mg/kg/day PO divided q8h; if over 12, treat with phenoxymethyl penicillin, 50 mg/kg/day PO divided q6h.

**(3)** Pneumonia. Order a chest x ray if there are symptoms of chest infection such as tachypnea, cough, or wheeze. If there are infiltrates on the x ray, obtain blood for CBC and culture and treat with chloramphenicol, 75 mg/kg/day IV divided q6h, and ampicillin, 100 mg/kg/day IV divided q6h.

(4) Bone and joint infection. If there is suspicion of septic arthritis or osteomyelitis, consult an orthopedic surgeon (see Chap. 24, Osteomyelitis).

(5) Meningitis. Consider a lumbar puncture (LP) in infants and young children under 18 months of age with high fever. Older children do not require an LP unless there are signs of meningismus (see Chap. 21, Bacterial Meningitis).

d. **Vasoocclusive crises**

(1) Adequate hydration is essential. Due to an inability to concentrate urine, sickle cell patients require 1–1.5 times maintenance fluid requirements, given IV or PO. Administer oxygen and monitor closely for fluid overload, especially in the severely anemic patient. If the child is acidotic, give bicarbonate, 0.5 mEq/kg IV and repeat prn.

(2) Treat with bed rest and acetaminophen, 10 mg/kg PO, and codeine, 0.5–1 mg/kg PO q4h for analgesia. Morphine may be required in severe cases. X rays should be performed in children with limp to look for aseptic necrosis.

e. **Splenic sequestration crises.** Aggressive fluid resuscitation is required in these children, usually with packed red cells (see Chap. 4).

f. **Megaloblastic crises.** Treat with folic acid, 1 mg/day.

g. **Aplastic crises.** These are usually self-limited. Transfuse if anemia is severe or if there is high-output cardiac failure.

h. **Follow-up.** Arrange for the child to see a hematologist within 12–24 hours.

3. **Disposition.** Admit all children with splenic sequestration, aplastic crisis, stroke, pulmonary infarction, suspected bacterial infection, priapism, unremitting vasoocclusive crisis, and children with vasoocclusive crises who do not respond to 2 hours of conservative treatment with analgesics and hydration.

E. **Glucose 6-phosphate dehydrogenase (G6PD) deficiency.** G6PD deficiency is an x-linked recessive disorder that is more severe in males and most common in Mediterranean, oriental, and black ethnic groups. Acute, rapidly progressive hemolysis can follow viral infection or ingestion of oxidants such as fava beans, naphthalene, or medications (Table 19-2). The peripheral smear shows anisocytosis, increased reticulocytes, and Heinz bodies on the reticulocyte stain. Affected children

**Table 19-2. Drugs provoking hemolysis in G6PD-deficient cells**

| | |
|---|---|
| Acetanilid | Para-aminosalicylic acid |
| Acetylsalicylic acid (aspirin) | Phenylhydrazine |
| $N^2$-acetylsulfanilamide | Primaquine |
| Antipyrine | Probenicid |
| Colamine | Pyramidon |
| Fava bean | Salicylazosulfapyridine |
| Furazolidone | Sulfacetamide |
| Isoniazid | Sulfisoxazole |
| Naphthalene | Sulfoxone |
| Nitrofurantoin | Synthetic vitamin K compounds |
| Pamaquine | Thiazosulfone |

Source: Wolfe, L. Blood Disorders. In J. W. Graef and T. E. Cone (eds.), *Manual of Pediatric Therapeutics*. Boston: Little, Brown, 1985.

frequently have a history of severe jaundice in the neonatal period. Diagnosis is confirmed by G6PD screen or assay.

1. **Management.** When anemia is severe, transfuse the patient with packed red cells, 5–10 ml/kg over 4 hours. Exchange transfusion may be required in the neonate. Caution the parents against oxidant drug administration.

2. **Disposition.** Admit all patients with acute hemolysis associated with G6PD deficiency.

3. **Key points**
   a. Children with acute onset anemia often require extensive workup and admission.
   b. Chronic anemia is usually due to iron deficiency; when suspected, treat empirically and repeat the reticulocyte count in 1 week.
   c. Early consultation with the blood bank is important in the management of children with hemolytic anemia.
   d. In most cases, painful sickle cell crises can be managed conservatively with fluids, bed rest, and analgesics.
   e. Consider the diagnosis of serious infection or sepsis in children with sickle cell disease and fever.

II. **Purpura and bleeding disorders**

A. **Purpura.** Extravasation of red blood cells into the skin or mucous membranes results in a discoloration called **purpura.** Petechiae are small purpuric lesions less than 2.0 mm in diameter; ecchymoses are greater than 2.0 mm in diameter. Purpura may be caused by (1) thrombocytopenia due to increased destruction (immune thrombocytopenic purpura [ITP], drugs) or decreased production (leukemia, aplastic anemia) of platelets; (2) platelet dysfunction, which may be congenital (von Willebrand's disease) or acquired (uremia, salicylates); (3) vascular disorders (Henoch-Schönlein purpura, drugs, meningococcemia). In contrast, fluid phase coagulation disorders such as hemophilia are more likely to cause **deep bleeding** (bruising, joint bleed) than superficial purpura. In conditions such as disseminated intravascular coagulation (DIC) there may be both purpura and a coagulation disorder.

1. **Diagnosis and assessment**
   a. **History.** Always exclude accidental or nonaccidental trauma as the cause of purpura. Determine onset, duration, previous episodes, and the site and type of bleeding (i.e., rectal bleeding, mucosal ooze). Ask about recurrent infections, medications, or underlying chronic illness (renal or liver failure). Determine if there is a family history of bleeding disorders or heavy bleeding with surgery, dental extractions, or trauma.
   b. **Examination.** In general, the **acutely ill patient** with purpura probably has an acquired disorder, whereas the **well-looking child** probably has a congenital coagulation disorder or ITP. The presence of petechiae or mucosal bleeding suggests decreased or dysfunctioning platelets. Deep muscle bleeds or hemarthrosis episodes are usually due to congenital coagulation disorders. When trauma is suspected, look for signs of child abuse (see Chap. 39). In all cases, perform a full neurologic evaluation, with funduscopy and cranial nerve, motor, and sensory testing, and compare sides for signs of focal dysfunction due to intracranial bleed.
   c. **Investigation.** Initially, obtain blood for CBC, differential count, platelet count, peripheral smear, prothrombin time (PT), partial thromboplastin time (PTT), and fibrinogen. If DIC is suspected, fibrin degradation products (FDPs) should also be measured. Other investigations may be ordered according to the working diagnosis, such as a bleeding time when von Willebrand's disease is suspected (Table 19-3).
2. **Management.** Acute bleeding disorders require prompt attention. Children who are sick or toxic with acute onset of purpura should be assumed to have sepsis due to agents such as *H. influenzae type b* or *Neisseria meningitidis*. In the child with unstable vital signs or toxicity follow recommendations in sec. **II.B,** below.

B. **Disseminated intravascular coagulation (DIC).** DIC is an acquired disorder in which there is consumption of coagulation factors and platelets, deposition of microthrombi, and activation of the fibrinolytic system. The most common cause of DIC is sepsis.
   1. **Diagnosis and assessment.** Bleeding and thrombosis result in purpura, peripheral cyanosis, hematuria, melena, and prolonged oozing from sites of trauma such as venipuncture sites. Diagnostic findings are usually related to the cause of DIC (Table

**Table 19-3. Diagnosis and treatment—common bleeding disorders**

| Diagnosis | Platelets | PT | PTT | Treatment | Comments |
|---|---|---|---|---|---|
| DIC | Decreased | Prolonged | Prolonged | See DIC, admit | Anemia, RBC fragments on smear, increased FDPs decreased fibrinogen |
| Vitamin K deficiency, liver disease | Normal | Prolonged | Prolonged | Vitamin K 5–10 mg IV, admit | Jaundice, hepatomegaly, history of antibiotic use |
| ITP | Decreased | Normal | Normal | Admit, prednisone 2.0 mg/kg/day if count decreases to $< 10 \times 10^9$/liter (10,000/mm$^3$) | Looks well; often recent viral illness |
| Factor VIII or IX deficiency | Normal | Normal | Prolonged | Factor replacement | Personal or family history |
| von Willebrand's disease | Normal | Normal | Prolonged | Cryoprecipitate, DDAVP, admit if severe | Positive history, increased bleeding time |
| Vascular disease | Normal | Normal | Normal | None | Henoch-Schönlein purpura, drugs, etc. |

**Table 19-4. Etiology of DIC**

| Cause | Examples |
|---|---|
| Infection | |
|   Bacterial | Gram-negative sepsis, *H. influenzae* type b, meningococcemia, *Streptococcus pneumoniae* |
|   Viral | Herpes simplex, varicella, cytomegalovirus, influenza |
|   Rickettsial | Rocky Mountain spotted fever |
| Severe trauma, shock | Intracranial trauma, burns |
| Leukemia | Acute promyelocytic leukemia |
| Large hemangioma | |
| Intravascular hemolysis (HUS) | |
| Toxins (snake, spider bite) | |
| Other | Heat stroke, complicated pregnancy, NEC, HMD, asphyxia |

Key: HMD = hyaline membrane disease, NEC = necrotizing enterocolitis

19-4). Laboratory findings are presented in Table 19-3.

2. **Management**
   a. **Resuscitation.** Assess and control airway, breathing, and circulation. Place the child on a cardiac monitor and administer oxygen. Obtain blood for CBC, platelet count, differential count, smear, cross-match, culture, and measurement of blood gases, BUN, creatinine, electrolytes, PT, PTT, FDPs, and fibrinogen. Collect a urine specimen for urinalysis.
   b. **Treat the underlying condition.** When the diagnosis is unknown, assume that the child is septic. Administer broad-spectrum antibiotics—ampicillin and gentamicin in the neonate, ampicillin and cefotaxime in infants from 4–12 weeks, ampicillin and chloramphenicol in children 12 weeks–6 years, and cefotaxime after 6 years (see Chap. 4). Give intravenous fluids or pressors as necessary (see Chap. 4).
   c. **Component therapy**
      (1) If there is significant hemorrhage, administer packed red blood cells and fresh frozen plasma (FFP) in aliquots of 10 ml/kg IV while monitoring circulatory status. If there is no response to FFP, cryoprecipitate may be given: 1 bag/3 kg body weight in infants, and 1 bag/5 kg body weight in children.
      (2) Give platelet concentrates, 1 pack/6.0 kg of

body weight if the platelet count is less than $20 \times 10^9$/liter (20,000/mm$^3$).

**d. Vitamin K.** Give vitamin K, 5 mg by intravenous push over 2 minutes. Vitamin K therapy is especially important in the child who has been on prolonged antibiotic therapy.

**e. Heparin.** Heparin may be used in selected patients such as those with promyelocytic leukemia. Consult a hematologist.

**f. Exchange transfusion.** Consider exchange transfusion for the treatment of unresponsive bleeding in neonates.

**C. Hemophilia.** Factor VIII and IX deficiencies are X-linked conditions. Patients at highest risk are those with severe disease who have factor levels less than 1% of normal. Deep bleeding commonly occurs in muscles (bruising) or joints (hemarthrosis). Intracranial hemorrhage is a major cause of mortality. **Severe** hemophilia occurs when factor levels are less than 2% of normal. In **moderate** disease factor levels are 2–5% of normal. **Mild** disease occurs when factor levels are 5–30% of normal.

**1. Diagnosis and assessment**

**a. History.** In the child with a suspected diagnosis of hemophilia, ask about a personal or family history of severe bleeding following trauma or surgery. Most severe hemophiliacs on home therapy present to the emergency room only when there is persistent bleeding or pain or concern about possible intracranial hemorrhage. Always determine if there has been trauma. Pain should be assumed to be secondary to bleeding until proved otherwise—the cause of lower quadrant abdominal discomfort is more likely to be a bleed than appendicitis.

**b. Examination.** When bleeding is suspected, examine the involved part carefully. Commonly affected joints are the knee, ankle, and elbow. There may be swelling, tenderness, and limited range of motion (see Chap. 24, Acute Arthritis). Muscle bleeding may result in a compartment syndrome, especially in the lower leg or forearm (see Chap. 24). Retropharyngeal bleeding may cause acute upper airway obstruction, a medical emergency. A full neurologic evaluation is required following any head injury, regardless of severity.

**c. Investigations**

**(1)** When hemophilia is suspected but has not been diagnosed, obtain blood for measurement of PT, PTT, and factor VIII and IX levels (see Table 19-3).

**(2)** In the known hemophiliac with protracted or severe bleeding, order a CBC and platelet count. Test inhibitor (Bethesda units) status

**Table 19-5. Treatment of bleeds in hemophilia**

| Type of bleed | Percentage of factor level required |
|---|---|
| Simple joint bleed | 20–40 |
| Deep muscle bleed (ileopsoas) | 40–60 |
| Oral bleeds | 40–60 |
| Hematuria | 40 |
| Head trauma (no CNS signs) | 50 |
| Intracranial bleed | 100 |
| Surgery | 80–100 |

Note: Factor VIII: 1 unit/kg raises level by 2%. Factor IX: 1 unit/kg raises level by 1%.

and consult a hematologist if bleeding has not been responding to treatment.

(3) If there is abdominal pain, check a urinalysis for hematuria and consider ultrasound examination or contrast studies to look for evidence of gastrointestinal, genitourinary, intraperitoneal, retroperitoneal, or ileopsoas bleeding.

(4) A CT scan is indicated in children with head trauma or abnormal or focal neurologic signs.

(5) X rays of joints following acute hemarthrosis are unnecessary in the emergency department unless a fracture is suspected.

2. **Management**
   a. **Resuscitation.** Control airway, breathing, and circulation. In children with severe hemorrhage, start two large-bore intravenous lines and resuscitate the child with intravenous fluid or blood.
   b. **Factor replacement.** Guidelines for specific factor replacement in hemophilia A and B are outlined in Table 19-5.
   c. **Other hemostatic measures**
      (1) Oral bleeds may benefit from additional treatment with antifibrinolytic agents such as transexaminic acid or aminocaproic acid (Amicar). Aminocaproic acid is administered as follows: **Loading dose:** 200 mg/kg PO (maximum 6 gm). **Maintenance dose:** 100 mg/kg/dose PO q6h (maximum daily dose 24 gm) for 2–5 days or until healing occurs.
      (2) Cryoprecipitate, 1 bag/6 kg body weight (80 factor VIII units/bag) can be given instead of heat-treated concentrate.
      (3) DDAVP, 0.3 μgm/kg in normal saline over 30 minutes, may be given to mild (>5% factor VIII and IX) patients to improve hemostasis.

DDAVP can also be given to children with severe bleeding due to von Willebrand's disease.

**d. General considerations**

   **(1)** Elevate and immobilize the affected joints for 24 hours and give acetaminophen to reduce pain.

   **(2)** Observe closely for signs of nerve entrapment or compartment syndrome (see Chap. 24).

   **(3)** Observe blood precautions—many hemophiliacs are hepatitis B or HIV positive.

   **(4)** Consult a hematologist and inform the blood bank of replacement needs.

**D. Immune thrombocytopenic purpura.** ITP is an idiopathic autoimmune disorder characterized by severe thrombocytopenia. It occurs in newborns delivered to mothers with ITP and in older children following a viral illness. Mortality ($< 1\%$) is usually due to CNS hemorrhage and generally occurs in children with platelet counts of less than $10 \times 10^9$/liter ($10,000/mm^3$). In general, children with ITP present with petechiae and ecchymoses but otherwise look well. There is no hepatosplenomegaly, which differentiates this condition from malignant marrow infiltrative diseases such as leukemia. Laboratory examination reveals an isolated thrombocytopenia, usually less than $50 \times 10^9$/liter ($50,000/mm^3$), with a normal Hb, WBC, and differential count.

   **1. Management**

   **a. Resuscitation**

      **(1)** In the child with ITP and life-threatening hemorrhage, headache, seizure, or intracranial bleed, assess and control problems in the airway, breathing, and circulation. Start an intravenous line, obtain blood for a crossmatch and order pooled platelets.

      **(2)** In the case of an intracranial bleed, obtain a CT scan and consult a hematologist and neurosurgeon immediately.

      **(3)** Give hydrocortisone 5 mg/kg intravenously q6h.

      **(4)** Intravenous gamma globulin may be useful in children who require a rapid elevation in platelet count. The dosage is 1 gm/kg IV administered over 4–6 hours; up to three doses may be given.

      **(5)** Transfuse packed red blood cells as indicated for hypovolemia secondary to bleeding.

      **(6)** If there is sudden deterioration in the clinical status of a child who is scheduled for neurosurgery, transfuse platelets continuously. Otherwise, withhold platelets for perioperative transfusion.

      **(7)** Splenectomy may be required.

   **b. Stable, platelet count more than $10 \times 10^9$/liter ($10,000/mm^3$).** The child who is stable with a platelet count above $10 \times 10^9$/liter (10,000/mm³) should be evaluated by a hematologist. Obtain blood for CBC, platelet count, differential count, and blood smear. Perform a careful neurologic examination including funduscopy, looking for signs of intracranial bleeding. Admission and treatment will depend on whether or not there is bleeding.

   c. **Stable, platelet count less than $10 \times 10^9$/liter (10,000/mm³).** The child with a platelet count below $10 \times 10^9$/liter should be admitted. The patient with a bone marrow biopsy consistent with ITP should be treated with prednisone, 2.0 mg/kg/day PO divided q12h for 2–3 weeks, then tapering the dose over 5–7 days. This usually results in an earlier rise in the platelet count (usually in 48–72 hours). Alternative therapy is with intravenous gamma globulin, 0.2–0.4 gm/kg IV daily for 2–5 days.

**E. Disposition.** Admission to hospital is required for patients with the following conditions:

   **a.** Head trauma, acute headache, spinal cord bleed.
   **b.** Retroperitoneal or ileopsoas hematoma.
   **c.** Compartment syndrome or high risk of same.
   **d.** Gastrointestinal bleeding.
   **e.** Poor compliance.
   **f.** All patients with ITP who have complications or platelet counts less than $10 \times 10^9$/liter (10,000/mm³).

**F. Key points**

   **1.** Consider the diagnosis of sepsis in all patients with acute onset of purpura.
   **2.** Administer broad-spectrum antibiotics to children with DIC of unknown etiology.
   **3.** In most cases, the diagnosis of purpura or bleeding disorder can be made by analysis of the PT, PTT, and platelet count.
   **4.** The hemophiliac with a head injury requires a minimum 50% factor replacement, CT scan, and admission.
   **5.** Intracranial hemorrhage is the major severe complication of ITP.
   **6.** In the patient with ITP and a platelet count under $10 \times 10^9$/liter (10,000/mm³), treat with PO prednisone or IV gamma globulin.

**III. Emergencies in oncology patients**

**A. Fever and infection**

   **1. Diagnosis and assessment.** Neutropenia in oncology patients is usually secondary to chemotherapy. These children are immune compromised, and fever should be considered due to infection until proved otherwise. Alternatively, severe infection may occur without fever or other signs of inflammation. Children with indwelling central lines are at particular risk for bacteremia and sepsis. Immune dysfunction increases the risk for opportunistic infections such

**Table 19-6. Risk of infection with neutropenia**

| Absolute neutrophil count | Infection |
|---|---|
| $< 1.0 \times 10^9$/liter (1,000/mm³) | Skin infection |
| $< 0.5 \times 10^9$/liter (500/mm³) | Pulmonary infection, fungal infection, sepsis |
| $< 0.2 \times 10^9$/liter (200/mm³) | Life-threatening sepsis |

as *Pneumocystis,* disseminated fungal infection, and severe viral infection (herpes simplex, herpes zoster, chickenpox, cytomegalovirus infection, atypical measles).

**2. Management**

**a.** Look for a focus of infection, including sites where the mucosal barrier or skin may be broken (oral, anal, blood-taking sites).

**b.** Perform a septic workup with a blood culture, urine culture, throat swab, and a chest x ray. Consider a lumbar puncture if there are neurologic signs or if the child is extremely irritable.

**c.** The susceptible child who has been **exposed to varicella virus** should be treated with varicella-zoster immune globulin (VZIG), 1 vial/10 kg (maximum dose 5 vials) IM, within 4 days of contact. **Chickenpox or herpes zoster disease** should be treated with intravenous acyclovir, 5 mg/kg/dose q8h.

**d.** In the child with an absolute neutrophil count (ANC) of less than $0.5 \times 10^9$ (500/mm³) and fever or other signs of infection, implement broad-spectrum antibiotic coverage with intravenous tobramycin, 5.0 mg/kg/day divided q8h, ampicillin, 200 mg/kg/day divided q6h, and cloxacillin or oxacillin, 200 mg/kg/day divided q6h, or another suitable antistaphylococcal agent.

**e.** The child with interstitial pneumonia should receive trimethoprim-sulfamethoxazole, 20 mg/kg/day as trimethoprim PO divided q8h for possible *Pneumocystis* infection.

**B. Bleeding.** Ineffective hemostasis is most commonly due to thrombocytopenia. Spontaneous mucosal hemorrhage may occur when the platelet count is less than $20 \times 10^9$/liter (20,000/mm³). Administration of 1 unit of platelet concentrate/m² of body surface area raises the count by $10–15 \times 10^9$/liter (10–15,000/mm³) in the nonsensitized, nonseptic patient. When possible, irradiate all blood products prior to administration. Avoid drugs such as salicylates that inhibit platelet function.

**C. Other complications**

**1. Superior vena cava syndrome/upper airway obstruction.** Obstruction of the superior vena cava (headache, neck vein distension, dyspnea, orthopnea, cardiovascular collapse) or upper airway can occur in children with Hodgkin's disease (HD) or non-Hodgkin's lymphoma (NHL). The chest x ray reveals a middle or anterior mediastinal mass. If possible, diagnosis should be made by biopsy prior to therapy; bone marrow or superficial node biopsy may be adequate.

   **a. Management**
      **(1)** Intubation is occasionally required in NHL.
      **(2)** In NHL there is usually a good response to treatment with prednisone, 60 mg/m$^2$/day PO divided q12h.
      **(3)** In HD primary treatment is by emergency radiotherapy. Consult an oncologist.
   **2. Acute spinal cord compression.** Acute spinal cord compression is seen in patients with primary or metastatic spinal tumors. The child usually has back pain that is maximal over the point of compression and weakness and sensory changes in the legs or disordered bladder or bowel function. Consult a neurosurgeon and oncologist immediately for CT scan and possible treatment with radiotherapy, chemotherapy, or surgery.

**D. Key points**
   **1.** Children with absolute neutrophil counts of less than $0.5 \times 10^9$/liter (500/mm$^3$) and fever should be presumed to be septic.
   **2.** Oncology patients exposed to varicella should receive varicella zoster immune globulin within 96 hours of contact. Those with signs of varicella or zoster disease require admission for IV acyclovir.

**Bibliography**

Corrigan, J. C. Jr. (ed.). *Hemorrhagic and Thrombotic Diseases in Childhood and Adolescence*. London: Churchill Livingstone, 1985.

Oski, F. A., and Nathan, D. G. (eds.). *Haematology of Infancy and Childhood* (3rd ed.). Philadelphia: W. B. Saunders, 1987.

Pearson, H. A. Sickle cell diseases: Diagnosis and management in infancy and childhood. *Pediatr. Rev.* 9:121, 1987.

Schulman, I. Idiopathic (immune) thrombocytopenic purpura in children: Pathogenesis and treatment. *Pediatr. Rev.* 5:173, 1983.

# 20

# Disorders in Infants

## Crying and Colic in Infants
### Gregory A. Baldwin

Crying is perceived as a sign of distress in the infant. In most cases of infant crying that are brought to the emergency department, no organic cause is found. An **organic cause** is more likely to be found in the child over 3 months of age or if the crying is of recent onset or occurs around the clock and the child cannot be consoled.

I. **Diagnosis and management of common causes.** All babies with crying of sudden onset need a thorough head-to-toe examination, to look for organic causes (Table 20-1).

   A. Vomiting, diarrhea, fever, lethargy, and poor feeding are always abnormal and should be regarded as signs of potentially serious disease.

   B. **Child abuse** may present as infant colic. Search carefully for signs of child abuse such as bruising, mouth injury, retinal hemorrhages, and injury to the extremities.

   C. **Hunger** may be diagnosed by a trial of feeding. Hunger commonly occurs in the breast-fed baby when the milk supply is inadequate. If the baby appears healthy and settles with feeding, counsel the mother to continue breast feeding and supplement her feeds with formula. Arrange for follow-up with a family doctor or pediatrician.

   D. For treatment of otitis media, mouth ulcers, and thrush, see Chap. 14.

   E. Most infants under the age of 3 months are obligate nose breathers. If the child has nasal stuffiness, instruct the parent to treat him or her with saline nose drops, 1–2 drops before feeds and prn to each nostril, followed 1–2 minutes later by gentle suction with a nasal aspirator to remove the mucus. A cool mist vaporizer placed in the child's sleeping area may also help.

   F. For diagnosis and treatment of anal fissures and constipation, see Chap. 16, Constipation.

   G. **Infant colic** is a condition of unknown etiology that occurs in the first 3 months of life—it is always a diagnosis of exclusion. The baby with colic is perfectly well between episodes. There are paroxysms of unexplained crying or fussiness of sudden onset, usually in the evening from 6 to 10 P.M. The baby characteristically draws the legs up, turns red, and cries.

II. **Management.** When infant colic is diagnosed, the primary task is to help the parents cope with the stress and rule out or prevent child abuse. Parents should be reassured that there is no serious disease. Encourage them to seek support from family, friends, and their family doctor. Counsel the mother against alteration of formula in the bottle-fed infant. Gentle swaddling, rocking, frequent burping while

**Table 20-1. Organic causes of crying that have physical findings**

Common causes
  Otitis media
  Stuffy nose
  Mouth ulcers, thrush
  Constipation, gastroenteritis
  Anal fissure
  Urinary tract infection
Uncommon causes
  General—failure to thrive, fetal alcohol syndrome
  Skin—any pruritic or painful rash
  Eyes—glaucoma, corneal abrasion, foreign body
  Ear, nose, and throat—pharyngitis
  Cardiovascular—CHF, SVT, any cause of coronary
    insufficiency
  Gastrointestinal—intususception, inguinal hernia, GE
    reflux, volvulus, acute abdominal conditions, pinworm
    infestation
  Genitourinary—urinary tract obstruction, meatal ulcer,
    torsion of testis or ovary
  Skeletal—fracture, subperiosteal hematoma, osteomyelitis,
    Caffey's disease, hair or thread twisted around digit
  Neurologic—increased ICP

Key: CHF = congestive heart failure, SVT = supraventricular
tachycardia, GE = gastroesophageal, ICP = intracranial pressure
Source: Adapted from B. D. Schmitt, Colic: Excessive crying in
newborns. *Clin. Perinatol.* 12:441, 1985.

feeding, and use of a pacifier may help. Although many physicians advocate use of medications such as simethicone
drops, 0.25–0.5 ml PO with or after each meal, there is no
conclusive evidence that they are effective. Do not prescribe
sedative or anticholinergic agents.
**III. Disposition.** Admit the infant when there is suspicion of
serious disease or evidence of child abuse, or when the parents are unable to cope with a crying child.
**IV. Key Points**
  **A.** Rule out organic causes in infants who present with excessive crying to the emergency room.
  **B.** Colic is more common in victims of child abuse; search
  for signs of nonaccidental injury.
  **C.** Avoid the use of anticholinergic medications.

### Bibliography

Schmitt, B. D. Colic: Excessive crying in newborns. *Clin. Perinatol.* 12:441, 1985.
Hewson, P., Oberklaid, F., and Menahem, S. Infant colic, distress, and crying. *Clin. Pediatr.* 26:69, 1987.

# Cyanosis in the Infant
Michael Seear

I. **Types of cyanosis.** Apparent cyanosis is often seen around the mouth or on the forehead in normal infants. It is due to the presence of rich venous plexuses in these areas.

A. **Central cyanosis.** Central cyanosis is defined as the presence of more than 5 gm reduced hemoglobin/100 ml of blood. Above this level, a bluish discoloration of the lips and fingernails is obvious. Minor desaturation in an anemic patient may not be clinically obvious (e.g., 20% desaturation with a hemoglobin of 10 produces only 2 gm/100 ml of reduced hemoglobin). Central cyanosis is always a sign of severe pathology.

B. **Peripheral cyanosis.** Peripheral cyanosis is a bluish appearance of the fingers and toes caused by poor perfusion. The lips and tongue remain pink. It is common and usually benign, although it may be an early sign of serious conditions such as hypoglycemia or sepsis.

II. **Diagnosis and assessment.** Most cases of cyanosis require urgent action, leaving little time for a detailed history and physical examination. The following scheme can be completed rapidly and will provide a broad diagnosis in most instances. Before starting the investigation, the child should be receiving 100% oxygen.

A. **History.** If the patient is a newborn infant, take a detailed pregnancy history including maternal drug abuse. Ask about the condition of the child at birth, APGAR scores, time to first breath, and whether forceps or anesthetic agents were used at the delivery. Determine if the child has ever been pink and whether there has been stridor, respiratory distress, or sweating. Ask about the feeding pattern. The family history should rule out rare hemoglobinopathies and familial malformations of the heart or lungs. In the child with tetralogy of Fallot, intermittent episodes of respiratory distress and increasing cyanosis usually represent hypercyanotic spells (Tet-spell) with infundibular spasm of the pulmonary artery.

B. **Examination.** Note whether the cyanosis is peripheral or central and whether the child's color changes to pink with oxygen administration. Measure the core temperature and note the general appearance of the child—e.g., meconium stained, small for gestational age. Look for signs of respiratory distress (accessory muscle use, tachypnea, indrawing). Listen for stridor, and carefully auscultate the chest. Measure the head circumference, feel the fontanel, and note the respiratory pattern and rate. In the cardiovascular examination, feel all the pulses, note the position of the apex beat and the size of the liver, and perform auscultation to detect any murmurs, dysrhythmias, or gallop rhythm.

C. **Investigations**

1. Order a chest x ray to look for evidence of pulmonary or cardiac disease.

    **2.** Perform the hyperoxic test: With the child receiving 100% oxygen, draw a blood sample for arterial blood gas measurement or perform pulse oximetry measurement; if the saturation rises to 95% or if there is an arterial $PO_2$ above 100, then cyanotic heart disease is unlikely.

**III. Causes.** Cyanosis is a common presenting sign in a wide range of diseases affecting the lungs, heart, or brain. The diagnosis can usually be made by the history, examination, and a few simple investigations. The easiest way to remember the groups of causes is to consider the path that oxygen takes from the nose to the peripheral tissues.

    **A. Oxygen supply.** In the neonate, hypoxia may be due to birth asphyxia. Beyond the newborn period, hypoventilation may be associated with neonatal apnea, seizures, intraventricular hemorrhage, and poisoning with respiratory depressants such as narcotics or sedative-hypnotics.

    **B. Conducting airway.** The infant airway is small and easily obstructed by congenital conditions such as choanal atresia, laryngomalacia, subglottic hemangioma, and tracheoesophageal fistula. Other diseases of the conducting airway include diaphragmatic hernia, congenital emphysema, and pneumothorax.

    **C. Diffusion.** Any serious lung disease can cause a diffusion gradient. Bacterial and viral pneumonia, hyaline membrane disease, and pulmonary edema are examples. Cyanosis due to a diffusion abnormality usually responds to oxygen.

    **D. Ventilation and perfusion mismatch.** Intrapulmonary shunting may be caused by any serious diffuse lung disease (see sec. **III.C** above). Intracardiac shunting is usually due to congenital heart defects such as transposition of the great arteries, pulmonary atresia, tricuspid atresia, total anomalous pulmonary venous drainage, tetralogy of Fallot, or persistent fetal circulation. Cyanosis caused by an intracardiac shunt will not respond to oxygen administration.

    **E. Oxygen carriage.** There must be an adequate amount of normal hemoglobin to carry oxygen. Abnormalities of oxygen carriage include methemoglobinemia, anemia (tissue hypoxia, but not usually cyanosed), and rare M hemoglobinopathies.

    **F. Oxygen delivery.** Conditions causing peripheral vascular shutdown with poor capillary flow can produce peripheral cyanosis. This group includes hypovolemia and shock, hypoglycemia, acidosis, cold stress, vasomotor instability, acrocyanosis, and polycythemia.

**IV. Management.** Definitive management depends on the underlying problem, but a few clinical situations require urgent treatment.

    **1.** Patients who are hypoventilating require intubation and mechanical ventilation regardless of the disease process.

    **2.** Any infant who is acidotic, febrile, or in respiratory distress should be assumed to be septic. Following a full septic workup (blood, urine, CSF cultures), the child should be treated with intravenous antibiotics (see Chap. 21, Fever).

**3.** A prostaglandin infusion is relatively safe and can be tried in any cyanotic or acidotic child in whom the diagnosis of duct-dependent congenital heart lesion is suspected. The dose is 0.05–0.1 µg/kg/minute. The major side effect of the drug is central apnea, which occurs in about 20% of cases. This usually responds to stimulation, but some infants require intubation and ventilation.

**4.** If a Tet-spell is suspected, place the child in the knee-chest position, and give morphine, 0.05 mg/kg IM or SC. If this is ineffective, administer propranolol, 0.1 mg/kg slowly intravenously. Infants under 1 month of age may respond to prostaglandin $E_1$. Refer all cases to a cardiologist.

**5.** If methemoglobinemia is suspected (chocolate-colored arterial blood, normal $PaO_2$), order a test of the methemoglobin level. Treatment is with methylene blue, 0.1–0.2 ml/kg IV over 5–10 minutes as a 1% solution mixed with normal saline.

**V. Disposition.** Admit all patients with central cyanosis to an intensive care unit.

**VI. Key points**

   **A.** In the infant cyanosis may be due to systemic disease such as hypoglycemia or sepsis.

   **B.** Any centrally cyanotic child who is hypoventilating should be intubated and ventilated.

   **C.** The cyanosed child who is stable should immediately be placed in 100% oxygen. This serves both therapeutic and diagnostic purposes.

**Bibliography**

Lees, M. H., and King, D. H. Cyanosis in the newborn. *Pediatr. Rev.* 9:36, 1987.

Yabek, S. M. Neonatal cyanosis. *Am. J. Dis. Child.* 138:880, 1984.

---

# Infant Apneic Spells
Gregory A. Baldwin

---

Apnea is an absence of breathing for 15 seconds or longer, or an absence of breathing associated with bradycardia, cyanosis, or pallor. Young infants often have periodic breathing, a rhythmic alteration of respiratory rate with short pauses of 3–10 seconds, which should not be confused with apnea.

**I. Diagnosis and assessment**

   **A. History.** Determine timing of the event, onset, and whether there is any relationship to feeds, choking, or gagging. Ask if the baby was conscious (eyes open?), cyanosed, or pale during the episode. Inquire about asso-

**Table 20-2. Some causes of apnea**

| Type | Examples |
| --- | --- |
| CNS | Breath-holding spell |
| | Seizure |
| | Infection (encephalitis, meningitis) |
| | Increased intracranial pressure |
| | Idiopathic (CNS immaturity) |
| | Intraventricular hemorrhage (newborn) |
| | Congenital anomaly (Arnold-Chiari) |
| | Poisoning (including CO) |
| | Trauma |
| Upper airway | GE reflux |
| | Feeding problem (incoordination, cleft palate) |
| | Infection |
| | Congenital anomaly |
| Lower airway | Infection (RSV, *Chlamydia,* pertussis, bacterial) |
| | Congenital anomaly |
| Other | Sepsis |
| | Metabolic (hypocalcemia, hypoglycemia) |
| | Dysrhythmia |
| | SIDS |
| | Infant botulism |
| | Congenital heart disease |

Key: GE = gastroesophageal, RSV = respiratory syncytial virus,
CO = carbon monoxide, SIDS = sudden infant death syndrome
Source: S. B. Torrey. Apnea. *Pediatr. Emerg. Car* 1:220. © by Williams
& Wilkins, 1985.

ciated movements, alteration of posture or tone, resuscitative attempts, and response to resuscitation. A mother will often be able to distinguish between an obstructive episode in which the baby is awake, trying to breathe, and distressed, and an episode of syncope or seizures with loss of consciousness and tone or abnormal movements. Inquire about upper respiratory infection, infectious contacts, medications, toxins, prematurity, family history of sudden infant death syndrome, and congenital malformations of the lungs or cardiovascular system (see Table 20-2). Breath-holding spells can usually be diagnosed by history.

**B. Examination.** If the vital signs are stable, the examination should focus on the positive elements of the history and rule out serious systemic disease. Poor feeding, irritability, sleepiness, fever, or hypothermia may be evidence of sepsis and infection in the neonate. If there is tachypnea, the problem may be respiratory or metabolic in nature. Note the tone and level of consciousness, and examine the fontanels and fundi for signs of increased intracranial pressure. Look for retinal hemorrhages as evidence of nonaccidental injury. Infantile botulism, a rare cause of infant apnea, may present with the additional symptoms of constipation, hypotonia, and ptosis (a late sign).

   **C. Investigations.** In the infant with true apnea, obtain blood for complete blood count (CBC), differential count, measurements of glucose, electrolytes, and blood gases. A full septic workup with lumbar puncture should be done if there is any suspicion of sepsis. If pulmonary disease is suspected, order a chest x ray, and if dysrhythmia or congenital heart disease is suspected, obtain a chest x ray and electrocardiogram (ECG).

**II. Management**

   **A.** Assess and support the airway, breathing, and circulation. If respirations resume spontaneously or with stimulation, administer oxygen and place the patient on a monitor.

   **B.** The child with recurrent severe apnea or the child suspected of serious underlying disease such as sepsis, meningitis, or trauma should be intubated and ventilated (see Chap. 1).

**III. Disposition.** All infants with a history of apnea of unknown or serious etiology should be admitted to hospital for continuous cardiac and respiratory monitoring.

**IV. Key points**

   **A.** In many cases, the history will distinguish between obstructive and nonobstructive apnea.

   **B.** Consider the diagnosis of sepsis in the infant with apnea.

**Bibliography**

Camfield, P., et al. Infant apnea: A prospective evaluation of etiologies. *Clin. Pediatr.* 21:684, 1982.

Torrey, S. B. Apnea. *Pediatr. Emerg. Care* 1:219, 1985.

---

# Jaundice in the Newborn
Gregory A. Baldwin

---

Most newborns develop jaundice in the first few days of life; the incidence is higher in the preterm infant. The child with a very high serum bilirubin level—usually more than 340 μmol/liter (20 mg/dl) in the term baby, variable in the preterm baby—is at risk for kernicterus. Occasionally, jaundice is a sign of serious disease such as sepsis or Rh isoimmunization.

**I. Diagnosis and assessment**

   **A.** Every baby with jaundice should have a full physical examination including determination of liver size and consistency. Pallor, petechiae, severe tachycardia, blood pressure instability, or congestive heart failure suggests sepsis or Rh-hemolytic disease.

   **B.** In all cases, initial blood work should include a CBC with smear and reticulocyte count, indirect and direct

**Table 20-3. Features of physiologic and pathologic jaundice**

| Feature | Physiologic jaundice | Pathologic jaundice |
|---|---|---|
| Onset | > 24 hours | < 24 hours |
| Duration | < 1 week (full-term)<br>< 2 weeks (preterm) | > 1 week (full-term)<br>> 2 weeks (preterm) |
| Peak total | < 220 μmol/liter (full-term) (< 12.9 mg/dl)<br>< 260 μmol/liter (preterm) (< 15 mg/dl) | > 220 μmol/liter (full-term) (> 12.9 mg/dl)<br>> 260 μmol/liter (preterm) (> 15 mg/dl) |
| Rate of increase of total bilirubin | < 85 μmol/liter/day (< 5 mg/dl/day) | > 85 μmol/liter/day (> 5 mg/dl/day) |
| Peak direct bilirubin | < 25 μmol/liter) (< 1.5 mg/dl) | > 25 μmol/liter (> 1.5 mg/dl) |

Source: Adapted from M. J. Maisels. Jaundice in the newborn. *Pediatr. Rev.* 3:305, 1982.

bilirubin measurements, blood type and Rh factor in mother and infant, and a direct Coombs' test on the infant. If sepsis is suspected, a full septic workup including lumbar puncture should be performed.

**II. Types of jaundice** (see Table 20-3)

    **A. Physiologic jaundice.** Most jaundice in the newborn period is physiologic and does not require treatment. Physiologic jaundice is indirect, starts on the second or third day of life, peaks at the fifth day, and resolves by the seventh day. Maximum levels are usually 200 μmol/liter (12 mg/dl).

    **B. Pathologic jaundice. Early (first 24 hours) indirect jaundice** may be due to hemolytic (Rh, ABO) disease. There may be a history of hydrops or evidence of heart failure or severe anemia. Polycythemia may also result in early indirect jaundice. Sepsis can cause mixed jaundice at any age. **Late-onset (> 5 days) indirect hyperbilirubinemia** is most often seen in healthy breast-fed babies. Rare causes of late indirect jaundice include hypothyroidism, bowel obstruction, enzyme deficiencies such as Crigler Najjar syndrome, and rare forms of hemolysis including G6PD deficiency and pyruvate kinase deficiency. **Early direct hyperbilirubinemia** (> 25 μmol/liter = 1.5 mg/dl) is usually due to sepsis or congenital infection (torch syndrome [toxoplasmosis, rubella, cytomegalovirus, herpes simplex], hepatitis, human immunodeficiency virus [HIV]). **Later onset direct jaundice** may be seen with biliary tract obstruction due to biliary atresia or cyst, or in metabolic diseases such as galactosemia, hereditary fructose intolerance, and alpha-1-antitrypsin deficiency.

### III. Management
  **A.** Babies with physiologic jaundice who appear well may be discharged, with follow-up arranged in 24 hours.
  **B.** The child with evidence of severe hemolytic disease (anemia, suggestive peripheral smear, or positive direct Coombs' test) should be admitted and considered for exchange transfusion. The presence of anemia or a rapidly rising bilirubin level ($> 0.5$ mg/dl/hour or 8.5 µmol/liter/hour) indicates the likely need for exchange transfusion.
  **C.** The treatment of other causes of jaundice depends on birthweight, age, bilirubin levels, and the etiology (e.g., sepsis, hypothyroidism). Consult a neonatologist when in doubt. Breast milk jaundice will resolve spontaneously; there is no need for a trial of formula feeding. Arrange for a follow-up examination and repeat test of bilirubin level in 2–3 days.
### IV. Disposition. Consider hospital admission in babies with pathologic jaundice.
### V. Key points
  **A.** Jaundice is a common problem in the newborn. History, physical examination, and basic laboratory tests including CBC, blood smear, reticulocyte count, blood type, Rh factor, and Coombs' test will rule out nearly all serious causes of pathologic jaundice.
  **B.** Late-onset indirect hyperbilirubinemia is usually related to breast feeding.
  **C.** Suspect sepsis, metabolic disease, or biliary tract obstruction in direct hyperbilirubinemia.

### Bibliography

Gartner, L. M. Cholestasis of the newborn (obstructive jaundice). *Pediatr. Rev.* 5:163, 1983.

Maisels, M. J. Jaundice in the newborn. *Pediatr. Rev.* 3:305, 1982.

Osborn, L. M., Reiff, M. I., and Bolus, R. Jaundice in the full-term neonate. *Pediatrics* 73:520, 1984.

# 21

# Infectious Disease

## Fever
David Scheifele

Interleukin 1 (leukocyte pyrogen), released from mono-nuclear phagocytes, stimulates the anterior hypothalamus, triggering heat-retaining reflexes and a subsequent rise in core body temperature above the normal range (37 ± 0.5°C). Fever is valuable as an indicator of illness, but in children its magnitude is often out of proportion to the stimulus, and it may be high with mild illnesses. Parents often misunderstand this phenomenon and are unduly alarmed. Neonates or patients in shock may not manifest fever during acute infection.

I. **Diagnosis and assessment.** Although the "hand on the brow" is remarkably accurate in detecting a high fever in the infant, it is no substitute for a thermometer. Oral temperature measurement requires cooperation by the patient, especially if a glass thermometer is used, and should be avoided in young or obtunded patients. Rectal measurement is a satisfactory alternative. Axillary measurements should be viewed as approximations. Fever may result in headache, muscle aches, nausea, and increased evaporative water losses. During rapid increases in fever, patients may look pale and experience chills and shivering. Many children tolerate fever to 39.0°C with remarkable ease. Fever with infection seldom exceeds 40.0°C and poses negligible risk of brain injury. However, temporary neuronal dysfunction may occur with high fever, resulting in delirium. Fever may trigger convulsions in those with a seizure disorder or a constitutional predisposition. In children with prolonged fever, consider other disorders including juvenile rheumatoid arthritis and Kawasaki syndrome (see Chap. 24, Kawasaki syndrome).

II. **Management**
   A. **Stabilization.** Promote comfort by removing excess blankets and clothing. Encourage oral hydration. Lower the hypothalamic "thermostat" by administering an antipyretic medication. Acetaminophen, 10–15 mg/kg PO (or PR) q4–6h, is preferred because of its convenient formulation, minimal toxicity in low doses, and lack of association with Reye's syndrome. For patients with delirium or risk of seizure, high fever may be reduced more rapidly by supplementing antipyretic therapy (as above) with measures to promote heat loss, such as use of a fan or sponging with tepid water. Drastic measures such as cold baths or alcohol sponging are contraindicated.
   B. **Further evaluation.** Having addressed the symptom of fever, one must determine its cause and the need for any specific therapy. Consider the possibilities of bacteremia and meningitis in all children (see later sections of this

chapter, Bacteremia, and Bacterial Meningitis). In children the most common causes of high fever are:
1. Acute viral infection including adenovirus, influenza, enterovirus, and measles
2. Acute otitis media
3. Pneumonia
4. Pyelonephritis
5. Iatrogenic: overwrapping of infants with mild fever
6. Bacterial enteritis

**III. Disposition.** Children who are delirious from high fever should be attended to promptly by emergency room staff.

**IV. Key points**
A. Among the many children with high fever due to viral or focal bacterial infection, there are a few with serious, bloodstream infection who require special attention.

**Bibliography**

Blanco, L., and Veltri, D. Ability of mothers to subjectively assess the presence of fever in their children. *Am. J. Dis. Child.* 138:976, 1984.

Kluger, J. D. Fever. *Pediatrics* 66:720, 1980.

McCarthy, P. L. Controversies in pediatrics: What tests are indicated for the child under 2 with fever? *Pediatr. Rev.* 1:51, 1979.

McCarthy, P. L., Lembo, R. M., Baron, M. A., et al. Predictive value of abnormal physical findings in ill-appearing and well-appearing febrile children. *Pediatrics* 76:167, 1985.

Schmitt, B. D. Fever phobia—misconceptions of parents about fevers. *Am. J. Dis. Child.* 134:176, 1980.

Yaffe, S. J. Comparative efficacy of aspirin and acetaminophen in the reduction of fever in children. *Arch. Int. Med.* 141:286, 1981.

# Bacteremia
David Scheifele

Bacteremia is a laboratory-diagnosed condition without distinctive clinical manifestations. Effective methods of recognizing bacteremic patients are not yet available. One difficulty is the variation in severity of bacteremia. Some infected patients have a few, readily cleared organisms (e.g., after dental work), others have moderate numbers of organisms that may clear with or without metastatic infection, and still others have overwhelming numbers of organisms that threaten survival. Some bacteremias complicate focal infections, whereas others occur primarily. A further difficulty is that significant bacteremias occur most commonly in children between 6 and 24 months of age, when subjective history is limited and other febrile illnesses are frequent. The current strategy is to anticipate bacteremia in situations associated with increased risk, using blood cultures to supplement clinical appraisal.

**I. Diagnosis and assessment.** The diagnostic test for bacteremia is a blood culture. The skin should be carefully disinfected prior to obtaining the sample. A single blood sample of 1–2 ml is usually satisfactory, divided between aerobic and anaerobic culture bottles if possible. Culture broths ideally should contain resins to adsorb antibiotics in the blood and agents to inactivate leukocytes and complement. Blood cultures should be considered in the following situations:

**A. Infants under 12 weeks of age with fever.** Young infants and neonates localize infection poorly and readily develop bacteremia.

   **1.** Experienced clinicians who are able to recognize benign causes of fever may decide to withhold treatment and admit the patient for symptomatic treatment and observation. If there is deterioration or suspicion of serious disease, follow recommendations in sec. **I.A.2** below.

   **2.** When there is any concern about serious infection, assume that the child is septic. Perform a complete blood count (CBC) and differential count, blood culture, urinalysis and urine culture, chest x ray, and lumbar puncture (see Chap. 21, Bacterial Meningitis) and begin empiric intravenous antibiotic treatment (see sec. **II.B** below). This is required even when focal bacterial infection is detected (e.g., otitis media, urinary infection).

**B. Immune-compromised children with fever.** Bacteremia should be suspected in any immune-compromised child with unexplained fever, especially those with neutropenia, immunoglobulin or complement deficiency, asplenia, or central venous catheters. Besides blood culture, perform a urinalysis, urine culture, and other appropriate cultures and begin empiric intravenous antibiotic therapy. For management of patients with oncologic disease and fever see Chap. 19.

**C. Infants 3–24 months old with high fever and leukocytosis.** In infants with fever of more than 39.0°C and no detectable focus of infection on physical examination, obtain blood for CBC and differential count. Those with a leukocytosis of more than $15 \times 10^9$/liter (15,000/μl) have a risk of bacteremia of between 3 and 8%. Blood culture is recommended in such patients. Except in the child with pneumonia, febrile infants are unlikely to have bacteremia secondary to focal infections. It should be emphasized that patients with a fever of less than 38.9°C who are not on antipyretic therapy and patients with a white blood cell count of less than 10.0 $\times 10^9$/liter (10,000/μl) are very unlikely to have bacteremia (accuracy > 99%).

**D. Toxic-appearing children of any age with unexplained illness.** Physical signs indicative of bacteremia are seldom present but include acute splenomegaly, macular or petechial rash, and hypotension. Patients with cellulitis or epiglottitis should be considered to have bacteremia. After obtaining blood for a culture begin empiric treatment with intravenous antibiotics (see sec. **II.B**).

## II. Management

### A. Investigations.
In addition to blood culture, other investigations of potential value include examination of Gram's-stained buffy coat of blood, examination of Gram's-stained fluid from pustular or petechial skin lesions, and tests of serum or urine for bacterial antigens. Antigen tests are most helpful when infection due to group B streptococcus or *Haemophilus influenzae* type b is suspected, the tests for antigens of other species being less sensitive.

### B. Intravenous antibiotics.
Treatment in hospital should be considered for ill-looking patients at risk for bacteremia. For neonates and young infants (< 12 weeks), a combination of ampicillin with either an aminoglycoside (tobramycin or gentamicin) or cefotaxime is usually appropriate. For children, cefuroxime, 150 mg/kg/day divided q8h has an appropriate spectrum of activity, as does the combination of ampicillin, 200 mg/kg/day divided q6h and chloramphenicol, 75 mg/kg/day divided q6h.

### C. Oral antibiotics.
Treatment with oral antibiotics in anticipation of bacteremia is not recommended, unless a focus of infection is detected. Efficacy of "blind" therapy has not been established. Follow-up examination after 24 hours for children at risk for bacteremia is recommended. A lumbar puncture should be considered if a high fever persists.

### D. Reevaluation.
Reevaluation of patients with positive blood cultures is essential. In all cases, obtain a repeat blood culture.

  1. Those with persistent fever of any magnitude or metastatic infection (e.g., septic arthritis, meningitis) should be admitted to hospital for appropriate treatment. The possibility of meningitis should be carefully considered and lumbar puncture performed if necessary. Hospitalization is usually appropriate for bacteremic neonates, immune-compromised patients, and those with troublesome organisms such as *Meningococcus, H. influenzae* type b, and *Salmonella*.

  2. Oral antibiotic therapy may be satisfactory for normal children who on reevaluation are afebrile and entirely well, having apparently recovered spontaneously from bacteremia. Recovery should be documented by repeating the blood culture.

### E. Chemoprophylaxis.
Therapy with rifampin should be considered for household members of patients who are found to be bacteremic with *H. influenzae* b or *Neisseria meningitidis* (see Chap. 21, Bacterial Meningitis).

## III. Disposition.
Patients with bacteremia should be treated in hospital. Those with septic shock should be admitted to an intensive care unit. Respiratory isolation precautions should be observed during the care of patients suspected to have meningococcal or *H. influenzae* type b bacteremia.

## IV. Key points

A. Identify children at high risk for bacteremia: children under 12 weeks of age, children 3–24 months of age with high fever and a high white blood cell count, and immunocompromised and toxic children.

### Bibliography

Cates, K. L. Host factors in bacteremia. *Am. J. Med.* 75(1B):19, 1983.

Crain, E. F., and Shelov, S. P. J. Febrile infants: Predictors of bacteremia. *J. Pediatr.* 101:686, 1982.

McLellan, D., and Giebink, G. S. Perspectives on occult bacteremia in children. *J. Pediatr.* 109:1, 1986.

Sullivan, T. D., LaScolea, E., and Neter, E. Relationship between the magnitude of bacteremia and the clinical disease. *Pediatrics* 69:699, 1982.

Teele, D. W., Pelton, S. I., Grant, M. J., et al. Bacteremia in febrile children under 2 years of age: Results of cultures of blood of 600 consecutive febrile children seen in a "walk-in" clinic. *J. Pediatr.* 87:227, 1975.

Waskerwitz, S., and Berkelhamer, J. E. Outpatient bacteremia: Clinical findings in children under two years with initial temperatures of 39.5°C or higher. *J. Pediatr.* 99:231, 1981.

---

# Bacterial Meningitis

David Scheifele

---

Pyogenic meningitis is usually a complication of bacteremia. Both phenomena occur most frequently in children aged 6–24 months. Lack of a subjective history in such infants can make early diagnosis difficult, but timely intervention is nevertheless vital for optimal outcome. The distinctive signs of meningitis (stiff neck, tense fontanel, somnolence) are indicative of advanced meningeal inflammation; early diagnosis rests on more subtle clues. *Haemophilus influenzae* type b (60–65%), meningococci, and pneumococci account for most cases of acute bacterial meningitis in children over 2 months of age. In neonatal meningitis, group B streptococci and gram-negative enteric bacteria predominate.

## I. Diagnosis and assessment

A. **Infants.** In infants the early symptoms and signs are nonspecific and include fever, irritability, anorexia, and vomiting. Undue lethargy is the most consistent sign of early meningitis. A high-pitched cry, full fontanel, and convulsion are more specific but later clues to meningeal inflammation. Neck and back stiffness indicate advanced inflammation but are not always present in affected infants, especially those under 18 months of age. In a cooperative, sitting infant, look for avoidance of flexion of the neck when an interesting object is placed in the child's lap. Apparent discomfort with passive flexion of the neck may be noted before the onset of neck stiffness.

**B. Children.** In older children a history of fever, severe headache, and soreness in the neck and back with movement readily suggest the diagnosis of meningitis. Meningeal signs are more easily elicited because the patient will complain if manipulations cause pain.

**C. Concurrent infections.** It is important to bear in mind that patients with meningitis may have several concurrent infections:

   **1. Surface colonization.** Surface colonization usually occurs within the nasopharynx and precedes invasive infection. Cold symptoms precede meningitis in about one-third of cases, suggesting that virus infection facilitates invasion by bacteria. Infection may spread to other persons from the colonized surface.

   **2. Respiratory tract infection.** A "portal of entry" infection such as otitis media or pneumonia may exist within the respiratory tract, providing a focus of high-grade infection from which bacteria invade the bloodstream. It is helpful to recognize such foci because they may facilitate the etiologic diagnosis (e.g., tympanocentesis for Gram's stain and culture) or require specific intervention (e.g., drainage of a large pleural effusion).

   **3. Bacteremia.** Bacteremia precedes meningitis and may cause injury to the vascular system. High-grade bloodstream infection may produce shock, disseminated intravascular coagulation, and a rash. The rash may be macular, petechial, or ecchymotic and is not unique to any particular pathogen but occurs most commonly with meningococcal, pneumococcal, and *H. influenzae* b infections.

   **4. Metastatic foci.** Metastatic foci may develop in tissues other than the meninges. The most common foci are pneumonia, septic arthritis, and pericarditis. Repeated examination is warranted to search for joint infections, especially of the hip, because these may require drainage to preserve the articular surfaces from damage (see Chap. 24, Acute Arthritis).

**D. Investigations**

   **1. Lumbar puncture.** The diagnosis can be established only by cerebrospinal fluid (CSF) examination. A lumbar puncture should be performed as soon as the diagnosis is suspected.

   **a.** Prior to the procedure, obtain blood for measurement of glucose and other studies (see sec. **I.D.2** below).

   **b.** In the child with coma, rapidly deteriorating level of consciousness, papilledema, or focal neurologic signs, a lumbar puncture should be deferred pending CT scan exam and consultation with a neurologist. Treatment must not be delayed in these children but should be commenced immediately following the blood culture.

    **c.** In patients with bacterial meningitis, the CSF is characteristically cloudy with more than 100 × $10^9$ white blood cells/liter, predominantly neutrophils, and the pressure is increased. The total protein level is elevated, glucose is low (less than half of the pre-lumbar puncture blood glucose concentration), and organisms are present in the Gram's-stained smear (see Appendix IV). Some of these findings are often absent, and any of these abnormalities should be viewed with concern particularly the presence of neutrophils. Prior oral antibiotic therapy may prevent detection of organisms by Gram's stain but usually does not interfere sufficiently with other parameters to mask infection. A positive CSF culture provides the definitive diagnosis and is often positive in those who have had prior treatment with oral antibiotics. When there is a bloody spinal tap and suspicion of infection, treat empirically until antigen, Gram's stain, or culture results are available.

  **2. Other investigations.** Other worthwhile investigations include blood cultures, smears and cultures from purpuric lesions, cultures of other body fluids (middle ear, abscess, joint, urine, stool), and measurements of serum electrolytes, BUN, and blood glucose levels, optimally drawn prior to the lumbar puncture. Rapid etiologic diagnosis may be possible using methods that detect bacterial polysaccharide antigens. Currently available agglutination tests for antigens of *H. influenzae* b and group B streptococcus are particularly sensitive, especially when applied to both CSF and urine samples.

**II. Management**

  **A. Resuscitation.** The seriously ill child with meningitis may require airway protection if he is comatose, circulatory support if he is in shock, seizure management if there are convulsions, and metabolic support if he is hypoglycemic. Hypoglycemia is of particular concern in young infants, whose limited glycogen stores are quickly depleted by poor intake and the stress of infection. If there is apnea, coma, status epilepticus, or a decreasing level of consciousness, suspect increased intracranial pressure and treat accordingly. See Chaps. 20, Infant Apneic Spells, and 22, Status Epilepticus, Coma, and Increased Intracranial Pressure.

  **B. Therapy**

    **1. Initial antibiotics.** Initial treatment should be started immediately after bacteriologic specimens have been obtained. The initial choice of antibiotics is based on the patient's age, taking into account the CSF Gram's-stained smear and any unusual features. Widely used regimens include (Table 21-1):

      **a.** Neonates: ampicillin and either an aminoglycoside (tobramycin or gentamicin) or cefotaxime

**Table 21-1. Dose schedule for antibiotics in bacterial meningitis**

| Drug | Daily dose | Interval (hours) |
|------|-----------|------------------|
| Ampicillin | 200–400 mg/kg | 4 |
| Penicillin G | 200,000 units/kg | 4 |
| Chloramphenicol* | 75–100 mg/kg | 6 |
| Gentamicin* | 5–7.5 mg/kg | 8 |
| Cefuroxime | 200–250 mg/kg | 6 |
| Ceftriaxone | 100 mg/kg | 12 |
| Cefotaxime | 200 mg/kg | 6 |

*Dosage should be adjusted according to peak blood levels. Dosages do not apply to neonates.

     **b.** Young infants (4–12 weeks): ampicillin and cefotaxime
     **c.** Young children (3 months–6 years): ampicillin and chloramphenicol *or* either cefuroxime, ceftriaxone, or cefotaxime
     **d.** Older children (over 7 years): ampicillin or penicillin G
  **2. Supportive care.** After correction of hypoglycemia or shock, restrict fluids to 50% of maintenance with 6-hourly monitoring of serum electrolytes in the first 48 hours of treatment. This action is necessary to reduce the consequences of inappropriate antidiuretic hormone (ADH) release and water retention. Closely monitor vital signs and the level of consciousness. Give anticonvulsant therapy if seizures occur and implement measures to reduce brain swelling if increased intracranial pressure is suspected (see Chap. 22).
  **3. Chemoprophylaxis.** Treatment with rifampin of household members and other close contacts may be required when the infective agent is *H. influenzae* type b or *N. meningitidis*. Relative contraindications to rifampin therapy include pregnancy and liver disease. Beware of interactions with oral contraceptives, oral anticoagulants, and plastic contact lenses. The regimens for each infection differ as follows:
     **a.** *N. meningitidis:* All household members are considered to be at risk for secondary infection, as are medical personnel who had intimate contact with the patient's respiratory secretions. Rifampin (10 mg/kg, maximum 600 mg/dose) is given PO twice daily for 2 days. Report cases to the public health authorities.
     **b.** *H. influenzae* b: Only household members 4 years of age or younger and not previously given HIB vaccine are considered at risk. If such an individual exists, all household members should receive rifampin (including the index case and any im-

munized children) unless a contraindication exists. Rifampin dosage is 20 mg/kg/day (maximum 600 mg) PO in a single daily dose for 4 days. Report cases to public health authorities, especially if the index case attends a day care facility.

**4. Lumbar puncture**

**a. Other prior investigations.** Blood for a serum glucose measurement should be drawn prior to the lumbar puncture.

**b. Contraindications.** A lumbar puncture should not be attempted in children with a bleeding diathesis nor in those in whom there is suspicion of raised intracranial pressure (ICP), including those with focal neurologic signs, status epilepticus, coma, or direct evidence of raised ICP (including papilledema, bulging fontanel, or split sutures).

**c. Equipment**

(1) Lumbar puncture tray containing:

(a) Appropriate infant (22-gauge short) or child (22-gauge long) lumbar puncture needle with stylet

(b) 1% lidocaine for use in children over 18 months

(c) Three sterile CSF specimen tubes

(2) 0.5% tincture of chlorhexidine, or povidone-iodine antiseptic solution

(3) Gloves, gown, mask

(4) Pressure manometer and stopcock

**d. Method** (see Fig. 21-1)

(1) Have an assistant restrain the child in the lateral decubitus position, achieving maximum flexion. Take care not to obstruct the airway.

(2) Locate the superior edge of the iliac crest—a line drawn through the iliac crests intersects the L4–L5 intervertebral space. This site or one interspace rostral to it (L3–L4) may be used.

(3) Wash the skin 3 times with aseptic technique using sterile gloves and tincture of chlorhexidine or other antiseptic solution. Local anesthesia with injected 1% lidocaine should be used for children over 18 months of age.

(4) Advance the needle bevel up, perpendicular to the coronal plane.

(5) Resistance will increase and then give way with a "pop" as the needle passes through the dura into the subarachnoid space.

(6) Remove the stylet and check for CSF drainage. If none is present, advance the needle further, remove the stylet and check again. Let the CSF drain into each of the three tubes. If desired, CSF opening pressure may be measured by attaching the stopcock and

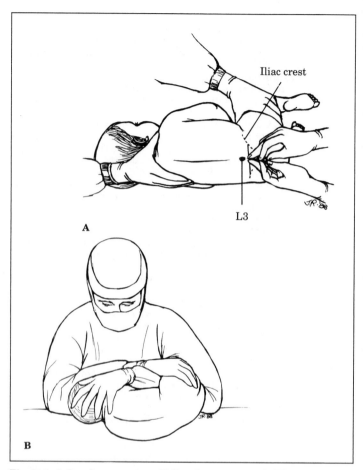

**Fig. 21-1. A. Lumbar puncture. B. Lumbar puncture holding technique.**

manometer to the needle hub. About 1 ml is needed in each tube for standard studies (cells, protein, glucose, Gram's stain and culture, antigen studies).

(7) Replace the stylet and remove the needle. Put pressure on the site for 1–2 minutes.

   e. **Complications**
      (1) Cerebellar or brainstem herniation
      (2) Infection
      (3) Epidermal cyst
      (4) Headache, limp, leg pain.

**III. Disposition.** All patients with meningitis should be admitted to a single hospital room, and respiratory isolation precautions should be exercised during the first 24 hours of antibiotic therapy. Patients in shock and those with acute onset of petechiae, severely depressed level of consciousness, or other complications should be admitted to an intensive care unit.

**IV. Key points**

**A.** In infants under 24 months, and especially in those under 18 months with meningitis, neck and back stiffness is not always present. Early signs and symptoms are nonspecific and include fever, irritability, anorexia, and vomiting.

**B.** Defer the lumbar puncture in children suspected of meningitis who have coma, rapidly deteriorating level of consciousness, papilledema, or focal neurologic signs. Obtain a blood culture, begin antibiotic therapy, and consult with a neurologist.

**Bibliography**

Klein, J. O., Feigin, R. G., and McCracken, G. H. Report of the task force on diagnosis and treatment of meningitis. *Pediatrics* 78:959, 1986.

Levy, D. R. Lumbar puncture and the diagnosis of meningitis. *South. Med. J.* 74:28, 1981.

Yogev, R. Advances in the diagnosis and treatment of childhood meningitis. *Pediatr. Infect. Dis. J.* 4:321, 1985.

---

# Encephalitis
David P. Speert

Encephalitis presents a number of diagnostic and therapeutic challenges. Clues to the specific etiology are often subtle, and existing therapies are imperfect. Early diagnosis is essential to identify candidates for specific antimicrobial therapy.

**I. Diagnosis and assessment.** Encephalitis is an inflammation of the brain and is often associated with an element of meningeal inflammation (meningoencephalitis). Disease limited to the central nervous system is most often caused by herpes virus, arbovirus, or enterovirus. Seasonal and geographic factors influence the occurrence of some etiologic agents (e.g., arboviruses). Other viral agents include adenovirus, mumps, rubella, measles, varicella, and rabies. Among the viral causes, only infection with Herpes simplex responds to antiviral therapy. Other illnesses that may mimic viral meningoencephalitis include brain tumor, lead encephalopathy, Reye's syndrome, drug intoxication, intracranial hemorrhage, brain abscess, arteriovenous malformation, and other causes of aseptic (nonsuppurative) meningitis such as tuberculosis and cryptococcosis.

**A. History.** Ask about antecedent illness, recent immunizations, insect or animal bites, and recent illnesses in family members, schoolmates, and playmates. Specific details about the current illness should be obtained, including evidence of an intercurrent infectious illness, the nature of any seizures, and medications prescribed to the patient or family members. Patients often present with symptoms of cerebral dysfunction such as an altered level of consciousness and focal neurologic signs or seizures. Neck stiffness is variable. Associated nonspecific symptoms include fever, headache, and vomiting.

**B. Physical examination.** When encephalitis is suspected, perform a full neurologic examination including assessment of cranial nerves (see Chap. 22). Signs of respiratory infection, rash, and insect or tick bites (arbovirus) should also be sought.

**C. Investigations.** Investigations should be initiated promptly in order to identify treatable causes of the central nervous system dysfunction, **especially meningitis.**

1. **Blood tests.** Obtain blood for complete blood count (CBC) and differential count, measurement of glucose level, culture, and viral serologic examination. If there have been seizures, order a BUN and measurement of electrolytes.

2. **Lumbar puncture** (see Chap. 21, Bacterial Meningitis). In encephalitis the CSF cell count may be normal, but there is usually a modest pleocytosis with a predominance of mononuclear cells. Early in the course of the disease there may be a predominance of neutrophils. The CSF protein level is usually modestly elevated, and the glucose concentration is normal or slightly decreased. In general, prior treatment with oral antibiotics does not cause the CSF of patients with meningitis to appear aseptic (see Chap. 21, Bacterial Meningitis).

**D. Herpes simplex encephalitis.** Herpes simplex encephalitis is rapidly progressive, with high morbidity and mortality. Affected children rarely have cutaneous herpetic lesions and often give no history of prior disease or contact with infected individuals. There is usually focal neurologic involvement, as evidenced by a mass lesion on CT scan, focal electroencephalographic (EEG) abnormalities, or focal seizures. Virus is rarely recovered from the CSF; definitive diagnosis is by brain biopsy. Effective antiviral therapy is available (see sec. **II.B** below).

**II. Management**

**A. General measures.** Assess and maintain the airway, breathing, and circulation. Treat seizures (see Chap. 22, Seizures). If there is increased intracranial pressure, aggressive therapy should be instituted with intubation and ventilation (see Chap. 22, Increased Intracranial Pressure).

**B. Suspected herpes encephalitis.** Whenever herpes simplex infection is suspected, begin therapy with acyclovir, 10 mg/kg/dose (500 mg/m$^2$/dose) q8h IV. A neurosurgeon should be notified if a brain biopsy is anticipated, and the patient should be assessed by a neurologist.

C. **The stable patient with encephalitis**
   1. Under certain circumstances, when there is an epidemic of meningoencephalitis in the community and the diagnosis is fairly certain, the patient need not be admitted to the hospital. If the illness is mild, the child can be discharged and reassessed the following day.
   2. If the diagnosis of aseptic meningoencephalitis is not certain, the patient should be admitted to the hospital for observation and repeat CSF examination within 24 hours.

III. **Disposition.** In general, admit all patients to hospital. Depending on the severity of the illness, the patient should be admitted to the intensive care unit or a general medical ward.

IV. **Key points**
   A. Herpesvirus infection may be the cause of sudden onset of focal neurologic dysfunction; consider therapy with acyclovir.
   B. Lumbar puncture is necessary to rule out other treatable causes of CNS dysfunction.

**Bibliography**

Griffith, J. F., and Ch'ien, L. T. Herpes simplex encephalitis, diagnostic and therapeutic considerations. *Med. Clin. North Am.* 67:991, 1983.

Whitley, R. J., Soong, S., Hirsch, M. S., et al. Herpes simplex encephalitis. Vidarabine therapy and diagnostic problems. *N. Engl. J. Med.* 304:313, 1981.

---

# Pneumonia

David P. Speert

The list of potential etiologic agents of pneumonia in childhood is extensive, but there are few clinical clues or diagnostic tests that can rapidly distinguish among them. Cough and tachypnea, the hallmarks of pneumonia, may also be due to congestive heart failure, asthma, gastroesophageal reflux, and foreign body aspiration.

I. **Diagnosis and assessment.** Pneumonia is diagnosed by physical examination and confirmed radiographically. The majority of cases are of viral etiology. *Streptococcus pneumoniae* is the most common bacterial pathogen.
   A. **History.** The common presenting complaints are cough, fever, dyspnea, chest pain, and, in the infant, difficulty with feeding. Older children and adolescents may produce sputum. Other symptoms include malaise, headache, and, in patients with lower lobe pneumonia, abdominal pain. In infants suspected of pneumonia, ask about paroxysmal coughing associated with color change, vomiting or apnea (pertussis, respiratory syncytial virus [RSV]), and a past history of lung disease or

prematurity. These infants are at risk for severe infection with respiratory failure.

**B. Examination.** Assess hydration and perform a complete cardiorespiratory examination in all cases. Signs of pneumonia include tachypnea (most reliable), inspiratory chest retractions, and, if severe, signs of respiratory failure (see Chap. 1). Auscultation and percussion are often normal in the young child with impressive x-ray evidence of disease. When rales, dullness to percussion, and bronchial breathing are found, the child has pneumonia until proved otherwise.

**C. Investigation.** Bacterial cultures of the throat or nasopharynx are of no benefit and usually reveal the resident flora of the upper respiratory tract.

1. **Chest x-ray.** A chest x ray helps to define the specific syndrome and narrow the etiologic possibilities. Radiographic findings of pneumonia are quite varied; the chest x ray may even be normal in the early stages. Therapy should be initiated on clinical grounds alone.

2. **Blood tests.** A complete blood count (CBC) and blood culture should be obtained when a bacterial etiology is considered. Blood cultures are positive in up to 25% of patients with pneumococcal pneumonia. Obtain measurements of blood gases when respiratory distress is moderate or severe. The cold agglutinin titer can be helpful in establishing the diagnosis of nonbacterial pneumonia; it is elevated in *Mycoplasma* and some viral infections but may be normal early in the disease.

3. **Other investigations.** Sputum samples may be obtained from older, cooperative children and are evaluated by Gram's stain and culture. Sputum should contain neutrophils; saliva does not. If RSV or pertussis infection is suspected, obtain a specimen of the nasopharyngeal secretions (see sec. **II.D** and **F** below). Culture of specimen of a pleural effusion is helpful in establishing an etiologic diagnosis; these specimens should be obtained by an experienced physician. A tuberculin skin test with appropriate controls should be applied when tuberculosis is suspected.

**II. Pneumonia syndromes.** The common causes of pneumonia are listed in Table 21-2. Clinical and radiographic manifestations for each type are not absolute—wide variations exist. In all cases, assess and control the patient's airway, breathing, and circulation. In children with signs of respiratory failure, give high-flow oxygen, start an intravenous line, and obtain blood for cultures and measurement of blood gases, glucose, and electrolytes (see sec. **I.C.2** above and Chaps. 1 and 3).

**A. Afebrile pneumonia of infancy (Chlamydia)**

1. **Diagnosis.** Babies with infection caused by *Chlamydia trachomatis* present at about 6 weeks of age with staccato cough, tachypnea, and notable absence

**Table 21-2. Common causes of pneumonia**

| Etiologic agent | Antimicrobial agent(s) of choice |
| --- | --- |
| Viruses | |
| Respiratory syncytial | Ribavirin |
| Influenza A | Amantadine |
| Influenza B | NA |
| Parainfluenza | NA |
| Adenovirus | NA |
| Bacteria | |
| *Streptococcus pneumoniae* | Penicillin |
| *Haemophilus influenzae* | Ampicillin or cefuroxime |
| *Staphylococcus aureus* | Cloxacillin or oxacillin |
| Group A streptococcus | Penicillin |
| Other | |
| *Chlamydia trachomatis* | Erythromycin |
| *Mycoplasma pneumoniae* | Erythromycin |
| *Mycobacterium tuberculosis* | Isoniazid, rifampin |

Key: NA = no antimicrobial agent available.

of fever or other systemic signs of toxicity. The differential white blood cell count may show eosinophilia ($> 0.3 \times 10^9$/liter or 300/mm$^3$). The chest x ray reveals hyperexpansion with diffuse interstitial and alveolar infiltrates.

2. **Management.** Treat with erythromycin, 35–50 mg/kg/day PO in three or four divided doses. Concomitant conjunctivitis needs no additional therapy. When the diagnosis has been verified, the mother should also be treated (see Chap. 21, Sexually Transmitted Diseases).

**B. Bronchopneumonia**

1. **Diagnosis.** Although typically viral in etiology, bronchopneumonia may also be caused by bacteria and mycobacteria. A viral etiology is likely if family members also have an acute respiratory illness. These children may have a dry, nonproductive cough, often with evidence of upper respiratory tract infection. The x ray finding of patchy areas of pulmonary infiltration, often with air trapping or hyperinflation, is characteristic. There is usually no frank lobar consolidation.

2. **Management.** Children who are toxic or who are suspected of having bacterial disease should be treated empirically with antibiotics (see sec. **II.C**). Amantadine, 5–8 mg/kg/day PO divided bid, is effective in the early stages of influenza A infection but is of no value in the therapy of other viral diseases.

**C. Lobar pneumonia**

1. **Diagnosis.** Frank lobar consolidation is characteristic of bacterial pneumonia. Physical examination may reveal evidence of consolidation localized to

a specific lobar distribution. Etiologic agents include *Streptococcus pneumoniae,* group A streptococcus, *Haemophilus influenzae, Staphylococcus aureus,* and *Mycoplasma pneumoniae.* A pleural effusion may be present with disease caused by any of these pathogens. A productive cough is often present; children old enough to cooperate should be encouraged to produce a sputum specimen for Gram's stain and culture.

   **2. Management**
      **a.** Children who are stable and do not require admission may be treated as outpatients:
         **(1)** If less than 6 years old give amoxicillin, 35–50 mg/kg/day PO divided q8h.
         **(2)** If 6 years or older give penicillin, 25–50 mg/kg/day PO divided q6h *or* erythromycin, 35–50 mg/kg/day PO divided q6–8h.
      **b.** If the child is sick or toxic admit for intravenous therapy with cefuroxime, 75–150 mg/kg/day divided q8h.

**D. Bronchiolitis.** This illness is usually caused by RSV and leads to lower airway obstruction with wheezing and cough. For details on diagnosis and management see Chap. 7.

**E. Pneumonia in the immune-deficient child.** Besides common bacteria and viruses, immune-deficient patients may present with opportunistic infections due to such agents as *Legionella,* cytomegalovirus, fungi, and *Pneumocystis.* These patients should be admitted for diagnosis and treatment (see Chap. 19).

**F. Pertussis**
   **1. Diagnosis.** Infection due to *Bordetella pertussis* has three characteristic stages: The **catarrhal stage,** with signs and symptoms of an upper respiratory infection, lasts 1–3 weeks. The second or **paroxysmal stage** (2–4 weeks' duration) consists of fits of coughing that may be associated with vomiting and, in severe cases, with cyanosis and apnea. The final or **convalescent stage** is characterized by mild cough only. Older children may make the characteristic whooping sound at the end of a paroxysm of coughing, but this does not always occur in infants. Young infants may present with apnea or respiratory failure. The chest x ray may be normal or reveal perihilar infiltrates or a "shaggy" heart border. The diagnosis is primarily clinical but may be supported by a raised white blood cell count with an absolute lymphocytosis and by a positive immunofluorescence test performed on nasopharyngeal secretions. A syndrome similar to classic pertussis may be caused by parapertussis or adenovirus infection.
   **2. Management.** Outpatient therapy with erythromycin, 30–50 mg/kg/day PO divided q6h for 10 days, decreases infectivity but does not alter the clinical course; it should be instituted following the catar-

rhal stage. All infants, and children with apnea, cyanosis, or respiratory distress should be given maximal oxygen and admitted for observation.

**III. Disposition.** Admit all patients with respiratory failure, suspicion of sepsis, or compromise of the immune system, and infants suspected of pertussis infection.

**IV. Key points**

    **A.** Pneumonia should be suspected in the child with fever and tachypnea at rest.

    **B.** Most patients can be treated as outpatients following appropriate cultures.

    **C.** Suspect *Chlamydia* in the young infant with afebrile pneumonia.

**Bibliography**

Long, S. S. Treatment of acute pneumonia in infants and children. *Pediatr. Clin. North Am.* 30:297, 1983.

Tipple, M. A., Beem, M. O., and Saxon, E. M. Clinical characteristics of the afebrile pneumonia associated with *Chlamydia trachomatis* infection in infants less than six months of age. *Pediatrics* 63:192, 1979.

## Toxic Shock Syndrome
Christine A. Loock and Gregory A. Baldwin

Toxic shock syndrome is a potentially life-threatening disease due to *Staphylococcus aureus* enterotoxin (TSST-1). Although it has been documented in neonates and in patients over age 80, one-third of cases occur in patients between the ages of 15 and 19. Over 70% of instances are associated with menstruation; nonmenstrual cases have been related to such factors as surgical infections, influenza infection, and nasal packing.

**I. Diagnosis and assessment.** Toxic shock syndrome (see Table 21-3) affects multiple organ systems. Most cases start with a prodrome of fever, chills, and myalgias lasting 1–4 days. The typical presenting complaint is rash, classically a generalized, red, sunburnlike exanthem. There may be vomiting and diarrhea. By definition, all patients with toxic shock syndrome have hypotension or orthostatic blood pressure changes. CSF examination often reveals a raised white blood cell count with normal CSF chemistry. Laboratory findings may include hyponatremia, hypocalcemia, hypoalbuminemia, hypokalemia, and hypomagnesemia.

    **A. Differential diagnosis.** The differential diagnosis includes:

        **1.** Septic shock from any cause—erythroderma not present.

        **2.** Severe viral exanthems—do not present with hypotension.

        **3.** Meningococcemias (and other bacteremias)—erythroderma not present.

**Table 21-3. Criteria for diagnosis of toxic shock syndrome**

A. Temperature greater than 38.9°C
B. Diffuse erythematous rash, including palms and soles, which desquamates 1–2 weeks after onset
C. Hypotension or orthostatic changes in blood pressure ($\geq$ 15 mm Hg drop when moving from lying to sitting position)
D. The following cultures or titers, if taken, are *negative*:
   1. Blood, throat secretions, or CSF (blood may be positive for *S. aureus*)
   2. Rocky Mountain spotted fever (*Rickettsia rickettsii*), leptospirosis, or rubeola
E. Involvement of three or more of the following organ systems:
   1. Gastrointestinal: vomiting or diarrhea
   2. Musculoskeletal: severe myalgias or creative phosphokinase level twice normal
   3. Renal: BUN and creatinine twice normal or pyuria ($\geq$ 5 white blood cells per high-power field) in the absence of urinary tract infection
   4. Hepatic: total bilirubin, SGOT (AST), and SGPT (ALT) twice normal
   5. CNS: altered mental status without focal neurologic signs when fever and hypotension are absent
   6. Mucous membrane involvement: vaginal, oropharyngeal, or conjunctival hyperemia
   7. Hematologic: platelet count $< 100 \times 10^9$/liter (100,000/μl)

Source: Adapted from S. W. Wright, and A. T. Trott. Toxic shock syndrome: A review. *Ann. Emerg. Med.* 17:268, 1988.

4. Rocky Mountain spotted fever—does not present with hypotension.
5. Leptospirosis—different epidemiology, rarely severe.
6. Kawasaki syndrome—does not present with hypotension.
7. Stevens-Johnson syndrome—may closely resemble TSS.
8. Scarlet fever—does not present with hypotension
   B. **Investigations.** When toxic shock is suspected, perform a full septic workup, with cultures of blood, CSF, skin, urine, vagina, and cervix. Isolation of the organism is not a criterion for the diagnosis. Obtain blood for a complete blood count (CBC), differential and platelet counts, BUN, and measurement of electrolytes and blood gases. Order a chest x ray if there is respiratory distress.
II. **Management**
   A. **Resuscitation.** Assess and control problems in the airway, breathing, and circulation. Start two large-bore intravenous lines and correct volume deficit, hypotension, acid-base imbalance, and hypoxia. Pressors may be useful in patients who do not respond to volume replacement alone (see Chap. 4). Patients often require intubation and ventilation.

#### B. Other therapy

1. Remove tampons and nasal packing and drain and debride any abscesses or wound infections. Since enterotoxin is thought to be the cause, antibiotic treatment may not alter the early course of the disease.
2. Treat with intravenous cefuroxime, 150 mg/kg/day divided q8h, for possible infection with *Neisseria meningitidis, Haemophilus influenzae,* or *Streptococcus pneumoniae,* until culture results are available (see Chap. 4).
3. Advise patient that tampon use may be contraindicated in the future.

### III. Disposition. All patients with toxic shock syndrome should be admitted to an intensive care unit for treatment and monitoring.

### IV. Key points

A. Toxic shock syndrome can occur in patients other than menstruating women.
B. Aggressive fluid therapy is the mainstay of treatment.

#### Bibliography

Hirsch, M. L., and Kass, E. H. An annotated bibliography of toxic shock syndrome. *Rev. Infect. Dis.* 8 (Suppl. 1), 1986.

Reese, R. E., and Douglas, R. G. D. *A Practical Approach to Infectious Diseases* (2nd ed.). Boston: Little, Brown, 1986.

Wright, S. W., and Trott, A. T. Toxic shock syndrome: A review. *Ann. Emerg. Med.* 17:268, 1988.

---

## Sexually Transmitted Disease
### Shirley A. Reimer and Christine A. Loock

The diagnosis of sexually transmitted disease (STD) should prompt suspicion of sexual abuse or assault, even in the sexually active teenager. Syphilis, gonorrhea, and acquired immune deficiency syndrome (AIDS) are notifiable diseases. The patient should be advised to refrain from sexual activity for a minimum of 2–3 weeks following treatment.

### I. Patterns of sexually transmitted disease

#### A. Males

1. **Diagnosis. Heterosexual** males usually present with urethritis and complain of burning dysuria and discharge. A less common presentation is that of epididymitis with scrotal pain, fever, and epididymal tenderness; the treatment is similar to that for urethritis. Diagnosis is made by Gram's stain or culture. For urethritis, obtain a sample of the urethral discharge to search for *Gonococcus* and *Chlamydia.* If there is a history of discharge but none is obtained, insert a swab 2–3 cm into the urethra and test for *Trichomonas, Chlamydia,* and *Gonococcus.* The diagnosis is strongly suggested by the presence of more than 5 white blood cells per high-power field on a stained urethral smear. Sexually active males with

**Table 21-4. Organisms causing PID**

| Type | Example |
| --- | --- |
| Aerobes | *Gonococcus, E. coli, Streptococcus, Staphylococcus, diphtheroids* |
| Anaerobes | *Peptococcus, Peptostreptococcus, Bacillus fusiformis, Bacteroides* |
| Other | *Chlamydia* |

urethral discharge should be presumed to have infection with *Gonococcus* and *Chlamydia;* treatment should be commenced immediately (see Table 21-5). In **homosexual** males, be aware of rectal infection (*Gonococcus,* syphilis) bowel infection (*Giardia,* amoebae), or systemic disease (hepatitis B, HIV). Perform rectal, urethral, and pharyngeal swabs. In all cases, check serologic tests for syphilis.

2. **Management.** Treat empirically for gonorrhea and chlamydial infection in heterosexual males, and for gonorrhea in homosexual males. For details of therapy, see Table 21-5.

B. **Females.** Females with sexually transmitted disease are often asymptomatic. Complications include infertility and ectopic pregnancy.

   1. **Pelvic inflammatory disease**
      a. **Diagnosis.** Acute pelvic inflammatory disease (PID) is a disease of polymicrobial origin. The most commonly involved organisms are listed in Table 21-4. *Gonococcus* is the sole infective agent in one-third of cases; in another one-third *Gonococcus* is accompanied by one or more organisms. *Chlamydia* is present in 20–60%. When PID is suspected, perform a full examination (see Chap. 18) with Gram's stain and cultures, and obtain blood for complete blood count (CBC), differential count, erythrocyte sedimentation rate (ESR), and syphilis serologic examination.

         (1) The diagnosis of acute PID is based on the following criteria:
            (a) **All three of the following must be present:**
               (i) Lower abdominal pain and presence of lower abdominal tenderness with or without evidence of rebound
               (ii) Cervical motion tenderness
               (iii) Adnexal tenderness
            (b) **One of the following must be present:**
               (i) Temperature above 38.0°C
               (ii) Leukocytosis of more than $10 \times 10^9$/liter (10,000/mm$^3$)

           **(iii)** Culdocentesis yielding peritoneal fluid containing white blood cells and bacteria

           **(iv)** Elevated ESR ($> 25$ mm/hour)

           **(v)** Gram's stain from the endocervix yielding gram-negative diplococci or a monoclonal directed smear from the endocervix revealing *Chlamydia trachomatis*

**b. Management** (see Table 21-5). Hospitalization is strongly recommended for adolescents owing to poor compliance and the seriousness of sequelae.

    **(1) Inpatient therapy** is accomplished with cefoxitin, 2 gm IV q6h, and doxycycline, 100 mg PO bid. If the patient is penicillin allergic, use clindamycin, 600 mg IV q6h, and gentamicin, 2.0 mg/kg as a loading dose, followed by 1.5 mg/kg IV q8h for maintenance. Continue IV therapy for 4 days or until 48 hours after defervescence. Continue doxycycline or clindamycin (450 mg PO qid) for a total of 10 days. For the latest treatment guidelines consult recent Center for Disease Control (CDC) recommendations.

    **(2) Outpatient therapy** is as follows:

        **(a)** Amoxil 3 gm PO *or*

        **(b)** Ampicillin 3.5 gm PO *or*

        **(c)** Aqueous procaine penicillin G $4.8 \times 10^6$ IM units *or*

        **(d)** Cefoxitin 2 gm IM

        **(e) Plus** probenecid 1.0 gm PO

        **(f) Followed by:** doxycycline, 100 mg PO bid, *or*

        **(g)** Tetracycline, 500 mg PO q6h for 10–14 days

**2. Subacute PID (*Chlamydia*)**

  **a. Diagnosis.** Chlamydial infection results in an attenuated inflammatory response, reducing the magnitude of signs, symptoms, and laboratory findings. Untreated, infection can result in tubal infertility, ectopic pregnancy, and chronic pelvic pain. The manifestations vary with age. **Children** present with urethritis (boys) and vaginitis (girls). Sexual abuse must be ruled out. In **adolescents** the syndromes are similar to those seen in adults, with low-grade fever and moderate abdominal, adnexal, and cervical tenderness.

  **b. Management.** Treatment should be initiated if there is a positive diagnostic test, a high index of suspicion, or infection in contacts.

    **(1)** In children **less than 9 years** of age use:

        **(a)** Erythromycin, 40 mg/kg/day PO divided q6h (maximum 500 mg) for 7 days *or*

        **(b)** Sulfamethoxazole, 75 mg/kg/day PO in two divided doses (maximum 1 gm bid) for 10 days

**Table 21-5. Treatment of gonococcal cervicitis, urethritis, and prepubertal vaginitis**

| Children under 9 years | Children over 9 years |
|---|---|
| **Penicillin-sensitive gonorrhea** | |
| Amoxicillin 50 mg/kg (max. 3.0 gm) PO, **PLUS** probenicid, 25 mg/kg (max. 1 gm) PO in a single dose, **PLUS** erythromycin, 40 mg/kg/day PO divided q6h (max. dose 500 mg) for 7 days | Amoxicillin, 3.0 gm PO, **PLUS** probenicid, 1.0 gm in a single dose, **PLUS** tetracycline, 500 mg PO q6h for 7 days, **OR** doxycyline, 100 mg PO q12h for 7 days |
| **OR** | **OR** |
| Ceftriaxone, 125 mg IM in a single dose, **PLUS** erythromycin, 40 mg/kg per day PO divided q6h for 7 days | Ceftriaxone, 250 mg IM in a single dose, **PLUS** tetracycline, 500 mg PO q6h for 7 days, **OR** doxycycline, 100 mg PO q12h for 7 days |
| **Penicillin-resistant gonorrhea or penicillin-allergic patient** | |
| Spectinomycin, 40 mg/kg (max. 2 gm) IM in a single dose, **PLUS** erythromycin 40 mg/kg/day PO divided q6h for 7 days | Spectinomycin, 2.0 gm IM in a single dose, **PLUS** tetracycline, 500 mg PO q6h for 7 days, **OR** doxycycline, 100 mg PO q12h for 7 days |
| **OR** | **OR** |
| Ceftriaxone, 125 mg IM in a single dose, **PLUS** erythromycin, 40 mg/kg/day divided q6h PO for 7 days | Ceftriaxone, 250 mg IM in a single dose, **PLUS** tetracycline, 500 mg PO q6h for 7 days, **OR** doxycycline, 100 mg PO q12h for 7 days |

Note: **1.** Sexual abuse must be ruled out. **2.** Follow-up cultures are necessary to ensure effective treatment. These regimens include appropriate therapy for concurrent chlamydial infections (erythromycin, tetracycline). Contact tracing and treatment of contacts are important. **3.** Tetracyclines should *not* be given to pregnant or lactating women or to children under 9 years of age. Homosexual males are *not* frequently coinfected with chlamydia, and therefore tetracyclines should be given only if concurrent chlamydial infection is found.
Source: Adapted from 1988 Canadian guidelines for the treatment of sexually transmitted diseases in neonates, children, adolescents, and adults. *Can. Dis. Weekly Rep.* 1452:1, 1988.

**Table 21-6. Treatment of pharyngeal gonococcal infection**

| Children under 9 years | Children over 9 years |
|---|---|
| **Penicillin-sensitive gonorrhea**<br>Aqueous procaine penicillin G, 100,000 units/kg (max. 4.8 × $10^6$ units) in a single dose IM, **PLUS** probenicid, 25 mg/kg (max. 1.0 gm) PO in a single dose, **PLUS** erythromycin, 40 mg/kg/day PO divided q6h for 7 days | **Penicillin-sensitive gonorrhea**<br>Aqueous procaine penicillin G, 4.8 MU IM, **PLUS** probenicid, 1.0 gm PO in a single dose, **PLUS** tetracycline, 500 mg PO q6h for 7 days, **OR** doxycycline, 100 mg PO q12h for 7 days |
| **OR** | **OR** |
| Ceftriaxone, 125 mg IM in a single dose, **PLUS** erythromycin, 40 mg/kg/day PO (max. 500 mg/dose) divided q6h for 7 days | Ceftriaxone, 250 mg IM in a single dose, **PLUS** tetracycline, 500 mg PO q6h for 7 days, **OR** doxycycline, 100 mg PO q12h for 7 days, **OR** tetracycline, 500 mg alone PO qid for 7 days |
| **Penicillin-resistant gonorrhea**<br>Ceftriaxone, 125 mg IM in a single dose, **PLUS** erythromycin, 40 mg/kg/day PO (max. dose 500 mg) for 7 days | **Penicillin-resistant gonorrhea**<br>Ceftriaxone, 250 mg IM in a single dose, **PLUS** tetracycline, 500 mg PO q6h for 7 days, **OR** doxycycline, 100 mg PO q12h for 7 days, **OR** trimethoprim/sulfamethoxazole, 9 single-strength tablets daily for 5 days PO, taken as single daily dose |

Note: **1.** Sexual abuse must be ruled out. **2.** Ampicillin, amoxicillin, and spectinomycin are not effective for pharyngeal gonococcal infection. **3.** Follow-up cultures are necessary to ensure effective treatment. These regimens include appropriate therapy for concurrent chlamydial infections (erythromycin, tetracyclines). Contact tracing and treatment of contacts are important. **4.** Tetracyclines should *not* be given to pregnant or lactating women or to children under 9 years of age. Homosexual males are *not* frequently coinfected with chlamydia, and therefore tetracyclines should be given only if concurrent chlamydial infection is found.
Source: Adapted from 1988 Canadian guidelines for the treatment of sexually transmitted diseases in neonates, children, adolescents, and adults. *Can. Dis. Weekly Rep.* 14S2:1, 1988.

**(2)** In children **over 9 years of age** use:
 **(a)** Tetracycline, 40 mg/kg/day PO divided q6h (maximum 500 mg) for 7 days *or*
 **(b)** Doxycycline, 5 mg/kg/day (maximum 100 mg bid) PO divided q12h for 7 days

**(3)** In **adolescents** use:
 **(a)** Tetracycline, 500 mg PO q6h for 7 days *or*
 **(b)** Doxycycline, 100 mg PO bid for 7 days

**3. Abscess**

 **a. Diagnosis.** An abscess may result from acute or subacute PID, often after suboptimal, delayed, or incorrect antibiotic therapy. It may present as acute PID or, if rupture occurs, septic shock. Bimanual and pelvirectal examination may reveal bilateral, unilateral, or cul-de-sac masses. Usually fever and leukocytosis are present. Ultrasound examination is often helpful in making the diagnosis.

 **b. Management.** Treat with the following antibiotics for appropriate polymicrobial coverage:
  **(1)** Penicillin G, 2–3 million units IV q4h *and*
  **(2)** Clindamycin, 600 mg IV q6h *and*
  **(3)** Gentamicin *or* tobramycin, 2 mg/kg IV, then 1.5 mg/kg q8h

**4. Chronic PID**

 **a. Diagnosis.** This is caused by sequelae of previous acute disease and does not involve active bacterial infection. It may be asymptomatic or may cause dysmenorrhea and dyspareunia. There may be masses secondary to hydrosalpinx or a complex of bowel, ovary, fallopian tube, and omentum.

 **b. Management.** Avoid use of antibiotics unless there is active inflammation. Analgesics may be necessary. Refer to a gynecologist for diagnosis and management.

**5. Cervicitis and urethritis**

 **a. Cervicitis**
  **(1) Diagnosis.** Common causes of cervicitis are Herpes simplex virus (HSV), gonorrhea, and *Chlamydia*. Patients may be asymptomatic, or there may be vaginitis, dyspareunia, and mild discomfort. The cervix may appear red and inflamed with a friable surface, or there may be ulceration, erosions, or mucopurulent secretions. The finding of more than 5 white blood cells per high-power field in a stained cervical secretion is virtually diagnostic.
  **(2) Management.** When STD is suspected, treat empirically as outlined in Table 21-5. If any lesions are seen on the cervix, arrange for follow-up with a gynecologist.

 **b. Urethritis**
  **(1) Diagnosis.** In females, urethritis is usually due to *Chlamydia* or gonoccocal infec-

tion, although *Trichomonas, Candida, Urea-plasma urealyticum,* and some viruses can cause urethral inflammation. Children may present with abdominal pain and dysuria, whereas adolescents complain of urethral discharge, dysuria, itch, or urethral discomfort unrelated to urination. Many infections are asymptomatic. In all cases the urine culture is negative.

(2) **Management.** Obtain a urine sample for urinalysis and urine culture. If there has been a discharge but none is available for culture, perform a urethral swab (2–3 cm into urethra) and test for *Chlamydia* and gonorrhea. Treat empirically for gonorrhea and *Chlamydia.*

## II. Other forms of STD

A. **Syphilis.** Suspect syphilis in all patients with genital lesions. Take wet smears of the area for dark-field microscopy, and draw blood for a VDRL test (reactive within 3 weeks of chancre appearance) or an FTA-ABS test. Most cases can be treated with penicillin. See the latest CDC recommendations and Table 21-7 for treatment.

B. **Chancroid and lymphogranuloma venereum.** In North America these diseases are rare outside of the southeastern United States. The usual presentation is an ulcerative genital infection, often with fever, inguinal adenopathy, and malaise. Treatment is achieved with erythromycin, 50 mg/kg/day PO (maximum 2 gm) di-

**Table 21-7. Treatment of syphilis**

| Type of syphilis | Preferred treatment | Alternative treatment* |
|---|---|---|
| Primary, secondary, or latent of < 1 year's duration | Benzathine penicillin G 50,000 units/kg (max. 2.4 MU) IM in single dose | Tetracycline, 500 mg PO q6h for 15 days; in children under 9 years old desensitization and use of penicillin is preferred. **OR** erythromycin, 40 mg/kg/day (max. dose 500 mg) PO divided q6h for 15 days |

*For alternative drugs see latest CDC report.
Source: Adapted from 1988 Canadian guidelines for the treatment of sexually transmitted diseases in neonates, children, adolescents, and adults. *Can. Dis. Weekly Rep.* 14S2:1, 1988.

vided q6h or trimethoprim-sulfamethoxasole, 8 mg/kg/day (maximum 320 mg) PO as trimethoprim divided q12h.

**C. AIDS.** The child with STD is at increased risk for acquired immune deficiency syndrome. In the older child or adolescent, persistent fever, night sweats, weight loss of more than 10%, generalized lymphadenopathy, persistent cough, fatigue, diarrhea, or frequent or unusual infections (*Candida,* persistent pneumonia) should raise suspicion of AIDS. The diagnosis can often be supported by finding leukopenia on a differential count. Follow local hospital protocols for antibody testing and exposure prevention.

**D. Herpes simplex virus (HSV).** Vulvar infection causes burning pain followed by vesicles and a weeping red eruption. Pain may be intense. Cervicitis is often asymptomatic. In primary infections, viremia may cause constitutional illness with fever, headache, myalgia, and meningismus. Meningitis is a rare complication. Treat first infections with acyclovir, 200 mg PO 2–5 times daily in adolescents. Severe or complicated infections should be treated with intravenous acyclovir, 5 mg/kg q8h.

**E. *Chlamydia trachomatis* or *Ureaplasma urealyticum.*** See sec. **I.B.2** above.

**F. *Trichomonas vaginalis*** (see Chap. 18, sec. **II**). *Trichomonas* causes leukorrhea and irritation in the female. Both partners should be treated with single-dose metronidazole, 2 gm PO.

**G. Congenital and anal warts.** See Chap. 18, sec. **II.**

**III. Disposition.** Admit all patients with severe deep pelvic pain or evidence of peritonitis.

**IV. Key points**

**A.** Due to poor compliance, most adolescents with PID require hospitalization for therapy.

**B.** *Chlamydia* causes subacute pelvic infection that may result in subsequent infertility and ectopic pregnancy. Maintain a high index of suspicion.

**C.** Report cases to public health authorities to enable tracing and treatment of contacts.

### Bibliography

Huffman, J. W., Dewhurst, C. J., and Capraro, V. J. *The Gynecology of Childhood and Adolescence.* Philadelphia: Saunders, 1981.

Treatment of sexually transmitted diseases. *Med. Lett.* 30(757): 5–11, 1988.

Reese, R. E., and Douglas, R. G. D. *A Practical Approach to Infectious Diseases* (2nd ed.). Boston: Little, Brown, 1986.

# Neurologic Disorders

## Seizures
Kevin Farrell and Gregory A. Baldwin

Most seizures will have stopped by the time the child reaches the emergency department; in general, if the seizure persists, the child is, for operational purposes, in status epilepticus (see Chap. 22, Status Epilepticus).

## I. Diagnosis and assessment
**A. History.** Take the history from a witness. Determine the circumstances, prodrome, focality, duration, postictal state, and frequency of seizure(s). In the child with a previous history of seizures, ask about medications, recent blood levels, and compliance. In the child without prior seizures, inquire about headaches, recent immunization, head injury, toxic ingestion, infection, family history, perinatal history, development, and past medical history.

**B. Examination.** Perform a full physical examination including a complete neurologic assessment. Look for signs of acute disease including focal neurologic deficits, signs of increased intracranial pressure (see Chap. 22, Increased Intracranial Pressure), and neck stiffness. Measure vital signs and look for evidence of trauma or dysmorphic features. Examine the skin for neurocutaneous abnormalities (adenoma sebaceum, café-au-lait spots, ash-leaf spot, facial hemangioma or angiofibroma).

## II. Afebrile seizures
**A. Etiology.** In most children who present with a first afebrile seizure, no cause is found. In the **known epileptic,** poor medication compliance and intercurrent infection are common etiologic factors. **Congenital abnormalities** of the brain such as cerebral dysgenesis and perinatal hypoxic-ischemic brain injury should be suspected in the child with dysmorphic features, developmental delay, cerebral palsy, or a history of encephalopathy in the first days of life. Additional **less common causes** to be considered include accidental and nonaccidental trauma, hypertension, toxic ingestion, hypoglycemia, and electrolyte abnormalities (calcium, sodium, magnesium).

**B. Management**
1. In the **well child with no focal signs** obtain blood for Dextrostix examination and arrange for an outpatient electroencephalogram (EEG) and follow-up. Other tests, including a CT scan and blood for measurement of calcium, magnesium, electrolytes, BUN, CBC, culture, or anticonvulsant levels, can be ordered when indicated by the history or physical examination.

2. If the **seizure is prolonged (> 10 minutes) or focal, or if there are focal neurologic signs** following the seizure, consult with a neurologist.
3. Advise parents that many children have only a single afebrile seizure. The risk of subsequent seizures is higher in the child with a family history of epilepsy, a prolonged or focal first seizure, an abnormal neurologic examination, or epileptiform activity on the EEG. For advice on counseling of parents see sec. **IIIB.4.**

## III. Febrile seizures

**A. History.** Febrile seizures are common and usually occur early in the course of febrile illnesses. They occur most often in children between 6 months and 3 years of age and are rare after 6 years of age. There may be a family history of febrile seizures. The risk of recurrent febrile seizures is 50% if the child is less than 1 year of age at the time of the first seizure, and 30% if the child is older. Consider other causes of fever and seizure before assuming that the patient has a simple febrile seizure; **CNS infections including bacterial meningitis should be considered in every seizure patient, particularly if it is the first seizure.**

**B. Management**

1. **Fever control.** Control fever with acetaminophen, 10–15 mg/kg PO, and observe the child for a period in the emergency room. A child who is happily playing hours after the seizure is unlikely to have serious underlying disease.

2. **Examination.** Examine the child for a focus of infection. Signs of CNS infection include a decreased level of consciousness, irritability, and neck stiffness. Search for evidence of increased intracranial pressure or focal neurologic abnormality.

3. **Investigations**

   **a. Blood work.** The otherwise well child with a first febrile seizure requires a Dextrostix measurement only. Other blood work, including measurement of serum electrolytes, BUN, calcium, and magnesium, are seldom helpful unless they are indicated by history or physical examination. A CBC and blood culture should be obtained in the child under 2 years of age with a rectal temperature greater than 39.0°C and no detectable focus of infection, and in children who appear "toxic" (see Chap. 21, Bacteremia).

   **b. Lumbar puncture.** In general, lumbar puncture should be performed in children with a first febrile seizure in the following situations: (1) in patients aged less than 18 months, (2) when CNS infection is suspected. An experienced clinician may elect to forego the lumbar puncture in a child who appears perfectly well after a period of observation. If a lumbar puncture is not performed, parents must be counseled about the signs and symptoms of CNS infection, and follow-up should be arranged in 12–24 hours.

    **c. EEG.** An EEG is of little value in the management of the child with a febrile seizure—it is not predictive of the risk for recurrence of febrile or afebrile seizures.

  **4. Counseling.** Most parents are terrified by a first seizure and fear that their child will die. Reassure them that less than 3% of patients with febrile seizures will develop epilepsy, although about 30% will have a recurrence of the febrile seizure. Advise them to position the seizing child on cushions or pillows in the Trendelenburg position on the left side, away from hard or dangerous objects. They should not force the child's mouth open to control the airway or put anything in the mouth. If the seizure lasts less than 5 minutes, they should call their doctor for advice. If it persists beyond 5 minutes, the child should be taken to the hospital immediately. Counsel them about fever control with subsequent illnesses and instruct them to return to the hospital if there is a decreased level of consciousness, increased irritability, or neck stiffness. A written handout is often valuable in such circumstances.

**IV. Disposition.** Children with CNS infection (meningitis, encephalitis), toxic ingestion, head injury, or systemic or metabolic disease causing seizures should be admitted. Most children with febrile seizures who appear well may be discharged following counseling of the parents. Admit children with prolonged, atypical, or multiple seizures. On some occasions, children must be admitted to allay parental anxiety.

**V. Key points**

  **A.** In general, a Dextrostix measurement is the only immediate investigation required in children with a first simple febrile seizure.

  **B.** Consider the diagnosis of meningitis in all children with a first febrile seizure.

**Bibliography**

Bettis, D. B., and Ater, S. B. Febrile seizures: Emergency department diagnosis and treatment. *J. Emerg. Med.* 2:341, 1985.

Joffe, A., McCormick, M., and DeAngelis, C. Which children with febrile seizures need lumbar puncture? *Am. J. Dis. Child.* 137:1153, 1983.

Vining, E. P. G., and Freeman, J. M. Management of nonfebrile seizures. *Pediatr. Rev.* 8:185, 1986.

## Status Epilepticus
Kevin Farrell

Status epilepticus (SE) is defined as a prolonged seizure lasting 30 minutes or more or recurrent seizures without interictal recovery of consciousness. Tonic-clonic SE is the most common type, although other types of seizures may progress to SE. Tonic-clonic SE occurs in 1–5% of patients with epilepsy and has a mortality of up to 10%. Death may occur owing to medical complications, overmedication, or the underlying disease. Status epilepticus lasting longer than 30 minutes may be associated with a permanent neurologic handicap.

### I. Diagnosis and assessment
**A. History and examination** (also see Chap. 22, Seizures, above). The initial history and physical examination must not delay management. Important points in the history include the occurrence of previous seizures, head trauma, febrile illness, exposure to drugs and toxins, and antiepileptic medication compliance and timing of the last dose. Causes that are common or for which specific treatment is available include bacterial meningitis, encephalitis, a sudden reduction in antiepileptic drug dosage, and hypoglycemia.

**B. Investigations**
  **1. Blood.** Obtain blood specimens for Dextrostix evaluation and measurement of serum glucose, serum electrolytes, calcium, magnesium, liver enzymes, levels of antiepileptic drugs, blood gases, and a complete blood count.
  **2. Lumbar puncture.** The child is usually comatose immediately after an episode of status epilepticus, making it difficult to exclude the presence of raised intracranial pressure. If bacterial meningitis is suspected, begin antibiotic treatment immediately after drawing a sample for a blood culture (see Chap. 21, Bacterial Meningitis). The lumbar puncture should be postponed until there is an improvement in the level of consciousness and reasonable evidence exists that intracranial pressure is not increased.
  **3. X rays.** A CT scan should be considered in children with persistent focal neurologic abnormalities or signs of raised intracranial pressure.

### II. Management (see Table 22-1)
**A. Resuscitation**
  **1.** Assess vital signs, maintain the airway, and administer oxygen. In general, do not place an oral airway in the patient during a seizure; this may result in oral injury and vomiting. The child should be positioned head down on the left side to avoid aspiration.
  **2.** Start an intravenous line and obtain blood specimens (see sec. **I.B.1,** above).
  **3.** If the Dextrostix reading is less than 2.2 mmol/liter (40 mg/dl), give a bolus of intravenous dextrose: 2.5

**Table 22-1. Management of status epilepticus**

1. Assess vital signs and maintain airway
2. Establish an intravenous line and draw blood for Dextrostix evaluation and measurement of glucose, electrolytes, and calcium levels, liver enzymes, CBC, and antiepileptic drug levels
3. If Dextrostix reading is less than 2.2 mmol/liter (40 mg/dl) give IV dextrose as follows: newborn: 2.5 ml/kg of 10% D/W; child: 1.0 ml/kg of 25% D/W. Follow with dextrose infusion (see Chap. 13, Hypoglycemia)
4. IV diazepam/lorazepam
5. IV phenytoin
6. IV phenobarbital*
7. Paraldehyde/lidocaine*

*An anesthesist should be called if the patient has been in tonic-clonic status epilepticus for 25 minutes or more.

ml/kg of 10% dextrose in water in the newborn and 1 ml/kg of 25% dextrose in water in the child, followed by an infusion (see Chap. 13, Hypoglycemia).
  **B. Anticonvulsant treatment**
    **1. Principles of anticonvulsant therapy**
      **a.** Intravenous **diazepam** or **lorazepam** acts rapidly and should be used in the initial treatment of status epilepticus.
      **b.** Because of the short duration of action of diazepam, a longer acting medication such as phenytoin (preferred) or phenobarbital should be given immediately following its administration.
      **c.** If the seizure persists for more than 25 minutes, consult an anesthesiologist when possible for intubation and use of general anesthetic agents.
    **2. Medications** (see Table 22-2)
      **a. Diazepam.** If there is difficulty obtaining intravenous access, administer diazepam rectally with a syringe attached to a shortened 4F or 5F feeding tube. Peak serum concentrations of the drug are achieved immediately following its administration by the intravenous route and in 4–10 minutes following administration by the rectal route. Diazepam may be associated with respiratory depression—this is more likely to occur in infants, in children with increased intracranial pressure, and in patients who have received phenobarbital.
        **(1)** Dosage
          **(a)** Intravenous—0.3 mg/kg up to a maximum of 10 mg given over 2 minutes by slow push. This dose may be repeated once after 10 minutes.
          **(b)** Rectal—0.5 mg/kg up to a maximum of

**Table 22-2. Antiepileptic drugs for treatment of status epilepticus**

| Name | Loading dose | Route | Loading duration | Maintenance dose |
|---|---|---|---|---|
| Diazepam | 0.3 mg/kg | IV | 2 min | — |
|  | 0.5 mg/kg | rectal | bolus | — |
| Lorazepam | 0.05 mg/kg | IV | 2 min | — |
| Phenytoin | 18 mg/kg | IV | 20 min | Infant: 10 mg/kg/day Child: 8 mg/kg/day |
| Phenobarbital | 10–15 mg/kg | IV | 15 min | 5 mg/kg/day |
| Paraldehyde | 0.3 ml/kg | rectal | bolus |  |
|  | 2.0 ml/kg of 10% sol'n | IV | slow bolus | 0.5 ml/kg/hr of 4% solution |
| Lidocaine | 3 mg/kg | IV | <25 mg/min | 5–10 mg/kg/hr |

10 mg. This dose may be repeated once after 10 minutes.

**b. Lorazepam.** Lorazepam is distributed less rapidly than diazepam and has a longer duration of action—up to 8 hours. Peak serum concentrations are achieved immediately following intravenous administration. However, lorazepam parenteral solution is slowly absorbed when administered by the rectal route.

(1) Dosage

(a) Intravenous—0.05 mg/kg up to a maximum of 2 mg diluted in an equal volume of normal saline or 5% dextrose in water, given by IV push over 2 minutes. May be repeated once in 15 minutes.

**c. Phenytoin.** Phenytoin is preferred over phenobarbital as a long-acting anticonvulsant: in the therapeutic range it has no significant effect on higher mental function, and it is less likely to cause respiratory depression. Because it may precipitate in dextrose solution, phenytoin should be given in normal or half normal saline. It can cause cardiac dysrhythmias and hypotension in patients with cardiac disease. The therapeutic range for predose serum levels is 40–80 μmol/liter (10–20 μg/ml).

(1) Dosage

(a) The loading dose is 18 mg/kg, administered intravenously in normal saline over 20 minutes. The total dose should not exceed 1000 mg.

(b) Maintenance dose is 5–10 mg/kg/day IV or PO, given every 8 hours. Children under 1 year of age may require a larger dose. The serum level should be measured 1 hour after administration of the loading dose and the maintenance dose commenced when it is estimated that the serum level will have fallen to 60 μmol/liter (15 μg/ml). Blood levels should be monitored frequently.

**d. Phenobarbital.** Phenobarbital may be associated with respiratory depression when it is given intravenously, particularly if the child has received diazepam. It has a profound effect on mental status, making it difficult to interpret an altered level of consciousness. The therapeutic range for predose serum levels is 65–170 μmol/liter (15–40 μg/ml).

(1) Dosage

(a) The loading dose is 10–15 mg/kg given intravenously over 10–15 minutes. In patients already taking phenobarbital, the loading dose is 5 mg/kg. Serum levels should be measured 1 hour after loading.

        **(b)** Maintenance dose is 3–5 mg/kg/day given at 12-hour intervals.

    **e. Paraldehyde.** The pharmacokinetic characteristics of paraldehyde are not well understood in children. The rectal route is the safest method of administration. Intravenously administered paraldehyde may cause cardiorespiratory depression and thrombophlebitis. It is contraindicated in patients with renal, liver, or lung disease. Paraldehyde should not be given in plastic syringes or bags, and intravenous sets containing the drug must be protected from the light.

      **(1)** Dosage

        **(a)** Rectal—0.3 ml/kg (maximum 5 ml) of 1 gm/ml of paraldehyde solution mixed with an equal volume of mineral oil.

        **(b)** Intravenous

          **(i)** To give a **loading dose,** make up a 10% solution by diluting 1 gm/ml of paraldehyde solution 9 : 1 with normal saline. Administer 2 ml/kg slowly (200 mg/kg).

          **(ii)** For the **maintenance infusion,** make up a 4% solution by adding 20 ml of 1 gm/ml paraldehyde solution to 500 ml of normal saline. Begin the infusion at a rate of 0.5 ml/kg/hour (20 mg/kg/hour) and titrate according to clinical response.

    **f. Lidocaine.** Lidocaine may induce dysrhythmias and hypotension, and vital signs should be assessed frequently during administration. Lidocaine is not currently recommended for treatment of seizures in children in the United States.

      **(1)** Dosage. An intravenous bolus of 3 mg/kg is given at a rate no faster than 25 mg/minute. The effect of the bolus will last only 20–30 minutes, and a constant intravenous infusion at a rate of 5–10 mg/kg/hour may be required for up to 3 days. Blood pressure and heart rhythm should be monitored frequently during the infusion.

    **g. General anesthesia.** Permanent brain injury may occur if tonic-clonic status epilepticus persists for longer than 30 minutes. When possible, the intensive care unit and the anesthesia department should be informed when the duration of status epilepticus is 25 minutes or more. This may occur soon after arrival in the emergency department in children with a lengthy transport time. Following intubation and ventilation, muscle relaxants and a short-acting barbiturate such as pentobarbital or thiopental may be given.

**C. Treatment of the underlying cause** is especially relevant in cases of hypoglycemia, hypo- or hypernatremia, hypocalcemia, hypomagnesemia, toxic ingestion, meningitis, or herpes simplex encephalitis. See Chaps. 13, 21, 23, and 27.

**D. Prevention or correction of complications**

1. **Acidosis.** Severe metabolic acidosis is often present with prolonged status epilepticus. This may contribute to the difficulty of controlling the seizure and may aggravate cerebral damage. Acidosis should be partially corrected using intravenous sodium bicarbonate if the pH is 7.2 or less (see Chap. 23, Acid-Base Disturbances).

2. **Hypoglycemia.** Hypoglycemia may occur with prolonged status epilepticus; serum glucose level should be monitored and the patient maintained on an infusion of 10% dextrose in water.

3. **Positioning.** Prevent pulmonary aspiration and traumatic injury by placing the child in a bed with cushioned rails, in the Trendelenburg position on the left side.

4. **Other measures.** Rare complications of status epilepticus include cardiac dysrhythmias, hypertension, pulmonary edema, hyperthermia, disseminated intravascular coagulation, myoglobinuria, and renal failure.

**III. Disposition.** Admit all patients with status epilepticus to an intensive care unit.

**IV. Key points**

A. Seizures lasting for more than 30 minutes may require the skills of specialists in anesthesia and neurology; consult early when possible.

B. Most cases of status epilepticus occur in known epileptics with inadequate medication levels.

C. Treatment with intravenous diazepam and phenytoin is usually effective in terminating seizures.

**Bibliography**

Camfield, P. R. Treatment of status epilepticus in children. *Can. Med. Assoc. J.* 128:671, 1983.

Curless, R. G., Holzman, B. H., and Ramsay, R. E. Paraldehyde therapy in childhood status epilepticus. *Arch. Neurol.* 40:477, 1983.

Delgado-Escueta, A. V., Wasterlain, C., Treiman, D. M., et al. Current concepts in neurology: Management of status epilepticus. *N. Engl. J. Med.* 306:1337, 1982.

# Coma
Kevin Farrell

Coma is a state of psychologic unresponsiveness in which the subject lies with eyes closed. Coma may be caused by diffuse lesions of both cerebral hemispheres or by lesions involving the pons, midbrain, or thalamus.

I. **Diagnosis and assessment.** Determine the type of coma by clinical assessment (Table 22-3). Ninety-five percent of cases of coma in children are due to nonstructural insults. Supratentorial or subtentorial structural lesions are uncommon causes but usually require immediate treatment.

A. **History.** Ask about trauma, seizures, past medical history, and exposure to medications, alcohol, and toxins. Recent fever suggests CNS infection (meningitis, encephalitis) or postinfectious encephalopathy (Reye's syndrome, postinfectious encephalomyelitis).

B. **Physical examination.** The primary goal of examination of the comatose child is to differentiate between structural (subtentorial or supratentorial) causes of coma, which may require urgent surgery, and nonstructural insults that may be amenable to medical therapy.

   1. **Neurologic examination**
      a. Level of consciousness. Measure and follow the level of consciousness using the Glasgow coma scale (see Table 41-1). Rapid and progressive worsening of condition may indicate cerebral herniation from a structural lesion.
      b. Eye signs
         (1) Fundi. Examine the fundi for papilledema and hemorrhage. **The absence of papilledema does not exclude the presence of increased intracranial pressure.**
         (2) Pupils. A unilateral, fixed, and dilated pupil may be due to uncal herniation due to a hemispheric mass lesion. A neurosurgeon should be consulted immediately. Rarely, a fixed dilated pupil may be due to a seizure or the use of mydriatic eye drops. Symmetric small pupils that respond to light suggest a metabolic cause of coma.
         (3) Extraocular movements. Test the eye movements using the doll's head maneuver or the cold caloric test (the eyes should move toward the ear being irrigated). Sixth nerve palsy suggests raised intracranial pressure.
      c. Other signs. In the infant, palpate the fontanel with the trunk and head in the upright position. Examination of brain stem reflexes and the motor system can help to diagnose the type of coma (see Table 22-3). Lateralizing motor signs (asymmetric reflexes, tone, response to pain) suggest a structural lesion.
   2. **General examination**
      a. Vital signs. Observe the respiration pattern. Hyperventilation may occur with metabolic acidosis, salicylate toxicity, or Reye's syndrome. Cheyne-Stokes respirations suggest bilateral hemisphere dysfunction. Hypertension may be due to renal disease, intoxication, or raised intracranial pressure.
      b. General signs. Determine if there is fever, neck stiffness, or other signs of CNS infection (see

**Table 22-3. Causes of coma**

| Type of coma | Examples | Clinical features |
|---|---|---|
| **Nonstructural insult** | | |
| | Meningitis, encephalitis | Alteration of consciousness, absence of lateralizing signs, preservation of pupil response, absence of conjugate deviation of eyes or dysconjugate gaze |
| | Cardiorespiratory arrest, hypothermia, hypotension | |
| | Seizure or post seizure, Reye's syndrome, hemolytic uremic syndrome, poisoning, dehydration, electrolyte disturbance, organ failure (renal, respiratory, liver) | |
| | Inborn errors of metabolism | |
| **Structural lesions** | | |
| *Supratentorial lesions* | | |
| | Trauma (accidental and nonaccidental), tumor, abscess, hemorrhage, infarction | Alteration of consciousness Focal motor signs are highly suggestive Conjugate eye deviation or dysconjugate gaze Unreactive or unequal pupillary response to light. |
| *Subtentorial lesions* | | |
| | Tumor, infarction, hemorrhage (posterior fossa, subdural, arteriovenous malformation) | Early brain stem dysfunction Dysfunction of ocular motility Abnormal respiratory pattern |

Chap. 21). Examine the child for signs of trauma such as bruising, laceration, hematoma, and hemotympanum. Petechiae or bleeding suggests a bleeding disorder.

**C. X ray and laboratory investigations**

1. **Laboratory tests.** When a diffuse brain insult is suspected, obtain blood specimens for culture and measurement of serum glucose, electrolytes, blood urea nitrogen, AST (SGOT), ammonia, toxic screen, blood gases, and a complete blood count and platelet count. Obtain urine specimens for urinalysis, toxic screen, and culture. In the infant with undiagnosed coma, plasma amino acids and urine organic acids should be measured.

2. **Lumbar puncture.** It is difficult to exclude the presence of raised intracranial pressure in the comatose patient. **Do not perform a lumbar puncture prior to consulting a neurologist.**

3. **Electroencephalogram** (EEG). An EEG may show characteristic abnormalities in metabolic coma, poisoning, and herpes simplex encephalitis.

4. **CT scan.** A CT head scan is indicated when a supratentorial or subtentorial structural lesion is suspected. A normal scan does not exclude the presence of cerebral edema or raised intracranial pressure.

**II. Management of the comatose child.** A neurosurgical or neurologic consultation should be obtained if there is uncertainty about the diagnosis or management.

**A.** Maintain the airway and ensure adequate ventilation. If the child is hypoventilating or if there is evidence of increased intracranial pressure, intubate and ventilate the child (see Chap. 22, Increased Intracranial Pressure).

**B.** Consult a neurosurgeon immediately if a structural lesion is suspected.

**C.** Control blood pressure (see Chap. 23, Hypertension).

**D.** Start an intravenous line and draw blood for investigations (see sec. **I.C.1,** above).

**E.** Check a Dextrostix for blood glucose concentration. If the reading is low, administer an intravenous bolus of glucose: 2.5 ml/kg of 10% dextrose in water in the newborn and 1 ml/kg of 25% dextrose in water in the child, followed by an infusion (see Chap. 13, Hypoglycemia).

**F.** In the child in whom poisoning is suspected, administer intravenous naloxone, 0.01 mg/kg; if this is ineffective, repeat with 0.1 mg/kg (see Chap. 27).

**G.** If bacterial meningitis is suspected, draw a blood specimen for culture and commence antibiotic treatment (see Chap. 21, Bacterial Meningitis).

**H.** If herpes simplex encephalitis is suspected, obtain an EEG and begin antiviral therapy with acyclovir (see Chap. 21, Encephalitis).

**III. Disposition.** Admit all patients with coma.

**IV. Key points**

**A.** In children 95% of coma cases have a nonstructural etiology.

B. Do not perform a lumbar puncture in children with coma except under the supervision of a neurologist or neurosurgeon.

### Bibliography

Plum, F., and Posner, J. B. *The Diagnosis of Stupor and Coma.* Philadelphia: F. A. Davis, 1982.

## Headache
Kevin Farrell

Headache in most children is due to tension or migraine headache. Serious intracranial disorders, while uncommon, must always be excluded.

I. **Diagnosis and assessment**
   A. **History.** Determine the onset, location, severity, prodrome, and precipitating or relieving factors. Ask about a past history of headache, recent trauma, visual disturbance, nausea or vomiting, and family history. A headache that awakens the patient at night, is most frequent in the morning, and is relieved by vomiting suggests raised intracranial pressure. Posterior fossa tumors often cause occipital headache.
   B. **Examination.** Look for signs of raised intracranial pressure such as papilledema or sixth nerve palsy (see Chap. 22, Increased Intracranial Pressure). Determine whether there is neck stiffness and measure the vital signs including the blood pressure. Suspect an underlying structural lesion in the patient with focal neurologic signs or ataxia. In the afebrile child, headache with meningismus may be associated with subarachnoid hemorrhage, posterior fossa tumor, or leukemic meningitis. Examine the sinuses, teeth, and ears for a source of referred pain.
   C. **Investigations.** The majority of children with headache require no investigation. In other children, tests should be ordered according to the working diagnosis and may include a complete blood count (CBC), BUN, urinalysis, sinus x rays, and CT scan. In the afebrile patient with headache, lumbar puncture should not be performed prior to CT head scan or consultation with a neurologist or neurosurgeon. Order a CT scan if there are focal signs, ataxia, evidence of increased intracranial pressure, or suspicion of subarachnoid hemorrhage.
II. **Causes of headache**
   A. **Febrile illnesses causing headache**
      1. **Systemic febrile illnesses** such as bacteremia, streptococcal pharyngitis, and enteroviral or influenza infection often cause headache.
      2. **Extracranial infections** such as otitis media, sinusitis, and dental pain may be associated with headache (see Chaps. 11 and 14).
      3. **Intracranial infection** due to meningitis must be

considered in any child with headache and meningismus. Meningismus may also be a false localizing sign in the febrile child with pneumonia, pharyngitis, or pyelonephritis.

**B. Afebrile illnesses**

1. **Migraine.** Migraine is a throbbing headache that is often localized to one or both frontal areas. The headache is often accompanied by nausea or vomiting, may be aggravated by bright light or noise, and is often helped by sleep. Migraine rarely wakes the patient during the night. A careful history will often reveal a history of similar headaches in a parent, sibling, or grandparent. The term classic migraine refers to headaches that are preceded by a visual aura (blurring, scotoma).

2. **Tension headache.** Tension headaches occur almost daily and often last most of the day. They rarely wake the child from sleep. The underlying source often lies in problems at school or at home; this history should be taken from the parents alone.

3. **Subarachnoid hemorrhage** (SAH) should be suspected if the headache has a sudden onset, especially when it is accompanied by neck stiffness. When possible, a CT scan should be obtained prior to a lumbar puncture. In the absence of CT scan facilities a lumbar puncture can be performed in such a child if there are no signs of increased intracranial pressure. SAH is suggested by the presence of blood in the cerebrospinal fluid (CSF) and xanthochromia in a freshly centrifuged specimen.

4. **Raised intracranial pressure** (ICP) should be suspected if the headaches are of recent onset, are increasing in severity, occur mainly at night or on waking, or are relieved by vomiting. Papilledema or focal neurologic signs are highly suggestive. These children require immediate neurologic consultation and CT scan.

   a. Raised ICP with a **normal CT scan** may be due to benign intracranial hypertension (BIH), leukemic meningitis, or Reye's syndrome. Patients with BIH are alert, have no focal neurologic signs (except for a false-localizing sixth nerve palsy in some cases), and may experience visual obscurations. Children with leukemic meningitis or Reye's syndrome usually have other signs of the disease (see Chap. 22, Reye's Syndrome).

   b. In general, **brain tumors** do not present with acute headache unless there has been hemorrhage into the tumor or sudden development of hydrocephalus.

   c. **Hydrocephalus** should be suspected if the patient has a ventricular shunt or "sun-setting" eyes.

5. **Trauma.** Trauma can cause headache by a variety of mechanisms.

   a. An acute progressive headache following head

trauma may be due to an acute extradural or subdural hematoma.

**b.** Headache may be related to an underlying skull fracture.

**c.** Occasionally acute severe headache following minor trauma may be a manifestation of posttraumatic migraine; this is a diagnosis of exclusion and should not be made without neurologic or neurosurgical consultation or CT scan.

**6. Other causes**

**a.** Street drugs such as amphetamines may cause an acute headache (see Chap. 27).

**b.** Hypertension is a rare but important cause of acute headache in children (see Chap. 23, Hypertension).

**c.** Arteriovenous malformation in childhood usually presents with subarachnoid hemorrhage or seizures. Headaches are an uncommon feature.

**III. Management.** In general, treatment should focus on the disease causing the headache and on providing suitable analgesia. Children with migraine or tension headaches often benefit from rest in a quiet, dark room.

**IV. Disposition.** Admit children with a serious underlying cause of headache.

**V. Key points**

**A.** Migraine is a common cause of headache in children.

**B.** Do not perform a lumbar puncture in the afebrile child with headache before consulting with a neurologist or neurosurgeon.

**Bibliography**

Kandt, R. S., and Levine, R. M. Headache and acute illness in children. *J. Child Neurol.* 2:22, 1987.

---

# Ataxia
## Kevin Farrell

Ataxia is an abnormality of coordination and balance. It may be caused by dysfunction of the vestibular apparatus, cerebellum, central white matter, posterior columns, or peripheral nerve or muscle. Most cases are due to intoxication or viral infection.

**I. Diagnosis and assessment.** In all instances, ask about trauma, toxic ingestion, and signs and symptoms of recent viral infection. A careful neurologic examination should demonstrate the anatomic basis for the ataxia and look for signs of increased intracranial pressure.

**A.** Children with **vestibular dysfunction** and labyrinthitis often have vertigo. The child may appear very ill during an attack and refuses to move. Nystagmus is common.

**B. Cerebellar ataxia** may be associated with intention tremor, a wide-based staggering gait, and nystagmus.

C. An **intracranial tumor** may be associated with signs of increased intracranial pressure.

D. Children with **posterior column abnormalities** (Friedreich's ataxia) and **peripheral neuropathies** usually have an abnormal sensory examination, although some children with acute postinfectious polyneuropathy (Guillain-Barré syndrome) present with only weakness and decreased stretch reflexes.

## II. Causes of ataxia

### A. Acute onset ataxia

1. Postinfectious cerebellar ataxia is often preceded by a viral illness such as chickenpox. There is truncal ataxia, and the muscle tone is slightly decreased. There are no lateralizing motor or sensory findings, and mental function is normal.

2. Intoxication with drugs (e.g., anticonvulsants, ethanol, antihistamines, phenothiazines, hypnotics). For associated signs and symptoms, refer to toxicologic information relevant to each of these drugs. In most cases there is an altered level of consciousness.

3. Postinfectious polyneuritis (Guillain-Barré syndrome). These children have areflexia with weakness. The majority develop sensory abnormalities.

4. Acute labyrinthitis (serous or suppurative) and acute vestibular neuronitis present with an acute onset of vertigo, usually following a viral illness. Children may also develop acute ataxia and vertigo following labyrinthine trauma.

5. Less common causes of acute ataxia include head trauma, heat stress, CNS infection (meningitis, encephalitis), acute hydrocephalus (aqueduct stenosis and posterior fossa tumors), occult neuroblastoma, multiple sclerosis, and posterior fossa subdural or epidural hematoma.

### B. Acute intermittent ataxia

1. **Basilar migraine.** Suspect this disorder if the episodes are accompanied by headache or vomiting and there is a family history of migraine.

2. **Benign paroxysmal vertigo of childhood.** This condition presents with recurrent episodes of ataxia and vomiting of abrupt onset and occurs in children under 5 years of age. The duration of each episode is usually less than 5 minutes. For a further description of the clinical presentation see sec. **I.A,** above.

3. **Autosomal dominant familial cerebellar ataxia.** This is a rare disorder, and there is usually a positive family history.

4. **Metabolic disorders** (maple syrup urine disease, Hartnup's disease). These are rare diseases that present in early childhood.

5. **Myoclonic seizures.** Intermittent ataxia may precede the onset of the seizure.

### C. Chronic progressive ataxia. Chronic progressive ataxia is rare. The causes of this form of ataxia include posterior fossa tumor, system degeneration (Friedreich's ataxia),

ataxia-telangiectasia, hereditary neuropathies, and metabolic disorders.

### III. Management

**A.** If **acute ataxia** occurs in a patient with **raised intracranial pressure, cranial nerve abnormalities,** or **long tract signs** (extensor plantar response, hemiparesis), urgent investigation with CT scan is indicated to exclude a posterior fossa mass.

**B.** When **intoxication** (ethanol, barbiturates, phenytoin) is suspected, obtain serum and urine samples for a toxic screen.

**C.** In all cases of **persistent** ataxia, consult a neurologist and admit the patient to the hospital.

### IV. Disposition. Admit all patients with persistent or undiagnosed ataxia.

### V. Key points

**A.** Ataxia associated with vertigo is suggestive of vestibular dysfunction or labyrinthitis.

**B.** Always rule out increased intracranial pressure and a space-occupying lesion in children with ataxia.

### Bibliography

Fleisher, G., and Ludwig, S. (eds.). *Textbook of Pediatric Emergency Medicine.* Baltimore: Williams & Wilkins, 1983.

## Acute Hemiparesis

Kevin Farrell

The sudden onset of hemiparesis or hemiplegia in a child is uncommon. Hemiparesis may be a transient phenomenon associated with seizures (Todd's paresis) or migraine, or it may be persistent when it is due to cerebral infarction or hemorrhage.

### I. Diagnosis and assessment

**A. History.** Enquire about the speed of onset, recent infections or immunizations, past medical history (heart disease, arteritis, sickle cell disease), and whether the child has had a fever or seizures.

**B. Neurologic examination.** The immediate assessment of the patient should include a careful neurologic examination to define the site of the lesion. Neck stiffness suggests meningitis or subarachnoid hemorrhage (SAH) (see Chap. 22, Headache), whereas a cranial bruit may indicate an arteriovenous malformation. Cranial bruits are commonly present in normal children up to the age of 5. Measure vital signs and look for evidence of congenital heart disease such as cyanosis, murmurs, or surgical scars.

### II. Causes of stroke. The differential diagnosis of stroke in children is best approached by considering whether it is related to a hemorrhagic or ischemic infarction. Hemorrhage can be rapidly diagnosed by a CT head scan (Fig. 22-1).

**A. Hemorrhagic stroke.** The most common causes of hemorrhagic stroke in children are trauma, arteriovenous malformation, aneurysms, bleeding into a tumor, and bleeding diatheses.

**B. Ischemic stroke**

1. **Acute infantile hemiplegia (AIH).** This idiopathic form of stroke occurs in children under 2 years of age and is frequently associated with coma, fever, and prolonged seizures. AIH is a diagnosis of exclusion. The hemiplegia is of rapid onset. Neurologic morbidity may be related to the duration of the seizures. Prompt treatment of the seizures is important (see Chap. 22, Status Epilepticus).

2. **Trauma.** In these patients there is usually a definite history of head trauma. Apparently minor trauma may occasionally result in extracranial carotid dissection and ischemic stroke.

3. **Congenital heart disease (CHD).** Strokes associated with CHD are more common in children under 2 years of age. Patients with cyanotic CHD are at highest risk, particularly if they are polycythemic or iron deficient.

4. **Infection.** Meningitis in children is frequently complicated by ischemic stroke secondary to underlying vasculitis. Brain abscess should be suspected in the child with hemiplegia and cyanotic heart disease who is over 2 years of age. Encephalitis due to enterovirus or herpes simplex virus can also result in stroke.

5. **Hematologic disorders.** Thrombotic disorders (including sickle cell disease) and bleeding diatheses must be excluded in all patients who present with stroke.

6. **Neurooncology.** Strokes may be related to an underlying brain tumor or malignancy. The stroke is usually slow in onset, and there may be signs and symptoms of increased intracranial pressure. The effects of chemotherapy, radiotherapy, or opportunistic infections in the immune-compromised host can also result in stroke.

7. **Arterial disorders.** The arteriopathies (polyarteritis nodosa [PAN], systemic lupus erythematosus [SLE]) that cause stroke in childhood primarily involve the large arteries. Occasionally, involvement of the medium and small vessels occurs, resulting in ischemic stroke.

**III. Causes of transient hemiparesis**

**A. Seizures.** Postictal or Todd's paresis is the most common cause of a transient hemiparesis. The arm is more severely affected than the leg, and both limbs are usually hypotonic. The hemiparesis resolves completely in most children within 2 days. Occasionally, hemiparesis may be an ictal manifestation.

**B. Hemiplegic migraine.** Hemiplegic migraine is a diagnosis of exclusion. It is suggested by a prior history of migraine or a history of headache with characteristic

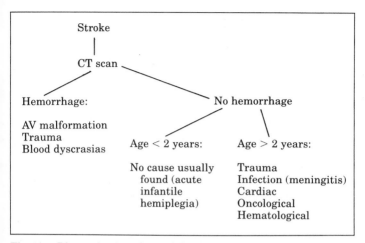

**Fig. 22-1. Diagnosis of stroke in children.**

features (see Chap. 22, Headache). There may be a family history of hemiplegic migraine.
  C. **Diabetes mellitus.** Children with diabetes may present with an acute hemiparesis that is transient. This often occurs during the night and may be related to a hypoglycemic episode.
IV. **Management**
  A. Assess and control the airway, breathing, and circulation and start an intravenous line.
  B. A CT scan should be performed to determine whether the patient has had a hemorrhagic or ischemic stroke. Initial laboratory investigations should include a complete blood count (CBC), platelet count, prothrombin time (PT), partial thromboplastin time (PTT), urinalysis, and measurements of electrolytes and serum glucose concentration. When indicated, draw blood for a sickle cell screen. Do not perform a lumbar puncture until a CT scan has been performed.
  C. In all cases, consult a neurologist or neurosurgeon and arrange for admission.
V. **Key points**
  A. Todd's or postictal paresis is the most common type of transient hemiparesis.
  B. Exclude cardiac abnormalities, hematologic disorders, and intracranial infection in all children with ischemic stroke.
  C. A CT head scan should be performed in all patients with a stroke.

**Bibliography**

Gold, A. P., and Carter, S. Acute hemiplegia of infancy and childhood. *Pediatr. Clin. North Am.* 23:413, 1976.

## Reye's Syndrome
Gregory A. Baldwin and Kevin Farrell

Reye's syndrome consists of an acute encephalopathy and fatty degeneration of viscera. It is frequently associated with varicella and influenza B infections in children. A statistical association between Reye's syndrome and salicylate ingestion during febrile illness has been shown.

I. **Diagnosis and assessment.** Typically the child has a history of severe vomiting, followed in 1–2 days by encephalopathy with stumbling gait, agitation, and combativeness. A decreasing level of consciousness is indicative of increased intracranial pressure (ICP). Progressive obtundation, coma, seizures, and hyperventilation may occur. The presentation in infancy is often different—seizures and respiratory symptoms (apnea, hyperventilation) are more common in this age group. Initial laboratory results usually show hypoglycemia, raised AST (SGOT), ALT (SGPT), and lactic dehydrogenase, a normal bilirubin level, a mixed metabolic acidosis and respiratory alkalosis, a serum ammonia level greater than 80 μmol/liter, and a prolonged prothrombin time (PT) and partial thromboplastin time (PTT). It is important to consider other metabolic disorders that may mimic Reye's syndrome; obtain blood specimens for measurement of plasma amino acids, lactate, and carnitine, and send a urine specimen for urinary organic acid measurement. Liver biopsy may be required for a definitive diagnosis.

II. **Management**
   A. Control problems in the airway, breathing, and circulation.
   B. Children with mild disease (lethargy, combativeness) require frequent monitoring. Start an intravenous line and give 10–20% dextrose in water to maintain a normal blood glucose level.
   C. Vital signs should be closely monitored for signs of increased intracranial pressure. Blood levels of glucose and gases should be measured hourly, and serum osmolality and PT should be determined every 12 hours. Serial neurologic assessment is important, including the Glasgow coma scale (see Chap. 41), pupil size and response, doll's eye response, caloric response, and respiratory rate. In most cases a CT scan and toxic screen are required to rule out other causes of a decreased level of consciousness.
   D. In the child with coma or suspected increased intracranial pressure, full brain resuscitation with intubation and hyperventilation is indicated (see Chap. 22, Increased Intracranial Pressure). Fluids should be restricted to 50% of maintenance while infusing a minimum of 0.4 gm/kg of dextrose per hour to maintain the serum glucose level and osmolality. The head should be elevated 30 degrees and positioned in the midline, and the child should be kept normothermic. Treat coagulop-

athy with vitamin K, 5–10 mg IV over 5–10 minutes, and fresh frozen plasma, 10 ml/kg IV. Treat seizures with intravenous phenytoin (see Chap. 22, Seizures).

**III. Disposition.** Admit all patients with suspected Reye's syndrome to an intensive care unit.

**IV. Key points**

**A.** Suspect Reye's syndrome in the child with acute encephalopathy.

**B.** Children with Reye's syndrome require careful management of raised intracranial pressure with fluid restriction, correct positioning, and often, intubation and hyperventilation.

**Bibliography**

Corey, L. Reye's syndrome: A clinical progression and evaluation of therapy. *Pediatrics* 60:708, 1977.

Hurwitz, E. S., et al. A national surveillance for Reye's syndrome: A five year review. *Pediatrics* 70:895, 1982.

Reye, R. D. K., et al. Encephalopathy and fatty degeneration of the viscera: A disease entity in childhood. *Lancet* 2:749, 1963.

---

# Increased Intracranial Pressure
David D. Cochrane

---

Increased intracranial pressure (ICP) is a neurologic emergency. Causes include head trauma (most common), meningitis, blocked shunt, space-occupying lesion (tumor, abscess, hemorrhage), Reye's syndrome, and benign intracranial hypertension. See Chaps. 19, 21, 22, and 41.

**I. Diagnosis and assessment**

**A. History.** The symptoms of increased ICP depend on the age of the patient and the speed of development of the lesion.

**1. In infancy,** because the skull can expand, the symptoms are nonspecific and usually develop gradually. There may be vomiting, mild fever, and alterations in behavior such as irritability, lethargy, or poor feeding. A bulging fontanel may be noted by the parents.

**2.** The child with a **closed fontanel** and elevated ICP may have a headache as well as irritability. Nausea and vomiting are common. Visual disturbances (blurring, strabismus), unsteadiness, and weakness may be present. Patients with aqueductal stenosis may present with Parinaud's syndrome (paralysis of conjugate upward movement of the eyes).

**3. Children with an intracranial tumor** often have a long history (weeks or months) of increasing vomiting, unsteadiness, and headache that is worse in the morning. Acute events such as hemorrhage from an arteriovenous malformation or tumor may present catastrophically with headache, vomiting, and altered level of consciousness.

4. In the **child with a shunt,** the family and old records are valuable sources of information. Inquire about the symptoms of previous episodes of shunt malfunction, the shunt type, and its components and location. Malfunction usually results in a decline in clinical status over a period of days, although hydrocephalus may cause a rapid deterioration. Infection should be suspected in the child with shunt malfunction, fever, and no detectable focus of infection.

5. Patients with **meningitis** often have fever or other signs of infectious disease (upper respiratory infection, rash). Older verbal children complain of neck stiffness and photophobia.

B. **Examination.** Perform a full neurologic examination. Test the patient for neck stiffness and cranial nerve function. Perform funduscopy to look for papilledema or absence of venous pulsations. Examine muscle strength and tone, sensation, and reflexes. Compare right and left sides, and look for eye signs or ataxia as evidence of a space-occupying lesion. Sudden deterioration or onset of focal signs may indicate brain herniation (see sec. **II.B,** below).

1. **The child.** Children with raised ICP may have an altered level of consciousness. Papilledema is often absent, but when seen it strongly suggests a diagnosis of tumor.

2. **The infant.** Tension in the fontanel is assessed with the child in an upright position. The head circumference should be recorded and compared with previous measurements or normal values for age.

3. **The child with a shunt.** Palpate the shunt tract. Subcutaneous fluid along the tract is always abnormal and may indicate a separation of the components or a distal obstruction. Occasionally, infants with newly inserted shunts have leakage of subgaleal fluid at the cranial insertion site—this does not necessarily indicate malfunction. Palpation or pumping of the reservoir is not a reliable test of function.

II. **Management.** For treatment of head trauma, Reye's syndrome, and meningitis, see Chaps. 41, 22, Reye's syndrome, and 21, Bacterial Meningitis. Management of the child with a shunt malfunction is presented in sec. **II.B.7,** below.

A. **The stable child**

1. Children who are not comatose, have no focal signs, and have stable vital signs are considered stable—papilledema is commonly present. Start an intravenous line and draw blood for a complete blood count (CBC), blood culture, and measurements of electrolytes and glucose level. Give oxygen by mask and keep the head elevated at 30 degrees in the midline. Place the child on a monitor and arrange for urgent computed tomography (CT) scan and neurosurgical consultation.

2. In the child with suspected shunt malfunction, per-

form a shunt tap (see sec. **II.B.7.a,** below). If there is evidence of infection on cerebrospinal fluid (CSF) laboratory examination (high protein level, white blood cell count often $> 100 \times 10^9$/liter, glucose level may be normal) or a strong suspicion of infection, treat the patient with intravenous vancomycin, 60 mg/kg/day divided q6h, and tobramycin, 5 mg/kg/day divided q8h. X rays of the shunt (skull, anteroposterior and lateral, chest and abdomen, anteroposterior) can help in the assessment of shunt integrity if the components are radioopaque. Consult a neurosurgeon in all cases of shunt malfunction.

**B. The unstable child.** Children with severe brain injury or suspected raised intracranial pressure and coma (including decerebrate and decorticate posturing), focal signs, seizures, or Cushing's triad (hypertension, bradycardia, slow or irregular breathing) require immediate therapy. When possible, get help from specialists in neurosurgery, intensive care, anesthesia, and neurology. A CT scan is mandatory.

1. **Hyperventilation.** Hyperventilation therapy is the most important aspect of treatment of the child with severely increased intracranial pressure. Controlled elective intubation should be performed under protection of atropine, pentothal, and muscular paralysis (see Chap. 1). Lidocaine, 1 mg/kg IV, should be given within 3 minutes prior to intubation, to blunt the associated rise in intracranial pressure. Keep the $PCO_2$ at 25–35 mm Hg, and the $PaO_2$ at 120–150 mm Hg.

2. **Paralysis.** Following intubation, maintain the child on a muscle relaxant such as pancuronium, 0.1 mg/kg IV q1–2h. Sedate with intravenous Valium (diazepam), 0.1 mg/kg IV 2–3h, and morphine 0.05 mg/kg IV q2–4h (or by infusion).

3. **Fluids.** Maintain circulating blood volume and blood pressure. If these are stable, restrict fluids to 50% of maintenance requirement (see Chap. 23, Fluids and Electrolytes). Monitor serum electrolytes every 4–6 hours and maintain normal serum osmolality. Insert a nasogastric tube (contraindicated in patients with basal skull fracture) and Foley catheter (for contraindications in patients with urethral trauma see Chap. 17).

4. **General considerations.** If spinal injury has been ruled out and circulatory status is controlled, elevate the head to 30 degrees and maintain it in the midline position. Maintain normothermia and treat seizures aggressively.

5. **Monitoring.** The child should be transferred to an intensive care unit for ventilation and monitoring. Consider installation of an intracranial pressure monitor.

6. **Mannitol.** Intravenous mannitol can be used to lower intracranial pressure temporarily if there is sudden deterioration in neurologic status. It is most

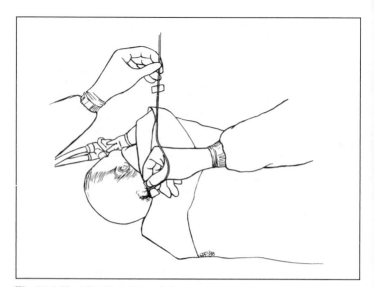

**Fig. 22-2. Ventriculoperitoneal shunt tap.**

effective in children with surgical lesions, shear hemorrhage, or contusion. Mannitol may worsen the condition of children with diffuse injury and brain swelling. The dose of mannitol is 0.25–1.0 gm/kg/dose IV. Insert a Foley catheter prior to administering mannitol.

7. **Shunt tap.** Severe acute shunt obstruction with advanced signs of increased ICP should be treated with rapid needle aspiration of the shunt reservoir in the case of a distal obstruction, or aspiration of one of the ventricles if there is a proximal obstruction.

  **a. Procedure** (Fig. 22-2)

    **(1) Ventricular shunt tap.** A shunt tap can determine the presence of infection as well as the patency and function of the system. Prior to the procedure, obtain all available information about the shunt. The reservoir is usually located in the posterior parietal, occipital, or posterior frontal regions.

    **(a) Equipment**

      **(i)** Lumbar puncture tray (see p. 251)

      **(ii)** 25 and 27 gauge butterfly needles with tubing

      **(iii)** Sterile gloves, gown, mask

      **(iv)** Povidone-iodine or 0.5% tincture of chlorhexidine antiseptic solution.

      **(v)** Razor

### (b) Method

(i) If necessary, have an assistant restrain the child. Parents are often comforting.

(ii) Palpate the location of the reservoir and tubing.

(iii) Shave a 3-cm diameter area around the reservoir. Using sterile technique, prepare the area over the reservoir 3 times with antiseptic solution and let dry. Place sterile drapes to isolate the puncture site.

(iv) Puncture the reservoir with a butterfly needle, entering the dome at least 45 degrees from the vertical. Be sure to remove the cap from the free end of the butterfly tubing.

(v) When the child has settled, hold the butterfly tubing vertically beside a ruler or attach it to a manometer to measure the pressure.

(vi) Patency of the system proximal to the point of puncture (ventricular catheter reservoir) is established by observing a free flow of CSF into the butterfly tubing.

(vii) Patency of the system distal to the puncture site is confirmed by finding an opening pressure within the limits of the valve (see the manufacturer's specifications). Distal patency can also be assessed by lowering the tubing until it fills with CSF, then raising it and observing runoff back into the shunt.

(viii) Obtain CSF specimens (0.5–1 ml each) for biochemical, cytologic, and bacteriologic analyses (see Lumbar Puncture - Meningitis).

(ix) Remove the needle, apply pressure and a Band Aid.

### (c) Complications

(i) Shunt or skin infection

(ii) Bleeding from scalp vessel

**III. Disposition.** Admit all patients with raised intracranial pressure to the intensive care unit.

**IV. Key points**

A. The signs of raised intracranial pressure in the infant are often subtle.

B. Children with raised intracranial pressure who are unstable require full brain resuscitation including intubation and ventilation.

C. Perform a shunt tap when malfunction or infection is suspected.

## Bibliography

Jennett, B., and Teasdale, G. *Management of Head Injuries.* Philadelphia: F. A. Davis, 1981.

Miller, J. D. Raised intracranial pressure and its effects on brain function. In A. Crockard, R. Hayward, and J. T. Hoff (eds.), *Neurosurgery, the Scientific Basis of Clinical Practice.* London: Blackwell Scientific Publications, 1985.

Pollay, M. Pathophysiology of cerebrospinal fluid circulation. In A. Crockard, R. Hayward, and J. T. Hoff (eds.), *Neurosurgery, the Scientific Basis of Clinical Practice.* London: Blackwell Scientific Publications, 1985.

Ward, J. D., Moulton, R. J., Muizelaar, J. P., et al. Cerebral hemostasis and protection. In F. P. Wirth, and R. A. Ratcheson (eds.), *Concepts in Neurosurgery* (Vol. 1). Baltimore: Williams and Wilkins, 1987.

# Renal Disorders

## Acute Renal Failure
David S. Lirenman

Acute renal failure may be defined as a sudden lowering or cessation of glomerular filtration rate (GFR) and subsequent loss of renal homeostasis (increased BUN and creatinine, acidosis, electrolyte abnormalities). Nearly all cases are reversible.

I. **Diagnosis and assessment.** The cause of acute decrease in GFR may be prerenal, due to impaired renal perfusion (the majority of cases), renal, due to direct insult to the kidney, or postrenal, due to obstructive uropathy (see Table 23-1). Normal urinary output in the child is approximately 2–4 ml/kg/hour. An output of less than 0.5 ml/kg/hour defines oliguria.

   A. **History**

      1. In children with **prerenal failure,** the cause is usually evident, as in trauma, gastroenteritis with dehydration, and septic shock.

      2. Children with **postrenal failure** may present with pyelonephritis or symptoms of obstruction (colicky flank pain, vomiting, poor urinary stream). Determine whether there is a family history of renal disease or renal calculi.

      3. In the child with **renal failure of unknown etiology,** a history of gastroenteritis, often with bloody diarrhea, and pallor suggests the diagnosis of hemolytic uremic syndrome. Ask about ingestion of renal toxins such as ethylene glycol or methyl alcohol. The child with a recent sore throat or impetigo, followed 2–3 weeks later by renal failure and dark or tea-colored urine probably has postinfectious glomerulonephritis. Flank pain, chills, fever, and pyuria may be due to acute pyelonephritis; in this case it is important to exclude associated urinary tract obstruction.

   B. **Physical examination.** Perform a complete physical examination. Children with prerenal failure may have mild signs of hypovolemia such as dry mucous membranes, tachycardia, and orthostatic changes in vital signs (see Chap. 23, Fluids and Electrolytes, sec. **II**). There may be shock with poor perfusion (cool limbs, decreased capillary refill), altered mental status, or hypotension (see Chap. 4). The presentation of postrenal or renal failure varies, depending on the etiology and duration. Renal insufficiency from any cause may present with nausea and vomiting, edema, hypertension, coma, seizures, and electrolyte abnormalities resulting in dysrhythmia or tetany.

**Table 23-1. Acute renal failure**

| Class | Examples | Treatment |
|---|---|---|
| Prerenal | Impaired renal perfusion:<br>Dehydration<br>Hemorrhage<br>Burn<br>Sepsis | Increase intravascular volume—isotonic fluid infusion |
| Renal | Trauma with severe hypovolemia<br>Hemolytic uremic syndrome<br>Toxins<br>Gastroenteritis with severe hypovolemia<br>Postinfectious glomerulonephritis<br>Acute pyelonephritis<br>Severe perinatal asphyxia | Supportive therapy |
| Postrenal (almost always associated with infection) | Posterior urethral valves<br>Ureteroceles<br>Bilateral ureteropelvic obstruction<br>Bilateral ureterovesical obstruction<br>Calculi | Relieve obstruction |

## C. Investigations

1. **Laboratory tests.** Obtain blood specimens for complete blood count (CBC), blood culture, BUN, and measurements of creatinine, electrolytes, calcium, phosphate, magnesium, glucose, and blood gases. Send a urine specimen for determination of pH, cells, Gram's stain, culture, specific gravity, osmolality, casts, and electrolytes. A number of biochemical parameters may be used to differentiate prerenal from renal failure (Table 23-2). They are not always reliable, especially in children who have been administered diuretics or an intravenous fluid bolus. The finding of severe metabolic acidosis with a large anion gap (see Chap. 23, Acid-Base Disturbances) suggests a toxic cause of renal failure or lactic acidosis (see Chap. 27).

2. **X rays.** A renal and bladder ultrasound examination is almost always required to exclude the diagnosis of postrenal failure. If ultrasound examination suggests obstruction, a voiding cystourethrogram and possibly a renogram will be required to locate the site of obstruction.

## II. Management

A. **Prerenal failure.** If prerenal failure is suspected, start an intravenous line and give a bolus of 10 ml/kg of normal saline. If there is no increase in urine output in 30

**Table 23-2. Biochemical parameters in acute renal failure**

| Age | Study | Prerenal failure | Intrinsic renal failure | Comment |
|---|---|---|---|---|
| **Child** | FEna (%) | <1 | >3 | May be low in acute glomerulonephritis or obstructive uropathy |
| | RFI | <1 | >1 | |
| | Una (mmol/liter) | <20 | >40 | Considerable overlap |
| | Uosmol (mOsm/liter) | >500 | <350 | |
| | U/P creatinine | >40 | <20 | Useful when Una or Uosmol not decisive |
| | U/P urea | >8 | <3 | Useful when Una or Uosmol not decisive |
| | U/P osmolarity | >1.3 | <1.3 | Unreliable in malnourished child |
| **Neonate (>35 weeks)** | FEna (%) | <3 | >3 | |
| | RFI | <3 | >3 | |
| | U/P osmolarity | >1 | <1 | As good as FEna in newborn |

Key: FEna = fractional excretion of sodium = $\dfrac{(Una \times Pcr)}{(Pna \times Ucr)}$, RFI = renal failure index = $\dfrac{Una}{Ucr/Pcr}$, U = urine, P = plasma, na = sodium, cr = creatinine.

Source: Adapted from D. Ellis, J. C. Gartner, and A. G. Galvis. Acute renal failure in infants and children: Diagnosis, complications, and treatment. *Crit. Care Med.* 9:607, 1981.

minutes, repeat the 10 ml/kg bolus and check blood and urine results (see sec. **I.C.1**, above). If there is a response, the diagnosis of acute prerenal failure is confirmed.

**B. Postrenal failure.** Children suspected of postrenal failure require urgent radiologic investigation with ultrasound, voiding cystourethrogram (VCUG), and in some cases a renogram. These children should be referred to a urologist.

**C. Principles in management of children with renal failure.** Once the diagnosis of renal failure is established, a number of management principles must be considered, including urgent consultation with a nephrologist.

   **1. Fluid balance.** Assess fluid balance and determine the child's weight. Obtain a chest x ray in children suspected of fluid overload (edema, increased weight, heart failure). Pulmonary edema is an indication for urgent dialysis. Children with renal failure require fluid restriction to 300 ml/m$^2$ of body surface area for insensible losses, plus a volume equivalent to their urine output; fluid requirements may vary with volume status, fever, and ongoing losses.

   **2. Dietary management.** Restrict intake of protein to a maximum of 1 gm/kg/day, potassium to 1 mEq/kg/day, and sodium to 1 mEq/kg/day. If the serum potassium concentration is greater than 6.0 mmol/liter (mEq/liter), remove potassium from the diet.

   **3. Hyperkalemia.** Hyperkalemia predisposes to life-threatening cardiac dysrhythmias.

      **a.** Mild to moderate hyperkalemia (6.0–7.0 mmol/liter or mEq/liter). Children with mild to moderate hyperkalemia may have peaked T waves on the electrocardiogram (ECG). If the serum potassium level is over 6.5 mmol/liter (6.5 mEq/liter), place the child on a cardiac monitor and treat with an ion exchange resin (see sec. **II.C.3.b.(1)** below).

      **b.** Severe hyperkalemia (> 7.0 mmol/liter or mEq/liter). A serum potassium level of over 7.0 mmol/liter (7.0 mEq/liter) or ECG evidence of severe hyperkalemia such as widened QRS complexes, flat P waves, or ventricular dysrhythmia requires aggressive management including any or all of the following:

         **(1)** Ion exchange resins. One g/kg (maximum dose 50 gm) of ion exchange resin such as sodium polystyrene (Kayexelate) or calcium resonium is mixed with 35% sorbitol (1 ml/gm) and is given by retention enema. This will reduce potassium by 0.5–2.0 mmol/liter (mEq/liter) within several hours.

         **(2)** Intravenous glucose. Give 5–10 ml/kg of 10% dextrose in water intravenously over 30 minutes; 1–2 ml/kg of 50% dextrose in water may be given in patients with hypervolemia. This will reduce the potassium level by 1–2 mmol/liter (mEq/liter) for several hours.

(3) Intravenous sodium bicarbonate, 1–2 mEq/kg given over 20–30 minutes acts within 1 hour to lower the serum potassium concentration. The effect is maximal in acidotic patients. This may not be feasible in the child with hypervolemia.

(4) Intravenous calcium gluconate. One ml/kg of a 10% solution should be given by slow push to children with signs of severe cardiac toxicity (dysrhythmias, widened QRS, flat P wave). Calcium gluconate should be administered only during continuous ECG monitoring. It does not lower serum potassium concentration.

(5) Dialysis.

4. **Acidosis.** Treat metabolic acidosis only if the pH is less than 7.2 and it is causing organ dysfunction (hypotension, dysrhythmia, myocardial dysfunction). To calculate the dose of sodium bicarbonate see Chap. 23, Acid-Base Disturbances. Dialysis may be necessary if volume overload prevents bicarbonate administration.

5. **Hypertension.** Treat hypertension if the systolic or diastolic values are above the ninety-fifth percentile for age and sex (Table 23-3). Treatment measures in-

Table 23-3. Classification of hypertension by age group

| Age group | Significant hypertension (mm Hg) | Severe hypertension (mm Hg) |
| --- | --- | --- |
| Newborn | Systolic BP $\geq$ 96 | Systolic BP $\geq$ 106 |
| 7 days | Systolic BP $\geq$ 104 | Systolic BP $\geq$ 110 |
| Infant (< 2 years) | Systolic BP $\geq$ 112<br>Diastolic BP $\geq$ 74 | Systolic BP $\geq$ 118<br>Diastolic BP $\geq$ 82 |
| Children (3–5 years) | Systolic BP $\geq$ 116<br>Diastolic BP $\geq$ 76 | Systolic BP $\geq$ 124<br>Diastolic BP $\geq$ 84 |
| Children (6–9 years) | Systolic BP $\geq$ 122<br>Diastolic BP $\geq$ 78 | Systolic BP $\geq$ 130<br>Diastolic BP $\geq$ 86 |
| Children (10–12 years) | Systolic BP $\geq$ 126<br>Diastolic BP $\geq$ 82 | Systolic BP $\geq$ 134<br>Diastolic BP $\geq$ 90 |
| Adolescent (13–15 years) | Systolic BP $\geq$ 136<br>Diastolic BP $\geq$ 86 | Systolic BP $\geq$ 144<br>Diastolic BP $\geq$ 92 |
| Adolescent (16–18 years) | Systolic BP $\geq$ 142<br>Diastolic BP $\geq$ 92 | Systolic BP $\geq$ 150<br>Diastolic BP $\geq$ 98 |

Source: Report of the Second Task Force on Blood Pressure Control in Children—1987. Reproduced by permission of *Pediatrics* 79(1):1–25. Copyright 1987.

clude intravenous diazoxide, oral nifedipine, and, in the child with volume overload, dialysis (see Chap. 23, Hypertension).

6. **Anemia.** Mild anemia is common secondary to hemodilution and ineffective erythropoiesis. If the hemoglobin drops rapidly or is below 70 gm/liter (7.0 gm/dl), cautious transfusion of 5–10 ml/kg over 3–4 hours of fresh, packed red blood cells is recommended.

7. **Medications.** If possible, avoid all nephrotoxic drugs. Drugs primarily excreted by the kidneys require modification of dose or lengthening of the dose interval.

8. **Dialysis.** The following are relative indications for urgent dialysis:
   a. Uncontrolled severe hyperkalemia.
   b. Severe acidosis with symptomatic volume overload.
   c. Evidence of severe volume overload, including pulmonary edema.
   d. Serum urea of over 40 mmol/liter (BUN > 110 mg/dl) or a serum creatinine over 400 μmol/liter (4.5 mg/dl) in infants, 600 μmol/liter (6.8 mg/dl) in toddlers, or 800 μmol/liter (9.0 mg/dl) in school-aged children.
   e. Removal of dialyzable toxins (see Chap. 27).

III. **Disposition.** Admit all children with acute renal failure. Those with evidence of pulmonary edema or cardiac toxicity secondary to hyperkalemia should be admitted to an intensive care unit.

IV. **Key points**
   A. Intrinsic renal failure must be distinguished from pre- and postrenal failure. Volume pushes of saline are frequently helpful in diagnosing prerenal failure, and radiologic investigation will help to establish the diagnosis of post (obstructive) renal failure.
   B. Management of renal failure requires control of fluid, sodium, protein, and potassium intake, as well as management of hyperkalemia, hypertension, and hypervolemia.

**Bibliography**

Barratt, T. M. Acute Renal Failure. In M. Holliday, T. M. Barratt, and T. Vernier (eds.), *Pediatric Nephrology* (2nd ed.). Baltimore: Williams and Wilkins, 1987.

Dobrin, R. S., Larsen, D., and Holliday, M. A. The critically ill child: Acute renal failure. *Pediatrics* 48:286, 1971.

Ellis, D., Gartner, J. C., and Galvis, A. G. Acute renal failure in infants and children: Diagnosis, complications, and treatment. *Crit. Care Med.* 9:607, 1981.

Gaudio, K. M., and Segal, N. J. Pathogenesis and treatment of acute renal failure. *Pediatr. Clin. North Am.* 34:771, 1987.

Trainin, E. B., and Spitzer, A. Treatment of Acute Renal Failure. C. M. Edelman Jr. (ed.), *Pediatric Kidney Disease.* Vol. 1. Boston: Little, Brown, 1978.

# Hypertension
James E. Carter

Severe hypertension exists when the average systolic or diastolic blood pressure is equal to or greater than the ninety-fifth percentile (see Table 23-3). Heart failure and hypertensive encephalopathy with headache, vomiting, visual disturbances, and seizures are life-threatening complications. Malignant hypertension—a severe rise in blood pressure associated with fundal hemorrhage, exudates, and papilledema—is rare in children. Mild hypertension in the emergency department may be due to a number of causes including anxiety; these children should be investigated on an outpatient basis.

I. **Diagnosis.** Blood pressure determination is part of the routine assessment of all children seen in the emergency department. The sphygmomanometer cuff must be wide enough to cover at least two-thirds of the length of the upper forearm. In infants Doppler ultrasound may be used to amplify the Korotkoff sounds. Alternatively, the capillary flush technique may be used to estimate the mean arterial pressure. This technique is performed by squeezing the arm for 1 minute, inflating the blood pressure cuff, deflating it slowly, and recording the point at which a capillary flush is visible in the hand. In children, most cases of severe hypertension are due to disease of the genitourinary system, such as acute glomerulonephritis or chronic pyelonephritis (reflux nephropathy; see Table 23-4).

A. **History.** Ask about a personal or family history of renal disease or hearing disorder (congenital nephritis). In the transplant patient ask about symptoms of rejection such as abdominal pain and fever. Determine if there has been abdominal pain, dysuria, frequency, or hematuria. Inquire about recent sore throat or skin infection (postinfectious nephritis), anemia, rash, or joint symptoms.

**Table 23-4. Causes of hypertension in children**

Reflux nephropathy

Renovascular disease

Essential hypertension

Acute postinfectious glomerulonephritis (poststreptococcal)

Other forms of nephritis (Henoch-Schönlein purpura)

Coarctation of the aorta

Chronic renal failure

Hemolytic uremic syndrome

Renal transplantation

Drugs (cocaine, amphetamines)

Pheochromocytoma

Adrenal hyperfunction

   **B. Examination.** Look for edema and signs of heart failure such as gallop rhythm, tachycardia, and hepatomegaly. Carefully examine the fundi for exudates, hemorrhages, and papilledema. Check the blood pressure in the legs— a differential of 20 mm Hg lower than the blood pressure in the arms is significant and suggests coarctation of the aorta. Palpate the abdomen for masses (Wilm's tumor, neuroblastoma, congenital renal anomaly) and listen for a bruit (renovascular disease). Look for signs of virilization as evidence of hyperaldosteronism.

   **C. Investigations.** Obtain blood for complete blood count (CBC), differential and platelet counts, BUN, and measurement of creatinine and electrolytes, and send a urine specimen for microscopic analysis and culture. In children with chronic renal failure, include measurements of phosphate and blood gases. A child with an abnormal urinalysis (red blood cells, white blood cells, casts) associated with elevation of BUN and serum creatinine probably has glomerulonephritis or pyelonephritis. Obtain an electrocardiogram (ECG) and chest x ray when there are symptoms of heart failure.

**II. Management**

   **A. Resuscitation.** Assess the airway, breathing, and circulation. Place the child with acute severe hypertension on a cardiac monitor, start an intravenous line, and give oxygen by mask. If available, use an automatic blood pressure measuring device (Doppler) for continuous monitoring every 15 minutes. If there are signs of hypervolemia with hypertension, treat with furosemide (Lasix), 2–3 mg/kg intravenously, given over 5–10 minutes. When renal failure is evident, arrange for urgent dialysis; hemodialysis is more effective than peritoneal dialysis.

   **B. Medications.** Severe hypertension requires immediate lowering of the blood pressure. Aim to decrease the blood pressure by one-third of the desired total in the first 6 hours. Care should be taken not to induce a precipitous fall in blood pressure when it has been chronically elevated. During treatment, monitor visual acuity and pupil reaction to light. A decrease in either parameter may be due to infarction from too rapid a drop in blood pressure; infuse normal saline, 10 ml/kg intravenously, until symptoms reverse.

   **1. Nifedipine.** Nifedipine is an effective agent for lowering blood pressure and can be given PO or sublingually (after puncturing the capsule with a needle). Nifedipine has not been approved for use in children; it is contraindicated in infants and should be used with caution in children with heart failure. Dosage: 5 mg in children aged 3–12 years and 10 mg in children over age 12. May be repeated once in 15 minutes.

   **2. Diazoxide.** Diazoxide is a potent vasodilator and may drop the blood pressure precipitously. It often causes hyperglycemia. Dosage: 3–5 mg/kg (maximum single dose is 300 mg) by rapid intravenous injection, administered with furosemide (Lasix), 1–2 mg/kg intravenously. May be repeated once in 30 minutes.

3. **Sodium nitroprusside.** A nitroprusside infusion should be initiated in children who are resistant to diazoxide and nifedipine. These patients should be monitored in an intensive care unit. A blood thiocyanate level must be checked in all children receiving nitroprusside for more than 48 hours. Dosage: 0.5–8.0 μg/kg/minute, titrating according to effect. (See Appendix V, part 3 for more information.)

4. **Hydralazine.** Hydralazine causes a reflex tachycardia. It is not always effective. Dosage: Begin with a dose of 0.1 mg/kg and increase q6h up to a maximum dose of 1.0 mg/kg of IM injection.

5. **Labetalol.** This is a combined alpha and beta blocker that is not yet approved for use in children. The dose is 1–3 mg/kg/hour given intravenously.

C. **Pheochromocytoma.** Hypertensive crises due to pheochromocytoma should be treated with alpha-adrenergic blocking agents (phentolamine, 0.1–0.2 mg/kg given over 20 minutes intravenously, or phenoxybenzamine, 1 mg/kg in 250 ml 5% dextrose in water given intravenously over 1 hour). These drugs should be administered during continuous monitoring in the intensive care unit.

D. **Stabilization**

1. Once the child is stable, order blood and urine tests (see sec. **I.C,** above) and assess cardiac status with an ECG and chest x ray. When blood pressure is controlled, the child should be started on propranolol, 0.5–1.0 mg/kg/day PO divided q6–12h to a maximum of 300 mg/day (contraindicated in patients with heart failure or asthma). Also, give a diuretic such as hydrochlorothiazide, 1 mg/kg/dose PO divided bid, or a vasodilator such as hydralazine, 0.75–7.0-mg/kg/day PO divided q6h. Consult a nephrologist for follow-up.

2. If coarctation is suspected, an echocardiogram should be obtained and a cardiologist consulted.

3. In children in whom hyperaldosteronism is suspected (virilized, cushingoid, low $K^+$, high $Na^+$), draw blood for measurement of cortisol, aldosterone, and 17-hydroxyprogesterone levels and consult an endocrinologist.

III. **Disposition.** Admit patients with severe hypertension and those with suspected glomerulonephritis. Children with complications (heart failure, encephalopathy) should be transferred to an intensive care unit. Patients with mild hypertension may be sent home with follow-up arranged in 24–48 hours.

IV. **Key points**

A. Most cases of severe acute hypertension in children are due to renal disease.

B. Life-threatening complications include heart failure and hypertensive encephalopathy.

C. Diazoxide and nifedipine are the initial medications of

choice for acute reduction of blood pressure in the child with severe hypertension.

### Bibliography

Mentser, M. Diagnosis and treatment of hypertension in children. *Pediatr. Clin. North A.* 29:933, 1982.

Report of the Second Task Force on Blood Pressure Control in Children—1987. *Pediatrics* 79(1):1–25, 1987.

## Hematuria

James E. Carter and Gregory A. Baldwin

Hematuria is defined as more than 5 red blood cells per high-power field of centrifuged urine, visible on at least two separate specimens. It may be visible to the naked eye or detectable only by chemical testing or microscopic analysis.

### I. Classification

**A. Apparent** hematuria, red-colored urine, is common and may be due to urates and ingestion of substances such as red dyes, beets, or blackberries. **Dipstick-positive urine without red blood cells** may be caused by hemoglobinuria (intravascular hemolysis, postexercise) or myoglobinuria (muscle damage). Hemoglobinuria can be distinguished by the presence of a pinkish tinge of the centrifuged sample. Heavy hemoglobinuria or myoglobinuria can cause renal damage; forced diuresis, alkalinization, and consultation with a nephrologist may be indicated (see Chap. 26, Electrical Burns).

**B. True** hematuria is urine that contains red blood cells and may be due to upper or lower urinary tract disease. Most cases seen in the emergency department are secondary to trauma or infection (see Chap. 17).

### II. Diagnosis and assessment

**A. History.** Determine the onset, pattern, and presence of associated genitourinary symptoms. Ask about trauma involving the back, abdomen, pelvis, or flank. Inquire about drug ingestion, travel, sickle cell disease, and extraurinary symptoms such as joint pain, fever, rash, or weight loss. A number of features in the history may be used to differentiate upper from lower tract sites of bleeding (see Table 23-5). Recurrent hematuria associated with urinary tract infections suggests Berger's disease (IgA nephropathy).

**B. Examination.** Measure the vital signs including blood pressure and perform a careful genital and abdominal examination, palpating the kidneys, bladder, and costovertebral angles. Look for signs of trauma to the abdomen, back, or flanks. If the child has pain, localize the site (see Table 23-6). Although rare, **bleeding disorders** such as hemophilia or thrombocytopenia should be suspected in the child with bruising, purpura, hemarthrosis, or a positive family history.

**1. Upper tract disease.** If upper tract disease is

**Table 23-5. Distinguishing features, upper vs
lower tract bleeding**

| Feature | Upper tract | Lower tract |
| --- | --- | --- |
| Onset | Gradual | Sudden |
| Pattern | Throughout stream | Terminal (end of voiding) |
| Color | Dark, cola-colored | Bright red, clots |
| Associated symptoms | Loin pain, fever, edema | Dysuria, frequency, lower abdominal pain |
| Family history | Positive (Alport's, benign familial hematuria) | Usually negative |
| Associated signs | Rash, arthralgia/ arthritis, edema, hypertension | |
| Proteinuria | $\geq 2^+$ in absence of gross bleeding | $\leq 2^+$ in absence of gross bleeding |
| Casts (urine < 4 hours old) | RBC (glomerular) Granular (less specific) | Usually absent |
| Red cell morphology (phase contrast microscopy)—can be performed only if heavy hematuria is present (>100 RBC/high-power field) | Crenated cells | Absent |

likely, look for signs of **nephritis,** including edema
and hypertension. The presence of a skin rash,
arthralgia, or arthritis also suggests nephritis. Carefully examine the abdomen for masses (Wilms' tumor, congenital malformation) and tenderness. Pallor and anemia may be due to **acute hemolysis** or
**chronic renal failure.**
2. **Lower tract disease.** In lower tract bleeding, rule
out preputial or meatal ulcer in boys, urethral foreign body in young girls, and trauma in both sexes.
C. **Investigations.** For investigation of the trauma victim,
see Chap. 17.
1. **First-line investigations.** In all cases obtain a
fresh urine specimen for gross examination, dipstick,
specific gravity (decreased in nephritis), culture, and
microscopy. A calcium : creatinine ratio may also be

**Table 23-6. Some causes of hematuria**

Infection

Trauma

Nephritis (acute, chronic, interstitial, hereditary, Berger's)

Idiopathic hypercalciuria

Exercise, fever, dehydration (microscopic)

Foreign body

Sickle cell trait

Benign recurrent hematuria

Renal malformations (cystic kidney, duplication)

UPJ obstruction

Tumor (Wilms', leukemia)

Tuberculosis

Nephrolithiasis

Bleeding disorder

Drugs (ASA, penicillins, sulfonamides)

Key: UPJ = ureteropelvic junction, ASA = acetylsalicylic acid
Source: Adapted from M. E. Norman. An office approach to hematuria and proteinuria. *Pediatr. Clin. North Am.* 34:1, 1987.

ordered. If bleeding is sufficiently heavy (more than 100 red blood cells per high-power field), an examination of red cell morphology by phase contrast microscopy may help to locate the site (see Table 23-6). Obtain blood samples for sickle cell screen in black children with undiagnosed hematuria.

2. **Second-line investigations.** In cases of heavy or prolonged bleeding obtain blood samples for a complete blood count (CBC), platelet count, prothrombin time (PT), and partial thromboplastin time (PTT). When upper tract bleeding is suspected, obtain blood for measurement of calcium, electrolytes, ASLO (antistreptolysin-O) titer, C3, C4, antinuclear antibody (ANA), BUN, creatinine, total protein, and albumin levels. Ultrasound examination or CT scan is indicated in cases of suspected tumor or congenital anomaly. For radiologic investigation of trauma, see Chap. 17.

III. **Management**

A. In the child with gross hematuria, always examine a freshly voided specimen. The absence of red blood cells implies hemoglobinuria or myoglobinuria.

B. Obtain a urine sample for microscopy, dipstick, and culture, and perform appropriate blood and x ray investigations as listed above in sec. **I.C.**

C. Children should be referred to a nephrologist for outpatient follow-up in the following situations:

1. Positive family history of nephritis or deafness.

2. Recurrent episodes of hematuria.

3. Systemic complaints including arthralgia/arthritis, rash, or fever.

4. Coexistent heavy proteinuria ($\geq 2+$ on dipstick) in the absence of gross hematuria.

**D.** Children with evidence of nephritis, renal failure, increased BUN, or creatinine levels should be admitted. Consult a nephrologist immediately.

**E.** Children with a renal mass and hematuria require ultrasound examination, and immediate consultation with a surgeon or oncologist is mandatory.

**F.** In cases of genitourinary trauma, consult a urologist (see Chap. 17).

**IV. Causes of hematuria.** Also see Chap. 23, Acute Renal Failure, Urinary Tract Infection; and Chap. 17.

**A. Acute glomerulonephritis.** This is a syndrome with multiple causes that results in cola- or tea-colored urine and decreased renal function with oliguria, increased BUN and creatinine, hypertension, and edema (periorbital edema early in the course).

1. **Diagnosis.** Children with nephritis may be asymptomatic or have abdominal pain, vomiting, and, in the presence of severe hypertension, encephalopathy and pulmonary edema (see Chap. 23, Hypertension). On urinalysis, red blood cell casts and proteinuria are present. Obtain a urine specimen for urinalysis and culture and blood samples for CBC, differential and platelet counts, measurement of electrolytes, calcium, BUN, creatinine, total protein, and albumin levels, ANA, C3, and C4. If poststreptococcal glomerulonephritis is suspected, a throat culture, ASLO titer, or anti-DNAase B titer should also be ordered.

   a. **Postinfectious** (streptococcal, viral, infective endocarditis, shunt infection) glomerulonephritis is the most common type. Poststreptococcal nephritis classically develops 1–3 weeks after a skin infection or pharyngitis in school-aged children.

   b. **IgA nephropathy** (Berger's disease) often occurs following an upper respiratory infection—there may be vague pain in the flanks or costovertebral angles.

   c. **Henoch-Schönlein purpura** causes nephritis in 30–40% of cases. Children usually have the classic signs and symptoms including abdominal pain, purpura, and arthralgia or arthritis.

   d. **Hemolytic-uremic syndrome** results in nephritis associated with bloody diarrhea, anemia due to microangiopathic hemolysis (burr, helmet, fragmented cells), thrombocytopenia, and occasionally neurologic symptoms (coma, seizures, blindness).

   e. **Other** rare forms of nephritis include primary nephritis (membranoproliferative), secondary nephritis (systemic lupus erythematosus), and nephritic-nephrotic syndrome with proteinuria, hyperlipidemia, and severe edema.

**2. Management.** See Chap. 23, Acute Renal Failure for the management of acute renal failure and its complications.

    **a.** Hypertension that is severe or is associated with seizures or pulmonary edema requires aggressive management (see Chap. 23, Hypertension).

    **b.** Children with poststreptococcal glomerulonephritis should be treated with penicillin G, 100,000 units/kg/day PO or IV divided q6h.

    **c.** Patients with hemolytic-uremic syndrome should be treated with ampicillin, 100 mg/kg/day IV divided q6h and, if the hemoglobin is less than 70 gm/liter (7.0 gm/dl), cautious transfusion with 5 ml/kg of washed packed red cells.

    **d.** Consult a nephrologist for ongoing management of glomerulonephritis.

**B. Acute hemorrhagic cystitis.** This is an acute, self-limited disorder that is most common in young males and is usually caused by adenovirus types 11 or 12. Onset occurs 1–2 weeks after a flulike illness. There are usually gross hematuria and symptoms of cystitis with dysuria, suprapubic pain, frequency, and urgency. Most cases resolve spontaneously in 1–2 weeks.

    **1. Management.** Treatment is symptomatic. Phenazopyridine (Pyridium) is a suitable urinary anesthetic. The dose is 100 mg PO q8h in children aged 5–14 (200 mg PO q8h in adults).

**C. Hypercalciuria. Idiopathic hypercalciuria** is a common disorder that can cause microscopic or gross hematuria, dysuria, frequency, enuresis, and suprapubic, abdominal, or urethral discomfort. Measurements of BUN, creatinine, electrolytes, CBC, C3, and C4 are normal. Other causes of hypercalciuria include type 1 renal tubular acidosis, diuretics (furosemide), hyperparathyroidism, juvenile rheumatoid arthritis, medullary cystic kidney, and high dietary calcium.

    **1. Management.** When hypercalciuria is suspected, obtain a urine specimen for urinalysis and a random calcium: creatinine ratio (significant if > 0.21). Refer to a nephrologist for follow-up.

**D. Benign recurrent hematuria.** Benign recurrent hematuria is a diagnosis of exclusion. It accounts for the majority of cases of asymptomatic hematuria in children. Patients have tea-colored urine, and there may be mild proteinuria on dipstick. There are no associated symptoms, and BUN, creatinine, electrolytes, CBC, C3, and C4 are normal. No treatment is necessary, and hematuria resolves spontaneously.

**V. Disposition.** Admit all patients with acute glomerulonephritis, bleeding disorder, and hematuria with abdominal mass.

**VI. Key points**

    **A.** Hematuria in children is usually due to infection.

    **B.** In patients with hematuria, measure the blood pressure and look for signs of nephritis.

**Bibliography**

Norman, M. E. An office approach to hematuria and proteinuria. *Pediatr. Clin. North Am.* 34:1, 1987.

Bergstein, J. M. Hematuria, proteinuria, and urinary tract infections. *Pediatr. Clin. North Am.* 29:55, 1982.

# Urinary Tract Infection
James E. Carter

Urinary tract infection (UTI) is common, affecting approximately 5% of females by age 15. It is of greatest significance in the child under age 3, when diagnosis is difficult and the risk of renal involvement and sequelae is high. The most common organisms are *Escherichia coli,* enterococcus, *Pseudomonas, Klebsiella,* and, rarely, *Staphylococcus epidermidis* and *Proteus.*

I.. **Diagnosis and assessment.** In all children presenting with urinary tract infection, check the blood pressure and examine the abdomen, flanks, and costovertebral angles. Urinary tract infection may be asymptomatic in all age groups.

A. **Older child.** The older child with **lower tract involvement** may present with any of the following: dysuria, frequency, urgency, incontinence, or nocturnal enuresis. When there is **upper tract involvement** (pyelonephritis), there may be a high fever, toxicity, loin pain (unilateral or bilateral), and vomiting.

B. **Young child.** Under the age of 3 it is unlikely that the child will be able to localize the discomfort; instead there may be vague abdominal pain, diarrhea or vomiting, and unexplained fever. Infants may present with nonspecific symptoms such as lethargy, poor feeding, and irritability. Bacteremia occurs in up to 30% of infants less than 3 months of age.

C. **Investigations**

1. **Urine.** Accurate diagnosis depends on the finding of a pure growth of organisms in an uncontaminated sample of urine—requisite colony counts vary with the method of sampling (Table 23-7). If possible, obtain a clean urine sample by midstream technique prior to commencing treatment. Alternative collection methods in the young child are suprapubic aspiration and catheter collection. Specimens must be cultured or refrigerated within 30 minutes. Until culture results are available a presumptive diagnosis of UTI can be made when one or more of the following is present:

a. Appropriate symptoms and signs referable to the genitourinary tract (see sec. **I.A** and **B** above).

b. Leukocyturia and pyuria ($> 5$ white blood cells per high-power field). The presence of white blood cell casts is strongly suggestive of pyelonephritis. Leukocyturia, pyuria, and hyaline and granular

**Table 23-7. Diagnosis of UTI—colony-forming units/ml**

| Method of collection | Infection | No infection |
|---|---|---|
| Midstream | $\geq 10^5$* | $< 10^3$* |
| Catheter (in and out) | $\geq 10^3$ | $< 10^3$ |
| Suprapubic | $\geq 10$ | $< 10$ |

*Colony-forming units/ml
Source: Adapted from A. B. Sedman. Urinary Tract Infection. In R. M. Barkin, and P. Rosen (eds.), *Emergency Pediatrics*. St. Louis: Mosby, 1986.

       casts may also be seen in children with dehydration and high fever.

    **c.** Bacteria seen on microscopy (Gram's stain of uncentrifuged urine).

    **d.** Positive nitrite test on dipstick.

  **2. Other investigations**

    **a.** A renal ultrasound examination should be arranged in young infants and when congenital anomalies or urinary obstruction are suspected.

    **b.** Obtain a blood culture in neonates and in children suspected of pyelonephritis.

    **c.** Consider a septic workup including lumbar puncture in infants less than 3 months of age when there is fever or suspicion of sepsis (see Chap. 21, Bacteremia).

    **d.** Blood for BUN, creatinine, and electrolytes should be drawn in children with hypertension, pyelonephritis, or recurrent UTIs.

**II. Management**

  **A.** If the child is less than 3 months old or is systemically ill, obtain a urine specimen and admit him for empiric intravenous therapy for presumed pyelonephritis: ampicillin, 150 mg/kg/day IV divided q6h, and gentamicin, 6 mg/kg/day IV divided q8h until culture and sensitivity results are obtained. Treat documented infections for 10 days.

  **B.** In the older child who is relatively well with a simple UTI, treat with amoxicillin, 30 mg/kg/day PO divided q8h, or trimethoprim-sulfamethoxazole (TMP-SMX), 6 mg/kg/day as trimethoprim PO divided q12h for 10 days. Advise the parent to push fluids and encourage frequent micturition.

  **C.** In the adolescent with cystitis, give single dose therapy with TMP-SMX, 3.0 gm PO. Ensure that the patient is not pregnant prior to beginning treatment.

  **D.** In all cases, arrange follow-up for repeat urine culture in 2–3 days, with ultrasound and voiding cystourethrogram examination in 3–4 weeks to exclude anomalies or genitourinary reflux.

**III. Disposition.** Admit children suspected of upper urinary tract infection or sepsis.

**IV. Key points**
   **A.** Children less than 3 years old with UTI often present with vague, nonspecific symptoms, including diarrhea and vomiting.
   **B.** Be suspicious of bacteremia and sepsis in the infant under 3 months of age with a UTI.

**Bibliography**

Bergstein, J. M. Hematuria, proteinuria, and urinary tract infections. *Pediatr. Clin. North Am.* 29:55, 1982.

Burns, M. W., Burns, J. L., and Kreiger, J. N. Pediatric urinary tract infection: Diagnosis, classification, and significance. *Pediatr. Clin. North Am.* 34:1111, 1987.

---

# Fluids and Electrolytes

Gregory A. Baldwin and James E. Carter

**I. Maintenance requirements.** An approximation of maintenance requirements for normal, healthy children is as follows:
   **A. Water**
      **1.** The true water requirement in the child is calculated on body surface area and equals 1500 ml/m$^2$. An easy to use approximation of the water requirement is shown in Table 23-8.
      **2.** Fluid needs are increased when there are insensible (fever, burn, tachypnea) or other losses (stool, urine) above normal.
      **3.** In the healthy term newborn, requirements are 60 ml/kg on the first day of life, gradually increasing to 120 ml/kg/day by 7 days of age.
   **B. Electrolytes**
      **1. Sodium**—40–60 mEq/m$^2$ **OR** 1–3 mEq/kg/24 hours.
      **2. Potassium**—30–40 mEq/m$^2$ **OR** 1–3 mEq/kg/24 hours.

**II. Dehydration.** The most common cause of dehydration in children is infectious gastroenteritis that results in diarrhea and vomiting. Children with increased insensible losses (high fever, tachypnea) or urinary losses (diabetic ketoacidosis, diabetes insipidus) are prone to dehydration if intake is insufficient. See Chap. 13, Diabetic Ketoacidosis, and Chap. 16, Acute Diarrhea.

**Table 23-8. Water requirements in children**

| Weight | Requirement |
| --- | --- |
| Less than 10 kg | 100 ml/kg/24 hours |
| 10–20 kg | 1000 ml + 50 ml/kg/24 hours |
| Above 20 kg | 1500 ml + 20 ml/kg/24 hours |

**A. Diagnosis and assessment**

  **1. History.** In all cases ask about preillness weight or weight loss as a measure of the severity of dehydration. Inquire when the child last passed urine and determine its color and odor. Dark, strong urine suggests moderate to severe dehydration.

  **2. Examination.** Measure vital signs and look for orthostatic changes in blood pressure (a drop of $> 15$ mm Hg moving from the supine to a sitting position is abnormal) and heart rate (an increase of $> 20$ beats/minute is abnormal). Orthostatic changes are not always reliable and are difficult to detect in children under age 5. Feel the fontanel, determine skin turgor, and note hydration of the mucous membranes, including tear formation.

  **3. Investigations.** In children with moderate or severe dehydration, obtain blood specimens for measurement of electrolytes, glucose, and BUN, and urine specimens for measurement of specific gravity (specific gravity of $\leq 1.015$ suggests a renal concentrating defect) and pH (alkalotic urine suggests renal tubular acidosis).

  **4. Severity of dehydration.** This can be determined directly by calculating the percentage of weight loss or indirectly by clinical assessment. Severity of dehydration can be classified as:

  **a. Mild volume depletion**—5% weight loss or less. There may be one or more of the following:

   **(1)** Tachycardia

   **(2)** Dry mucous membranes

   **(3)** Slight decrease in urine output

  **b. Moderate volume depletion**—10% weight loss. Look for

   **(1)** Increased severity of signs listed in sec. **II.A.4.a** above

   **(2)** Decreased skin turgor

   **(3)** Sunken fontanel

   **(4)** Sunken eyes (often best judged by the parent)

   **(5)** Increased BUN, urine specific gravity of more than 1.030

  **c. Severe volume depletion**—15% weight loss. The child with severe volume depletion is in shock (see Chap. 4). Signs of shock include

   **(1)** Decreased level of consciousness

   **(2)** Mottled skin

   **(3)** Cool extremities with decreased capillary filling

   **(4)** Oliguria or anuria, urine specific gravity of more than 1.035

   **(5)** Decreased blood pressure, a late sign

**B. Type of dehydration** (osmolality). Dehydration is classified as hypotonic, isotonic, and hypertonic based on the serum sodium level.

  **1. Isotonic dehydration—serum sodium concen-**

tration **130–150 mmol/liter** (mEq/liter). The majority of cases of dehydration are isotonic; about 65% of children with diarrhea and vomiting fall into this category. There is no water balance abnormality.

2. **Hypertonic dehydration—serum sodium concentration of more than 150 mmol/liter** (mEq/liter). In hypertonic dehydration there is a deficit of free water. About 25% of cases of dehydration in children are hypertonic. Evidence of hypovolemia may not occur until dehydration is severe. Children often have a characteristic "doughy" texture to the skin or tongue. See sec. **III.A,** below.

3. **Hypotonic dehydration—serum sodium concentration of less than 130 mmol/liter** (mEq/liter). In hypotonic dehydration there is an excess of free water. About 5–10% of dehydrated patients have the hypotonic variety. Losses occur primarily from the extracellular fluid (ECF) compartment, and circulatory insufficiency presents early. See sec. **III.B,** below.

C. **Management.** The major goal of treatment is to treat or prevent circulatory collapse by replacing water and electrolyte losses. When planning intravenous fluid replacement, include deficit replacement and maintenance requirements (see sec. **I** above) and make provision for ongoing losses. For treatment of specific disorders see appropriate chapters (e.g., Chap. 13, Diabetic Ketoacidosis, Chap. 16, Acute Diarrhea, Chap. 26).

1. **Initial treatment of severe dehydration (weight loss of 15% or more).** If the patient demonstrates a profound volume depletion or is assessed to have a body weight loss of 15% or greater, give oxygen, start an intravenous line, and administer normal saline or Ringer's lactate in aliquots of 10 ml/ kg until the patient is stable (see Chap. 4). Subsequent therapy is detailed below.

2. **Treatment of mild to moderate dehydration**

   a. **Isotonic dehydration.** In treatment of isotonic dehydration, intravenous infusion of a hypotonic dextrose solution containing 30–55 mEq of sodium per liter is usually adequate. Give 50% of the calculated fluid requirement (deficit plus maintenance) in the first 8 hours and the remaining 50% during the next 16 hours (see Table 23-9).

   b. **Hypotonic dehydration.** In general, this type of dehydration is treated in the same way as isotonic dehydration, allowing the serum sodium concentration to rise spontaneously over 24–48 hours. Be suspicious of other causes of hyponatremia, including Addison's disease and inappropriate antidiuretic hormone (ADH) secretion (see sec. **III.B,** below). If the child has neurologic symptoms (seizures, coma) and the serum sodium level is very low (< 120 mmol/liter or 120 mEq/

**Table 23-9. Sample calculation: fluid rehydration**

A 10-kg child who is 10% dehydrated with estimated losses of 400 ml per day requires:

*Maintenance:* 100 ml/kg × 10 kg = 1000 ml

*Deficit:* 10% (dehydrated) × 10 kg = 1 kg = 1000 ml

*Ongoing losses:* 400 ml

Total: 1000 ml + 1000 ml + 400 ml = 2400 ml

**First 8 hours give:** 1200 ml = 150 ml/hr

**Next 16 hours give:** 1200 ml = 75 ml/hr

Therefore, the order should read:
150 ml/hr × 8 hr, then 75 ml/hr × 16 hr

liter) or has dropped precipitously, rapid infusion of hypertonic saline is indicated (see sec. **III.B,** below).

   c. **Hypertonic dehydration.** If fluid replacement is too rapid in children with hypernatremic dehydration, a precipitous fall in serum sodium concentration may result in cerebral or pulmonary edema. Following initial resuscitation (see sec. **II.C.1** above), aim to replace calculated water losses over 48–72 hours, ensuring that the serum sodium level does not fall by more than 10 mM/day (10 mEq/day). A good initial rehydration solution is 5% dextrose half normal saline. Check serum glucose and calcium levels. See sec. **III.A,** below.

3. **Other electrolytes**

   a. Potassium. Maintenance potassium requirements of 20–40 mEq/liter of fluids can be added to the intravenous solution when there is evidence of adequate renal function (normal urine output, BUN, or creatinine level).

   b. Bicarbonate. Sodium bicarbonate therapy is not required unless there is organ dysfunction (myocardial dysfunction, dysrhythmia, hypotension) with severe metabolic acidosis (pH < 7.20) or a superimposed disorder aggravating acidosis (e.g., salicylate intoxication). For calculating dose see Chap. 23, Acid-Base Disorders.

4. **Stabilization and monitoring.** In moderate or severe dehydration monitor urine output, fluid intake, electrolytes, urine electrolytes, blood gases, and weight, and chart the data on a flow sheet.

5. **Oral rehydration therapy.** In cases of mild dehydration, oral rehydration is often suitable. A number of commercially prepared oral electrolyte preparations are available. For details see Chap. 16, Acute Diarrhea.

## III. Electrolyte abnormalities
### A. Hypernatremia (see Table 23-10)
#### 1. Causes
**a.** Increased intake. **Excessive sodium intake** is usually the result of hypertonic fluid administration in a dehydrated child with gastroenteritis. It may also occur following sodium bicarbonate administration and in victims of salt-water drowning. Rare causes include hyperaldosteronism and essential hypernatremia.

**b.** Water loss. Hypernatremia may also be due to a **negative free water balance** secondary to increased insensible losses (sweating, hyperventilation) or diabetes insipidus.

#### 2. Diagnosis and assessment. These children tend to present with neurologic signs: lethargy, irritability, hyperreflexia, hypertonia, muscle twitching, and convulsions. Circulatory function tends to be preserved until the deficit is severe, at which time the child's condition deteriorates suddenly into shock. Mortality and morbidity are considerable when concentrations exceed 160 mmol/liter (160 mEq/liter). Hypocalcemia and hyperglycemia may also occur with hypernatremia.

#### 3. Management. Following resuscitation, the free water deficit should be replaced over 48 hours, adjusting the rate of infusion to allow a slow steady fall in serum sodium concentration (10 mmol/day or 10 mEq/day maximum) to prevent cerebral edema. Measure the serum sodium level every 4 hours. To calculate the free water deficit:

$$\frac{\text{Actual serum sodium}}{140} \times \text{wt (kg)} \times 0.6$$
$$= \text{free water deficit}$$

Dialysis may be required in extreme cases.

### B. Hyponatremia (Table 23-10)
#### 1. Causes. Rarely, children may have apparent hyponatremia due to hyperglycemia, hyperproteinemia, or hyperlipidemia.
**a. Hyponatremia and dehydration** may occur with diarrhea in infants, renal failure, renal tubular acidosis, adrenal insufficiency, burns, or diuretic use.

**b. Hyponatremia with edema** may be seen with congestive heart failure, liver failure, nephrotic syndrome, and hypoalbuminemia.

**c. Hyponatremia** with normovolemia may be seen with factors causing inappropriate ADH secretion.

#### 2. Signs and symptoms. Severe hyponatremia may cause lethargy, confusion, nausea, muscle cramps, hypothermia, coma, seizures, and death. Coma or seizures are unlikely unless the serum sodium con-

**Table 23-10. Abnormalities of sodium and potassium**

| Abnormality | Type | Causes |
|---|---|---|
| Hypernatremia | Excessive sodium | Hypertonic fluid administration during gastroenteritis |
| | | $NaHCO_3$ administration |
| | | Salt water drowning |
| | | Hyperaldosteronism |
| | | Essential hypernatremia |
| | Water loss | Increased insensible losses: sweating, hyperventilation |
| | | Diabetes insipidus |
| Hyponatremia | Hyponatremia with dehydration | Diarrhea in infants |
| | | Renal failure |
| | | Renal tubular acidosis |
| | | Adrenal insufficiency |
| | | Burns |
| | | Diuretic use |
| | Hyponatremia with edema | Congestive heart failure |
| | | Liver failure |
| | | Nephrotic syndrome |
| | Hyponatremia with normovolemia | Inappropriate ADH secretion |
| Hypokalemia | | Anorexia nervosa |
| | | Protracted vomiting and diarrhea |
| | | Diabetic ketoacidosis |
| | | Renal tubular acidosis |
| | | Diuretics |
| | | Alkalosis (intracellular shift) |
| | | Hyperaldosteronism |
| | | Familial periodic paralysis |
| Hyperkalemia | | Acidosis |
| | | Hyperkalemic familial periodic paralysis |
| | | Hemolysis |
| | | Rhabdomyolysis |
| | | Potassium-sparing diuretics |
| | | Adrenal insufficiency |
| | | Renal failure |

Source: Adapted from R. Schrier. *Renal and Electrolyte Disorders* (2nd ed.). Boston: Little, Brown, 1985.

centration drops precipitously or is less than 120 mmol/liter (120 mEq/liter).

**3. Treatment** depends on the cause and on the status of the child.

  **a.** The child with signs of **acute hypovolemia** should receive normal saline in a 10 ml/kg bolus intravenously; this is repeated prn until the child is stable.

  **b.** Acute onset of neurologic signs and symptoms (coma, seizures) in the child with a sodium level of less than 120 mmol/liter should be treated with an infusion of hypertonic saline to raise the level to 125 mmol/liter (125 mEq/liter), as follows:

    **(1)** Milliequivalent Na required = (125 − actual Na) × 0.6 × wt (kg).

    **(2)** Give dose as 3% NaCl (513 mEq/liter) IV at 4–6 mEq/kg/hour.

    **(3)** In the child with a serum Na level of more than 120 mmol/liter (120 mEq/liter) and neurologic signs or symptoms following a precipitous drop in the serum sodium concentration, administer NaCl to raise the level by 5 mmol/liter (5 mEq/liter)—see formula in sec. **III.B.3.b.(1)** above.

  **c.** Many children with hyponatremia do not require urgent treatment but should be admitted to hospital for investigation. In children who are not obviously hypovolemic, restrict fluids to 50% of maintenance and give maintenance sodium (1–3 mEq/kg/day) until a diagnosis is made. Obtain blood specimens for measurement of electrolytes, serum albumin, BUN, creatinine, liver function tests, blood gases, and serum osmolality, and urine for measurement of electrolytes and osmolality.

**C. Hypokalemia** (Table 23-10)

  **1. Causes.** Hypokalemia may be seen with anorexia nervosa, protracted vomiting and diarrhea, diabetic ketoacidosis, renal tubular acidosis, use of diuretics, alkalosis (serum potassium is decreased by 0.5 mmol/liter or 0.5 mEq/liter for every 0.1 increase in pH), hyperaldosteronism, and familial hypokalemic periodic paralysis. Alkalosis can cause hypokalemia due to intracellular ion shift.

  **2. Signs and symptoms.** In general, the clinical signs of hypokalemia are subtle and include paralytic ileus with abdominal distention, muscle weakness and cramps, and diminished reflexes. Severe hypokalemia may lead to atrial and ventricular dysrhythmia, tetany, and encephalopathy. ECG signs include depressed T waves, U waves, and a prolonged QT interval. Familial hypokalemic periodic paralysis presents with a slow onset of weakness that lasts 48–72 hours and is associated with exercise or large meals.

  **3. Treatment**

    **a.** Most children with hypokalemia and intact renal

function can be treated conservatively, ensuring adequate oral or intravenous intake. Potassium, 20–40 mEq/liter of intravenous maintenance fluid, is adequate in most cases.

**b. Severe hypokalemia with dysrhythmia or tetany can be treated with potassium infusions at rates of up to 0.5 mEq/kg/hour via a central line; this infusion should be administered only in an intensive care unit while the child is on a cardiac monitor.**

c. Familial periodic paralysis is treated with potassium supplementation, 2–6 mEq/kg/day PO; follow-up should be arranged for monitoring serum potassium levels in 12–24 hours.

**D. Hyperkalemia**

1. **Causes. Pseudohyperkalemia** may be caused by tight tourniquet application, squeezing of the blood-taking site, or hemolysis, thrombocytosis, or leukocytosis of the blood sample. **True hyperkalemia** may be due to acidosis, hyperkalemic familial periodic paralysis, hemolysis, rhabdomyolysis, potassium-sparing diuretics, adrenal insufficiency, or renal failure.

2. **Signs and symptoms and treatment.** The severe effects of hyperkalemia are exacerbated when there is concurrent hyponatremia, acidosis, or hypocalcemia. For diagnosis and management, see Chap. 23, Acute Renal Failure.

**E. Hypocalcemia**

1. **Causes.** In the newborn, hypocalcemia may be seen in infants with severe stress, in infants born to mothers with hyperparathyroidism, and with congenital lesions such as DiGeorge's syndrome. In older children, hypocalcemia is often secondary to renal failure, hypoparathyroidism, rickets, or drugs (furosemide). **Apparent** hypocalcemia, in which there is a normal ionized level of calcium, occurs in children with hypoalbuminemia.

2. **Symptoms and signs.** When the level of ionized calcium is very low, tetany may result, with seizures and laryngospasm. Other signs of hypocalcemia include Trousseau's and Chvostek's signs, an altered level of consciousness, a prolonged QT interval (correct for rate) on ECG, carpopedal spasm, and jitteriness in the newborn.

3. **Treatment.** Obtain blood specimens for measurement of phosphate, alkaline phosphatase, magnesium, and an ionized calcium level. When hypocalcemia is symptomatic, start an intravenous line, place the child on a cardiac monitor, and administer 10% calcium gluconate, 2 ml/kg IV over 30 minutes. If there is concurrent hypomagnesemia, this must be corrected before the child will respond to the calcium infusion. Consult an endocrinologist in all cases.

**IV. Key points**

**A.** In the treatment of children with hypernatremia, ensure that the serum sodium level does not fall faster than 10 mM/day (10 mEq/day).

**B.** In cases of hypocalcemic tetany that are resistant to treatment, rule out concomitant hypomagnesemia.

**C.** Children with hyponatremia should be treated with NaCl infusion if they are symptomatic.

## Acid-Base Metabolism
Gregory A. Baldwin

**I. Definitions**

**A. Acidosis**—a tendency toward an acidemic pH, less than 7.35.

**B. Alkalosis**—a tendency toward an alkalemic pH, more than 7.45.

**II. Principles in management of acid-base disorders**

**A.** When there is a clinical suspicion of an acid-base abnormality, obtain a blood gas measurement (arterial, or a capillary or venous sample from a nonexercised extremity) and a plasma bicarbonate measurement.

**B.** Use the "rules" of acid-base metabolism (Table 23-11) or an acid-base map (Fig. 23-1) to determine the underlying abnormality.

**C.** In metabolic acidosis of unknown etiology, the differential diagnosis may be narrowed by determination of the **anion gap.** In metabolic alkalosis, measure the **urine chloride excretion** (see Table 23-12).

**D.** Treat the cause; this is especially relevant when the disorder is due to respiratory failure or volume depletion. **Treat the acid-base disturbance only if it is resulting in significant organ system dysfunction** (myocardial depression, dysrhythmia, hypotension); in otherwise healthy children, this is unlikely to occur unless the pH is less than 7.20 or greater than 7.55.

    **1. Respiratory acidosis** (see Chap. 1).

**Table 23-11. Rules of acid-base metabolism**

1. Metabolic acidosis: The $PaCO_2$ should fall by 1.0–1.5 times the fall in plasma bicarbonate concentration.

2. Metabolic alkalosis: The $PaCO_2$ should rise by 0.25–1.0 times the rise in plasma bicarbonate concentration.

3. Acute respiratory acidosis: The plasma bicarbonate concentration should rise by about 1 mmol/liter (1 mEq/liter) for each 10 mm Hg increment in $PaCO_2$ ($\pm$ 3 mmol/liter or 3 mEq/liter).

4. Acute respiratory alkalosis: The plasma bicarbonate concentration should fall by about 1–3 mmol/liter (1–3 mEq/liter) for each 10 mm Hg decrement in $PaCO_2$, and usually not to < 18 mmol/liter (18 mEq/liter).

Source: Reprinted from R. Schrier. *Renal and Electrolyte Disorders* (2nd Ed.). Boston: Little, Brown, 1985.

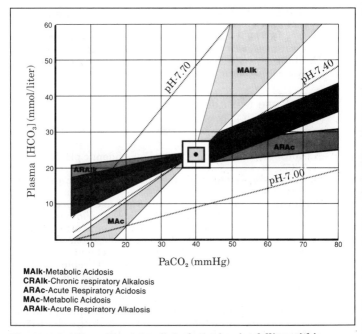

**MAlk**-Metabolic Acidosis
**CRAlk**-Chronic respiratory Alkalosis
**ARAc**-Acute Respiratory Acidosis
**MAc**-Metabolic Acidosis
**ARAlk**-Acute Respiratory Alkalosis

Fig. 23-1. Acid-base (map) for clinical use. A point falling within a band usually means that the indicated simple acid-base disorder is present. However, a mixed disorder could mimic a simple disorder as in the following example. A patient with metabolic alkalosis has a plasma [$HCO_3^-$] of 38 mmoles/L. He then develops acute respiratory acidosis (acute hypercapnia) with a $PaCO_2$ of 70mm Hg. His acid base variables alone suggest chronic respiratory acidosis. Therefore the clinical setting must always be considered in interpreting acid-base disorders. (Central square includes normal mean values for $PaCO_2$ and [$HCO_3^-$] ± 2 units; open part of the square expands this range to ± 4 units.) MAlk = metabolic alkalosis; MAc = metabolic acidosis; CRAc = chronic respiratory acidosis; ARAc = acute respiratory acidosis; CRAlk = chronic respiratory alkalosis; ARAlk = acute respiratory alkolosis. (By permission of W. D. Kachny and P. Gabow. From Pathogenesis and Management of Metabolic Acidosis and Alkalosis. In R. W. Schrier (ed.). *Renal and Electrolyte Disorders* (3rd ed.). Boston: Little, Brown, 1986.)

2. **Metabolic acidosis** is due to a decrease in plasma bicarbonate or an accumulation of $H^+$ ions. Severe metabolic acidosis (pH < 7.20) leads to hypotension directly and by way of decreased cardiac output. Cardiac dysrhythmias and deep rapid (Kussmaul's) respirations may also result. Calculate the anion gap using the formula:

Serum Na − (serum $HCO_3$ + serum Cl) = anion gap

The normal value is less than 12 in children and somewhat higher in newborns.

**Table 23-12. Causes of acid-base disorders**

| | |
|---|---|
| **Causes of metabolic acidosis**<br>Normal anion gap<br>　Diarrhea<br>　Renal tubular acidosis<br>　Sepsis<br>　Shock from any cause<br>Increased anion gap<br>　Diabetic ketoacidosis<br>　Lactic acidosis<br>　Inborn errors of<br>　　metabolism<br>　Salicylates<br>　Paraldehyde<br>　Alcohols (methyl,<br>　　ethyl, isopropyl)<br>　Ethylene glycol<br>　Renal failure<br><br>**Causes of metabolic alkalosis**<br>Sodium chloride<br>　responsive<br>　(Urine chloride < 10<br>　　mmol/liter or 10<br>　　mEq/liter)<br>　Vomiting, chloride<br>　　diarrhea<br>　Diuretics<br>　Cystic fibrosis<br>Sodium chloride<br>　resistant<br>　(Urine chloride > 10<br>　　mmol/liter or 10<br>　　mEq/liter)<br>　Potassium depletion<br>　Cushing's syndrome<br>Unclassified<br>　Alkali administration | **Causes of respiratory alkalosis**<br>Central stimulation<br>　Anxiety<br>　Head injury<br>　Salicylates<br>　Fever<br>　Reye's syndrome<br>Peripheral stimulation<br>　Lung disease<br>　Mechanical hyperventilation<br><br>**Causes of respiratory acidosis**<br>Neuromuscular disorder<br>　Spinal injury<br>　Botulism<br>　Toxic ingestion<br>　Guillain Barré syndrome<br>Airway obstruction<br>　Foreign body<br>　Aspiration<br>　Bronchospasm<br>　Croup/epiglottitis<br>Thoracic-pulmonary disorder<br>　Pneumothorax<br>　Traumatic injury<br>　Pneumonia<br>　Smoke inhalation |

Source: Adapted from R. Schrier. *Renal and Electrolyte Disorders* (2nd ed.). Boston: Little, Brown, 1985.

**a. Normal anion gap** (<12). Most cases of normal anion gap metabolic acidosis are due to dehydration following gastroenteritis. For other causes see Table 23-12.

**b. Increased anion gap** (>12). Metabolic acidosis with an increased anion gap occurs in a set of disorders known by the mnemonic MUDPIES: methanol, uremia, diabetic ketoacidosis, paraldehyde, and iron, isoniazid, ethanol, ethylene glycol, and salicylate ingestion—see Table 23-12.

         **c. Management.** When metabolic acidosis is severe and is causing organ dysfunction, give one-half of the dose of $HCO_3$ required to raise the pH to 7.20, then repeat the blood gas and plasma bicarbonate measurements: One-half $NaHCO_3$ replacement dose = Base deficit OR (desired $HCO_3$ − actual $HCO_3$) × 0.3 × wt (kg)

    **3. Metabolic alkalosis.** Metabolic alkalosis occurs when the pH is greater than 7.45 due to an increase in plasma bicarbonate. It usually results from excessive vomiting (pyloric stenosis) or gastric drainage. Metabolic alkalosis may present with paresthesias, muscle cramps, weakness, or muscular irritability secondary to a decrease in ionized calcium. When severe (pH > 7.60), cardiac dysrhythmias may occur. Measure the urine chloride concentration to determine the type of metabolic alkalosis present, and determine the serum potassium level in all cases.

        **a. Management**

           **(1)** Chloride-responsive disturbances (see Table 23-12) should be treated with an intravenous bolus of normal saline of 10 ml/kg.

           **(2)** If there is hypokalemia, replace potassium intravenously.

           **(3)** Other causes must be treated individually.

           **(4)** Patients with severe symptoms may require therapy with acetazolamide or ammonium chloride.

    **4. Respiratory alkalosis.** This is due to central or mechanical hyperventilation (see Table 36-5) and is uncommon in children. The plasma bicarbonate level is normal, the $PCO_2$ is decreased, and the pH is increased. The only possible treatment is that of the underlying disorder.

**III. Key points**

    **A.** When possible, treatment of an acid-base disorder should focus on the cause.

    **B.** In general, treatment of the acid-base disturbance is necessary only if there is significant organ dysfunction (usually pH < 7.20 or > 7.55).

**Bibliography**

Schrier, R. *Renal and Electrolyte Disorders* (2nd ed.). Boston: Little, Brown, 1985.

# Musculoskeletal Disorders

## Acute Arthritis
Ross E. Petty

Acute **arthritis** is the sudden onset of pain, swelling, heat, and limitation of motion in a joint. In contrast, **arthralgia** refers to pain in a joint without the other findings; arthralgia may precede arthritis by hours or days. Recent onset of arthritis in a single joint (monoarthritis) requires prompt investigation to rule out sepsis. For diagnosis and management of limp, osteomyelitis, and Kawasaki syndrome, see appropriate sections of this chapter.

### I. Diagnosis and assessment
#### A. History
1. **Onset and duration.** In young or nonverbal children, onset of arthritis is often dated from the time the parent first noted pain or crying with limb movement, systemic signs such as fever, or decreased use of the limb (limp, refusal to bear weight). A sudden onset suggests trauma; a gradual onset over hours suggests infection; a long duration or slow onset suggests malignancy, inflammation, or a mechanical abnormality.
2. **Trauma.** Although minor trauma is a common event in the life of a small child, it seldom causes monoarthritis. Be suspicious of nonaccidental trauma if there is a discrepancy between the history and physical findings or between histories obtained from different people.
3. **Preceding or concurrent illness**
   a. Fever. In the febrile child, consider the diagnoses of septic arthritis, osteomyelitis, reactive arthritis (including acute rheumatic fever), serum sickness, malignancy, systemic onset juvenile rheumatoid arthritis (JRA), and other connective tissue diseases.
   b. Rash. A purpuric rash concentrated in dependent areas (lower limbs, buttocks) suggests Henoch-Schönlein purpura (see Chap. 23). Other arthritides associated with rash include acute rheumatic fever (erythema marginatum), meningococcemia (petechiae, purpura), gonococcemia (maculopapular, vesicopustular), Lyme disease (erythema chronicum migrans), systemic onset JRA (fine pink-red macular rash), and nonspecific (presumably viral) infections.
   c. Upper respiratory tract infection (URI). Children with acute rheumatic fever and transient synovitis frequently have a recent history of URI or pharyngitis.
   d. Diarrhea or abdominal pain. A history of gastrointestinal complaints may be associated with

inflammatory bowel disease. Postinfectious arthritis may be related to *Yersinia, Campylobacter, Salmonella,* or *Shigella* enteritis.

   **e.** Genitourinary symptoms. Arthritis associated with genitourinary tract infection or sexually transmitted disease (STD) usually occurs in adolescents. Consider Reiter's syndrome (urethritis, arthritis, conjunctivitis) or gonococcal arthritis in these patients. Hematuria is associated with systemic lupus erythematosus (SLE), Henoch-Schönlein purpura, and serum sickness.

  **4. Hemophilia.** Acute arthritis in the hemophiliac is almost always due to intraarticular hemorrhage. There is usually an abrupt onset of pain and swelling, most commonly in the knee, ankle, or elbow (see Chap. 19).

**B. Examination**

  **1. General.** Perform a complete examination: Look at the skin for rash, listen to the heart for murmurs, and determine if there is lymphadenopathy, hepatomegaly, or splenomegaly.

  **2. Musculoskeletal.** In the child with polyarthritis, examine all of the joints, including those of the hands, feet, and spine. On inspection, note any erythema, swelling, or signs of trauma, and compare each side with the contralateral side. Note the position of the limb—a child with an effusion of the hip often holds the joint abducted, externally rotated, and flexed. Feel for warmth, swelling, and thickening. If the child will allow it, test the active range of motion and palpate for crepitus. Next, test the passive range of motion and power, and finally, observe the gait if the lower limb is involved.

**C. Approach to the child with suspected arthritis**

  **1. Localize the problem**

    **a.** Localized **soft tissue pain** or swelling is usually due to trauma.

    **b. Bone pain** on percussion or palpation suggests osteomyelitis, trauma, or malignancy.

    **c. Joint pain** on active and passive motion with resistance to movement is probably due to arthritis or hemarthrosis.

  **2. Determine the number of sites involved**

    **a. Acute monoarthritis** is septic until proved otherwise. Monoarthritis of the hip may also be due to toxic synovitis. The onset of JRA in a single hip joint is unusual.

    **b. Acute polyarthritis** with multiple painful or swollen joints makes the diagnosis of a septic process unlikely. Causes of polyarthritis include serum sickness, rubella (older teenager), juvenile rheumatoid arthritis, Kawasaki syndrome, Lyme disease, hemophilia, and SLE (see sec. **II,** below). Multiple painful or swollen soft tissue or bony lesions suggest the diagnosis of accidental or nonaccidental trauma. Multiple sites of bone pain, especially at the ends of long bones, may be due to malignancies such as leukemia or neuroblastoma.

## D. Investigations

1. **Arthrocentesis.** Arthrocentesis is an essential procedure in the child with acute ($<$ 72 hours) monoarthritis. Send aspirated material for Gram's stain, culture, rapid antigen testing, cell count, and chemical testing (see sec. **III,** below).

2. **Other investigations.** A blood culture should be performed when sepsis is suspected. In addition, obtain a complete blood count (CBC), and a differential count, an erythrocyte sedimentation rate (ESR), and, when there is diarrhea or abdominal pain, cultures of the stool. When sexually transmitted disease (STD) is suspected, obtain cultures of the urethra, cervix, rectum, and pharynx (see Chap. 21, Sexually Transmitted Disease). An antinuclear antibody titer (ANA) may be helpful in suspected JRA or SLE.

3. **X rays.** X rays should always be obtained if trauma or malignancy is suspected. Early radiographs of inflamed or infected joints are rarely helpful and show only nonspecific soft tissue swelling. A bone scan may be useful in documenting subclinical sites of infection in children with osteomyelitis.

## II. Specific causes of arthritis

**A. Septic arthritis.** This diagnosis should be suspected in any child with acute onset monoarthritis. Septic arthritis is usually secondary to hematogenous dissemination of *Staphylococcus aureus* (most common), *Haemophilus influenzae* type b (6 weeks–4 years age group), or group B streptococcus or gram-negative bacteria in neonates. Tuberculosis is a rare cause. Although any joint may be involved, the joints most commonly affected are the knee (40%), hip (25%), ankle (15%), and elbow (10%). Septic arthritis in a small joint (PIP, metacarpophalangeal) is rare. The child usually presents with sudden onset of pain, refusal to use the limb, fever, and signs of toxicity. The young infant may have nonspecific signs such as irritability and poor feeding with decreased limb movement. In nearly all instances, there is extreme pain on movement of the involved joint, which is held in a neutral position: abduction, external rotation, and flexion of the hip, flexion of the knee and elbow, and plantar flexion of the ankle. Most children with septic arthritis have a raised white blood cell count with a left shift and a raised ESR ($>$ 50 mm/hour).

1. **Management**

a. **If infection is suspected, obtain a blood culture, perform arthrocentesis to obtain synovial fluid** (see sec. **III,** below)**, and admit the child to hospital for treatment with intravenous antibiotics. Children with septic arthritis of the hip should be kept NPO—consult an orthopedic surgeon for drainage under general anesthesia.** Surgical drainage is always indicated in hip infection and is usually indicated in infections of the elbow, shoulder, or ankle, or when there is a poor response to 48 hours of antibiotic treatment.

**b.** When possible, therapy should be guided by the results of bacterial antigen tests or Gram's stain of joint fluid.

**c.** When the organism is unknown, treat empirically according to age:

    **(1)** Birth to 6 weeks. Suspect *S. aureus,* group B streptococcus, or gram-negative organisms. Use cloxacillin or oxacillin, 125 mg/kg/day divided q6h IV (or another suitable anti-staphylococcal agent) *and* gentamicin, 5 mg/kg/day IV divided q8h.

    **(2)** Over 6 weeks. Suspect *H. influenzae* type b or *S. aureus.* Use chloramphenicol, 75 mg/kg/day IV divided q6h *and* cloxacillin or ox-acillin, 125 mg/kg/day IV divided q6h or an-other suitable antistaphylococcal agent *or* cefuroxime, 100 mg/kg/day IV divided q8h.

**d.** Gonococcal arthritis

    **(1)** Children under 45 kg: Use aqueous penicil-lin 100,000 units/kg/day IV divided q6h *or* ceftriaxone, 80 mg/kg/day (Maximum 2 gm) IV divided q12h *or* cefotaxime, 150 mg/kg/day IV in divided doses q8h.

    **(2)** Children over 45 kg: Use aqueous penicillin G 100,000 units/kg/day IV divided q6h *or* ceftriaxone, 1 gm IV daily divided q12–24h.

**e.** In children with *H. Influenzae* b infection, rule out concurrent infections such as otitis media and meningitis.

    Antibiotics should be given IV for a minimum of 1 week and thereafter for 3–4 weeks PO pro-vided that peak serum bactericidal concentra-tions of at least 1 : 8 can be demonstrated (see Chap. 24, Osteomyelitis, for specific criteria for oral therapy). Repeated joint aspiration may be necessary for pain relief. Acetaminophen, 10 mg/kg PO divided q4h, acetylsalicylic acid (ASA), 20–30 mg/kg/dose PO q6h prn, and codeine, 0.5–1.0 mg/kg divided q6h, are useful analgesics. Pain re-lief can also be achieved by splinting, elevation, and the use of ice packs.

**B. Serum sickness.** Serum sickness is characterized by flitting (moves from one joint to another), fleeting (stays in one joint for hours to a few days) polyarthritis that primarily involves the large joints. Affected joints are exquisitely painful, hot, and sometimes red. It occurs most commonly in the 5–15 year age group, often follow-ing antibiotic use (erythromycin, penicillin, cefaclor, sulfonamide) or viral infection (herpes, adenovirus, Ep-stein-Barr virus [EBV]). Systemic signs including ade-nopathy, fever, and erythema multiforme rash are com-mon. See Chap. 12.

**Table 24-1. Revised Jones Criteria**

| Major criteria | Minor criteria |
| --- | --- |
| Carditis | Fever |
| Polyarthritis | Arthralgia |
| Chorea | Previous rheumatic fever or rheumatic carditis |
| Erythema marginatum | |
| Subcutaneous nodules | Elevated ESR, CRP, WBC |
| | Prolonged PR interval |

Note: Documentation of a preceding streptococcal infection is also needed: throat swab for rapid antigen test or culture, scarlet fever, or ASLO titer.
Key: ESR = erythrocyte sedimentation rate, CRP = C reactive protein, WBC = white blood cell count.

1. **Management.** In general, symptomatic treatment and reassurance of parents is all that is required. Skin lesions usually resolve over 1–2 weeks. Arthralgia improves with ASA, 20–30 mg/kg/dose PO q6h.
C. **Acute rheumatic fever.** This poststreptococcal illness occurs most commonly in the 5–15 year age group; it is rare in younger children.
   1. Diagnosis requires the presence of two major or one major and two minor Jones criteria as well as evidence of a preceding streptococcal infection (see Table 24-1). Early in its course, rheumatic fever may not fulfill these criteria.
   2. The arthritis usually affects large joints and is flitting (moves from one joint to another), exquisitely painful, and usually responds dramatically to aspirin.
   3. Carditis may present with a murmur (mitral regurgitation, aortic regurgitation), prolonged PR interval on ECG, heart failure, or evidence of pericarditis (friction rub, pleuritic chest pain).
   4. **Management.** When this diagnosis is suspected, draw blood for culture, antistreptolysin-O (ASLO) titer, ESR, CBC, and differential count. Obtain a chest x ray and ECG and consult a cardiologist. The child with acute rheumatic fever should be admitted to hospital and treated with ASA, 100 mg/kg/day PO divided q6h, maintaining serum levels of the drug between 1.4 and 1.8 mmol/liter (20–25 mg/dl). Give phenoxymethyl penicillin, 50 mg/kg/day PO divided q6h, or erythromycin, 30–50 mg/kg/day PO divided q6h for 10 days. Those with congestive heart failure or carditis should be given prednisone, 2 mg/kg/day PO divided q6h, in addition to specific therapy for heart failure (see Chap. 8). Following acute treatment, patients must be maintained on antimicrobial prophylaxis.

**D. Systemic lupus erythematosus.** Sudden onset of painful, symmetric polyarthritis in a teenage girl suggests the diagnosis of SLE. Photosensitive dermatitis, painless oral ulceration, pleural or pericardial effusions, alopecia, Raynaud's phenomenon, and abnormalities in laboratory tests (hematuria, hematocytopenia, positive Coombs' test, high ANA titer, anti-DNA test, hypocomplementemia) support the diagnosis.

  **1. Management.** If SLE is suspected, obtain blood specimens for CBC, differential count, ESR, platelet count, Coombs' test, ANA, renal function, and liver function, and a urine specimen for urinalysis. Depending on the condition of the patient, arrange for either admission or outpatient follow-up with a rheumatologist.

**E. Juvenile rheumatoid arthritis.** The arthritis associated with JRA usually presents as a persistent, progressive arthritis with morning stiffness. Severe complications include iritis, pericarditis, pleuritis, and myocarditis. The different types present as follows:

  **1.** In pauciarticular JRA there are 1–4 affected joints.

  **2.** In polyarticular JRA there are more than 4 affected joints.

  **3.** Systemic onset JRA is a polyarticular arthritis, with additional findings of hepatosplenomegaly, adenopathy, characteristic high afternoon spikes of fever, and a pink-red macular rash.

  **4. Management.** Obtain blood specimens for laboratory tests (see sec. **II.D,** above) and x rays of severely affected joints. Although iritis is usually asymptomatic, inquire about decreased visual acuity, eye pain, or photophobia. Examine the eyes for evidence of iritis (see Chap. 15). Initially, begin therapy with ASA, 70–100 mg/kg/day PO divided q6h. If iritis is suspected, consult an ophthalmologist. Children who are systemically ill or are severely debilitated should be admitted. Otherwise, arrange outpatient follow-up with a rheumatologist.

**F. Lyme disease.** This syndrome can mimic JRA except for the presence of the characteristic erythema chronicum migrans (ECM) rash following a tick bite. There is marked geographic variation in the prevalence of this disease (which is most common in northeastern United States, Wisconsin, California, and Oregon), but it is reported worldwide. ECM is usually found on the trunk or proximal limb, starts as a red papule, and spreads slowly to become a large red plaque 10–20 cm in diameter, clearing over 2–3 weeks. Arthritis occurs an average of 1 month after ECM appears and is pauciarticular, typically involving the knee (75%), shoulder (25%), elbow (20%), temporomandibular joint (20%), or ankle (12%). Complications include aseptic meningitis, neuritis, Bell's palsy, and dysrhythmia (atrioventricular block).

  **1. Management.** Obtain blood samples for CBC, differential count, ESR, Lyme titer, and liver function, and a urine specimen for urinalysis. If meningitis is suspected, perform a lumbar puncture (see Chap. 21, Bacterial Meningitis). Treatment is as follows:

   a. **Children 8 years old or under:** phenoxymethyl penicillin, 50 mg/kg/day PO, divided q6h, or erythromycin, 30 mg/kg/day PO, divided q6h.

   b. **Children over 8 years old:** tetracycline, 250 mg PO q6h. Antibiotic therapy should be maintained for 10–20 days. Malaise, arthritis, and fever can be treated with ASA, 70–100 mg/kg/day PO divided q6h.

## III. Arthrocentesis

   **A. Procedure.** Arthrocentesis is essential in the investigation of the child with acute onset monoarthritis; when possible it should be performed by an orthopedic surgeon or rheumatologist. Arthrocentesis of the hip should be performed by an orthopedic surgeon, if possible.

   **1. Equipment**
      a. Sterile drapes, gloves, gowns
      b. Antiseptic solution: povidone-iodine, alcohol
      c. Arthrocentesis tray containing:
         (1) Plain 1% lidocaine solution (3–5 ml)
         (2) 3-ml syringe with 25-gauge needle for local anesthesia
         (3) 10-ml syringe with 20-gauge needle for aspiration
         (4) EDTA blood tube for cell count and differential
         (5) Plain blood tube for glucose measurement
         (6) Sterile tube for Gram's stain and culture

   **2. Method**
      a. If necessary, restrain the child and have an assistant fix the limb above and below the joint.
      b. Wash the skin 3 times with antiseptic solution.
      c. Anesthetize the skin and subcutaneous tissue down to the joint capsule with 1% plain lidocaine. Wait 2–3 minutes for anesthesia to take effect.
      d. Insert a 20-gauge needle into the joint, then attach the 10-ml syringe and aspirate fluid. Place fluid in each of the three tubes (1–2 ml is sufficient for each).

   **3. Methods for each joint**
      a. **Knee** (Fig. 24-1). Aspirate from either the medial or lateral side: With the knee straight or slightly flexed, direct the needle downward at 35-degree angle, beneath the lateral pole of the biconvex patella.
      b. **Elbow.** Flex the joint to 90 degrees and aspirate laterally, in the middle of the triangle formed by the head of the radius, the lateral epicondyle, and the olecranon.
      c. **Ankle.** With the foot-leg angle at 90 degrees, enter the joint between the anterior tibialis tendon and the medial malleolus.
      d. **Shoulder.** Aspiration is easiest with the arm hanging externally rotated, the needle inserted just below and lateral to the coracoid process.

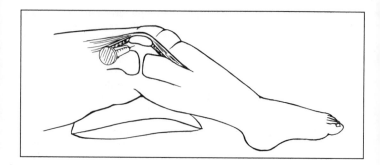

**Fig. 24-1. Knee joint aspiration.**

4. **Investigations**
   a. **Visually inspect** the fluid for color and turbidity:
      (1) **Yellow clear fluid** is normal and may be associated with a low-grade inflammation or infection.
      (2) **Yellow cloudy fluid** suggests infection or inflammation.
      (3) **Completely red fluid** is due to hemarthrosis from trauma or hemophilia.
      (4) **Greenish fluid** suggests sepsis.
   b. **Microbiology.** Send the fluid samples to the laboratory for Gram's stain, latex agglutination test, and culture in a sterile tube.
   c. **Hematology.** Send fluid sample in an EDTA tube for cell count and differential count.
      (1) **If white blood cells number less than 2 × 10⁹/liter (2000/mm³):** normal or low-grade inflammation is present.
      (2) **If white blood cells number more than 2 × 10⁹/liter (2000/mm³):** inflammation or infection exists.
   d. **Chemistry.** Send fluid in a plain-top tube for measurement of glucose level; if glucose is less than 1.1 mmol/liter (< 20 mg/dl), sepsis is likely.
5. **Complications**
   a. Introduction of infection
   b. Bleeding
IV. **Disposition.** Admit all patients with acute monoarthritis, septic arthritis, acute rheumatic fever, severe or complicated Lyme disease, JRA, or SLE. Children with septic arthritis of the hip require aspiration and arthrotomy under general anesthesia.
V. **Key points**
   A. Acute monoarthritis is due to sepsis until proved otherwise.
   B. X rays are often normal in the child with acute septic arthritis.

**C.** Children with sepsis of the hip require open arthrotomy.

**D.** Suspect serum sickness in the child with acute polyarthritis following viral infection or antibiotic medication.

### Bibliography

Cassidy, J. T., and Petty, R. E. *Textbook of Pediatric Rheumatology* (2nd ed.). New York: Churchill-Livingstone, 1989.

Fink, C. W., and Nelson, J. D. Septic arthritis and osteomyelitis in children. *Clin. Rheum. Dis.* 12:423, 1986.

Syriopoulou, V. P., and Sneath, A. L. Osteomyelitis and septic arthritis. In R. D. Feigin, and J. D. Cherry (eds.), *Textbook of Pediatric Infectious Diseases* (2nd ed.). Philadelphia: Saunders, 1987.

## Limp

Ross E. Petty

Limp is defined as an asymmetry of gait. It may result from structural asymmetry, muscle weakness, or pain. Trauma, including problems with footwear, is the most common etiology. Other common causes are as follows: (1) Under age 5: transient synovitis, and bone and joint infections; (2) in school-aged children: Legg-Perthe's disease, and transient synovitis; (3) in older children and adolescents: Osgood-Schlatter disease and slipped capital femoral epiphysis.

### I. Diagnosis and assessment

**A. History.** Determine the time of onset of limp and the events immediately preceding it, including febrile illness (toxic synovitis, reactive arthritis, septic arthritis), recent injection or immunization, strenuous physical activity (muscle strain), trauma, or new footwear. In young children, be wary of stress fractures following minor trauma to the tibia, fibula, metatarsals, or femur as a cause of gradually evolving limp.

   **1. If pain is absent,** consider leg length inequality, and muscle weakness caused by peripheral neuropathy or primary myopathy. Primary myositis is usually accompanied by muscle tenderness.

   **2. If pain is present,** determine the site of pain to narrow the differential diagnosis (Table 24-2).

**B. Examination**

   **1. Gait.** Ask the child to walk back and forth several times in a long hallway and observe the gait.

   **a.** Antalgic gait. Pain in the leg causes the child to minimize the duration of time he bears weight on the affected side.

   **b.** Circumduction gait. Loss of flexion at the hip, knee, or ankle causes the child to swing the leg out on the affected side.

   **c.** Ataxic gait. A broad-based gait occurs in children with muscle weakness or ataxia (see Chap. 22, Ataxia).

   **d.** Trendelenburg gait. Weakness of the gluteal

**Table 24-2. Painful causes of limp**

| Site | Examples |
|------|----------|
| Back pain | Trauma, spondylolysis or spondylolisthesis, inflammation (discitis, spondylitis), infection (osteomyelitis), tumors (osteoid, osteoma, malignancy) |
| Sacroiliac joint pain | Trauma, septic sacroiliitis, or inflammatory sacroiliitis |
| Hip pain | Transient (toxic) synovitis, Legg-Perthe's disease, slipped capital femoral epiphyses, chronic inflammatory synovitis (juvenile ankylosing spondylitis, JRA), muscle weakness (dermatomyositis), or congenital dysplasia or dislocation |
| Knee pain | Hypermobility, patellar dislocation, Osgood-Schlatter disease, inflammatory enthesitis, loose body (meniscus, cartilage), or chronic inflammatory synovitis |
| Ankle and foot pain | Hypermobility, trauma (including stress fracture and footwear problems), chronic inflammatory synovitis or enthesitis |

medius muscle causes excessive movement of the upper body to the weight-bearing side with "sagging" of the iliac crest level on the non-weight-bearing side.

**e.** Psoas limp. Weakness of the psoas muscle or an intraarticular hip lesion causes the hip to be flexed, abducted, and externally rotated.

**f.** Scissors gait. Tightness or spasticity of the hip adductors causes the knees to be held close together.

**g.** Leg length inequality. The long leg may be circumducted, and the child "dips" the pelvis when bearing weight on the short leg.

**h.** Steppage gait. Loss of foot dorsiflexion causes exaggerated lifting of the knee on the affected side.

**2. Examination of the painful area**

**a.** Find the source. Most children over age 3 can reliably localize the source of the pain. In the nonverbal infant or child, locate the source by gently squeezing the leg, moving from the foot up toward the hip while watching the infant's face for a grimace or cry. **Enthesitis** is an inflammation at the attachment of fascia, capsule, ligaments, or tendons to bone. Common sites are in the forefoot (insertion of the Achilles' tendon, insertions of the plantar fascia to the calcaneus, base of the fifth metatarsal, and heads of the metatarsals), and around the knee (tibial tuberosity, 6, 10, and 2 o'clock positions on the patella).

**b. Referred pain.** Absence of tenderness in the painful area suggests referred pain. Sacroiliac joint disease may cause pain in the buttocks or posterior thighs. Disease in the hip often causes pain over the inguinal ligament or the medial aspect of the knee.

**3. Joint and limb examination.** If the problem cannot be discerned from the gait and the pain cannot be localized, examine the joints carefully (see Chap. 24, Acute Arthritis). **Always exclude septic arthritis, osteomyelitis, and slipped capital femoral epiphysis.** Compare leg lengths by measuring distances from the anterior superior iliac spine to the ipsilateral medial malleolus. Inequality of 1 cm or more is considered significant.

**4. Neurologic examination.** If no musculoskeletal cause can be demonstrated, perform a thorough neurologic examination, evaluating symmetry of tone, muscle strength, sensation, and deep tendon reflexes to rule out lesions of the upper motor neuron pathways, spinal cord, anterior horn cell, posterior columns, or peripheral nerves.

## C. Investigations

**1.** When the cause of limp is **unknown,** or when more than minor traumatic injury is suspected, obtain an x ray of the affected part. In cases of nontraumatic limp draw blood for CBC, differential count, and ESR.

**2.** Other tests, including technetium-99 bone scan, aspiration of joint fluid, or aspiration of bone marrow may be obtained as indicated (see sec. **II** below).

# II. Specific disorders

## A. Discitis.
An inflammatory, possibly infectious disorder of the disc, most commonly located between L4 and L5 (45%) or between L3 and L4 (35%), discitis usually occurs in 1–3 year olds. The characteristic clinical presentation is low-grade fever, tripod posturing (leaning back on extended arms) while sitting, and refusal to walk. Abdominal pain may also be present. There is well-localized tenderness on palpation of the spinous processes over the affected area, pain on straight leg raising, and a decreased range of motion of the spine. Radiographs may show disc space narrowing, and technetium scan usually demonstrates a discrete area of increased uptake.

**1. Management.** Treatment is supportive, consisting of bed rest and analgesics. Consult an orthopedic surgeon.

## B. Transient synovitis of the hip.
This presumably viral disorder occurs most commonly in boys aged 3–10 years. Low-grade fever may be present. The hip is held in mild flexion, abduction, and external rotation with pain maximal directly over the inguinal ligament or referred to the medial aspect of the knee. Radiographs may either

be normal or show evidence of increased intraarticular fluid; technetium scan may be normal or show increased uptake on both sides of the joint space. The white blood cell and differential count are normal, and the ESR is normal or mildly elevated (< 40 mm/hour). Although rarely indicated, aspiration of the hip joint may be performed to rule out sepsis or provide symptomatic relief. Analysis of the aspirate reveals a mildly inflammatory, culture-negative fluid.

   **1. Management**
   **a.** The child with mild symptoms, an ESR of less than 40, and absence of fever may be managed at home with bed rest and analgesia (ASA, 20–30 mg/kg PO q6h) for 10–14 days.
   **b.** In other cases, admission to hospital for traction and analgesia are required. Refer the patient to an orthopedic surgeon.

**C. Legg-Perthe's disease.** Legg-Perthe's disease is an idiopathic aseptic necrosis of the femoral head. It is preceded by trauma in 20% of cases and is most common in 4–9-year-old boys. It may be bilateral. It presents with an insidious onset of limp and pain in the inguinal region or the medial aspect of the knee. Internal rotation and abduction are limited. In patients with **early** disease, the physical examination may be normal, but technetium-99 bone scan shows decreased uptake in the femoral head. The CBC and ESR are normal.

   **1. Management.** Immediate orthopedic assessment and treatment with bed rest are essential.

**D. Slipped capital femoral epiphysis.** This disorder is most frequent in 12 to 15-year-olds and is often bilateral. The onset may be abrupt, with severe pain in the inguinal area or the medial side of the knee. Physical examination reveals limitation of hip flexion and internal rotation. Frog-leg lateral radiographs of the hip show medial, downward, and backward displacement of the epiphysis.

   **1. Management.** Immediate orthopedic intervention is necessary. The patient should be kept in bed until assessed.

**E. Osgood-Schlatter disease.** Osgood-Schlatter disease is a traction injury of the apophysis of the tibial tubercle; it occurs in adolescents, who present with limp and tenderness over the site. Treat with ASA (see sec. **II.B.1.a,** above), and advise against strenuous activity until the symptoms settle in 3–6 weeks. Patients with persistent symptoms require immobilization in a cast and occasionally surgical intervention.

**F. Chondromalacia patella** (patellofemoral syndrome). Patellofemoral syndrome is a common cause of chronic knee pain in adolescents, particularly overweight females. Pain becomes worse with exercise and, in the classic case, when walking downstairs. Refer the patient to an orthopedic surgeon for follow-up.

**G. Osteochondritis dissecans.** Aseptic necrosis of the lateral portion of the medial femoral condyle results in fracture with chronic pain and tenderness, usually worse after exercise. Refer to a surgeon for immobilization in a cast.

**III. Disposition.** Most children with acute onset of limp do not require hospitalization. Cases of acute trauma, neurologic disease, and skeletal infection (osteomyelitis, septic arthritis) are examples of disorders that require admission.

**IV. Key points**

    **A.** Trauma is the most common cause of acute limp.

    **B.** Determine whether acute onset of limp is due to pain.

    **C.** CBC and differential count, ESR, and bone scan can help to make the diagnosis of infection. When sepsis is suspected, consult an orthopedic surgeon for bone or joint aspiration.

**Bibliography**

Cassidy, J. T., Petty, R. E. *Textbook of Pediatric Rheumatology* (2nd ed.). New York: Churchill-Livingstone, 1989.

Phillips, W. A. The child with a limp. *Ortho. Clin. N.A.* 18:489, 1987.

## Osteomyelitis

Gregory A. Baldwin and Ross E. Petty

Osteomyelitis usually follows hematogenous dissemination of infection in the child with bacteremia but can also result from direct spread of local infection. The overwhelming majority of cases are due to *Staphylococcus aureus*.

**I. Diagnosis and assessment**

    **A. History.** Most children present within a week of onset of symptoms. Older children are able to localize the pain to bone and often relate the onset to recent trauma. Younger children may have a history of fever and decreased use of a limb. Neonates often present with nonspecific symptoms such as irritability, poor feeding, lethargy, and pseudoparalysis of the limb.

    **B. Examination.** Carefully examine the joints, soft tissues, and bones of the extremity. Look for other foci of infection, including septic arthritis (most common in young infants). In general, osteomyelitis results in localized tenderness, swelling, and warmth over the metaphysis of the long bones. The most likely sites are the proximal tibia and distal femur. Erythema or cellulitis of the skin is unlikely unless the bone is subcutaneous or a subcutaneous abscess has developed. For examination of joints or the limping child, see Chap. 24, Limp; and Acute Arthritis.

    **C. Investigations**

        **1. Blood and cultures.** In children in whom osteomyelitis is suspected, obtain blood specimens for CBC, differential count, ESR, and blood culture (50%

are positive) in addition to Gram's stain and culture of other sites of infection.
   2. **X rays.** When bone infection is suspected, obtain x rays of the area. Bony changes are unlikely before 10–14 days after onset of infection; soft tissue swelling is an early radiographic sign of infection. Late changes include lysis of bone and elevation of the periosteum.
   3. **Bone scan.** Technetium-99 three-phase (immediate, delayed blood pool, and delayed bone uptake) bone scan may be helpful in the diagnosis of acute osteomyelitis, although it is not always reliable in detecting very early disease. Bone scans can be useful in the following situations: in localizing infection in the pelvis or spine; in looking for multiple sites in the neonate (often unreliable); and in differentiating infarction from infection in children with sickle cell disease.

## II. Management

A. Arrange investigations as outlined in sec. **I.C** above and consult an orthopedic surgeon for aspiration. Send the aspirate for Gram's stain, culture, and antigen analysis. Immobilize and elevate the limb and give analgesics.

B. Following aspiration, begin intravenous antibiotic therapy based on the Gram's stain. If the Gram's stain is negative or the organism is unknown, treat empirically as follows based on age and predisposing conditions:
   1. Birth to 2 months: Neonates are prone to infection from *S. aureus,* group B streptococcus, and gram-negative enteric organisms. Treat with:
      a. Cloxacillin or oxacillin, 100 mg/kg/day IV divided q6h or another suitable antistaphylococcal agent **and**
      b. Gentamicin, 5 mg/kg/day IV divided q8h.
   2. Over 2 months: Nearly all infections will be due to *S. aureus.* Treat with:
      a. Cloxacillin or oxacillin, 150 mg/kg/day IV divided q6h **or**
      b. Vancomycin, 50 mg/kg/day IV divided q8h (if child is penicillin allergic).

C. Surgical drainage may be required if:
   1. Pus is obtained from the aspirate.
   2. There are x-ray changes.
   3. There is no response to 24–48 hours of antibiotic therapy.

D. Sickle cell disease. *Salmonella* and *S. aureus* are common. Treat with:
   1. Chloramphenicol, 75 mg/kg/day IV divided q6h **and**
   2. Cloxacillin or oxacillin, 150 mg/kg/day IV divided q6h or another suitable antistaphylococcal agent.

E. *Pseudomonas* infection. This rare infection is usually seen in IV drug users (osteomyelitis) or patients with puncture wounds of the foot (osteochondritis). All cases require surgical debridement. Patients with osteochondritis also require 10 days of antibiotic therapy with:

  **1.** Ticarcillin, 200–300 mg/kg/day IV divided q6h **and**
  **2.** Tobramycin, 6 mg/kg/day IV divided q8h.
**F.** Except in cases of *Pseudomonas* infection, therapy
should include a minimum of 3 weeks of intravenous antibiotics. This regimen is followed by 3 weeks of intravenous or oral antibiotics. Oral antibiotic therapy may
be used only if the following criteria are met:
  **1.** Treatment in hospital only.
  **2.** Bacteria have been identified and are sensitive to
  oral medications.
  **3.** Patient responds to intravenous therapy.
  **4.** Serum bactericidal concentrations can be measured
  and peak levels maintained at 1 : 8 or greater.
**III. Disposition.** Admit all children with osteomyelitis.
**IV. Key points**
  **A.** Consider the diagnosis of osteomyelitis in the child with
  decreased use of a limb and fever.
  **B.** When osteomyelitis is suspected, obtain blood for culture, CBC, differential count, and ESR, and perform a
  bone scan.
  **C.** Most cases of osteomyelitis are due to *S. aureus*.

### Bibliography

Green, N. E., and Edwards, K. Bone and joint infections in children. *Orthop. Clin. North Am.* 18:555, 1987.

## Kawasaki Syndrome
Ross E. Petty and Gregory A. Baldwin

This systemic disorder usually occurs in the infant or very
young child. Accurate diagnosis requires the presence of
five of six clinical criteria (Table 24-3).

   In general, patients follow a triphasic course: (1) Stage 1
(1–10 days) is characterized by high fever and onset of the
diagnostic criteria listed in Table 24-3. (2) During stage 2

**Table 24-3. Criteria for diagnosis of Kawasaki disease**

1. Fever of 5 days' duration or longer (100%)
2. Polymorphous skin rash on trunk (80%)
3. Bilateral bulbar conjunctivitis (84%)
4. Acute nonpurulent swelling of cervical lymph node to >1.5
   cm diameter (73%)
5. Changes in hands and feet
   a. Edema of the hands (65%) or
   b. Red palms and soles (69%) or
   c. Desquamation of fingertips (80%), a late finding
6. Mucous membrane changes (92%)
   a. Dry, red, fissured, vertically cracked lips or
   b. Strawberry tongue or
   c. Diffuse reddening of the oropharynx

(11–24 days) there is defervescence, thrombocytosis (up to $1200 \times 10^9$/liter = 1,200,000/mm$^3$), desquamation of rash, and in some cases, the onset of cardiovascular complications. (3) In stage 3 (> 25 days) there is resolution of outward evidence of the disease, although cardiovascular complications may still occur or progress.

Most children with Kawasaki syndrome are extremely irritable. Less common findings include arthritis (19%), iritis, aseptic meningitis, urethritis with sterile pyuria, jaundice and hydrops of the gallbladder, and diarrhea and abdominal pain. With the rare exception of central nervous system vasculitis, disease of the coronary arteries constitutes the major cause of long-term morbidity and mortality. Cardiac disease is more common in males, in children under 1 year of age, and in patients with prolonged fever. It may result in dysrhythmia, congestive heart failure, pericarditis, and myocardial ischemia or infarction. Coronary artery aneurysms and their sequelae occur in 1–2% of patients. Diseases that resemble Kawasaki syndrome include toxic shock syndrome, scarlet fever, serum sickness, and Stevens-Johnson syndrome.

I. **Investigations.** Draw blood for a complete blood count (CBC), differential count, platelet count, erythrocyte sedimentation rate (ESR), blood culture, throat culture, and antistreptolysin-O (ASLO) titer, and obtain a urine sample for urinalysis. Lumbar puncture should be performed when meningitis is suspected.

II. **Management**
   A. Children with Kawasaki syndrome should be admitted to hospital. Consideration should be given to hydration status and restoration of fluid volume.
   B. Congestive heart failure should be treated (see Chap. 8).
   C. Give acetylsalicylic acid (ASA), 60–110 mg/kg/day PO divided q4h or q6h. When the fever falls or the platelet count rises at the end of the first stage, reduce the ASA dose to 5–10 mg/kg/day.
   D. Give intravenous gamma globulin to children who present in the first 10–12 days of the illness. The dose is 400 mg/kg daily for 4 consecutive days.
   E. Refer all cases to a rheumatologist and cardiologist; echocardiography should be performed at 10 days, 21 days, and 2 months.

III. **Disposition.** Admit all children with suspected Kawasaki syndrome.

IV. **Key points**
   A. Irritability, rash, mouth changes, and high fever should prompt suspicion of Kawasaki syndrome.
   B. Initial treatment is accomplished with ASA and, when indicated, gamma globulin.

**Bibliography**

Kato, H., Inoue, O., and Akagi, T. Kawasaki disease: Cardiac problems and management. *Pediatr. Rev.* 9:209, 1988.

Melish, M. E., Hicks, R. V., and Reddy, V. Kawasaki syndrome: An update. *Hosp. Pract.,* March, 1982.

Newburger, J. W., et al. The treatment of Kawasaki syndrome with intravenous gamma globulin. *N. Engl. J. Med.* 315:341, 1986.

# 25

# Psychologic Disorders

## Psychiatric Emergencies
Derryck H. Smith

Most pediatric psychiatric emergencies occur in adolescents. Priorities in management are to identify those patients in need of protection and to rule out serious medical or psychiatric illness.

I. **Psychiatric assessment**
   A. **History**
      1. **Interview.** Conduct the interview in a comfortable quiet room. Initially include all persons (family, social workers, police) who have accompanied the patient. When a basic understanding of the problem has been achieved, interview the patient alone. For most psychiatric disorders, the best single source of information is a direct interview with the child. Establish rapport and let the child know you are there to help—this is particularly important with an adolescent. Determine the chief complaint, onset and duration of symptoms, and precipitating or perpetuating factors.
      2. **Medical history and examination**
         a. **Mental status examination.** Note the patient's appearance and behavior, mood (depressed, manic, or anxious), orientation, judgment, and cognitive functioning. Ask about suicidal thoughts or actions and look for psychotic phenomena such as delusions, hallucinations, and impairment in reality testing.
         b. **Past history.** Determine the past medical and psychiatric history including medications and take a brief developmental history.
         c. **Family history.** Ask about the family psychiatric history, including depression, suicide, psychosis, substance abuse, and sociopathy.
         d. **Functional enquiry.** This inquiry should include a history of sleep disturbances such as insomnia (define as initial, mid, or terminal), nightmares, sleep walking, or nocturnal enuresis. Ask about appetite, and weight loss or failure to gain weight. A brief review of systems should be conducted.
         e. **Parent's history and family functioning.** A brief understanding of the parents' childhood often provides valuable clues to the current parenting skills.
         f. **Social functioning.** Ask about recent school performance—a sensitive measure of severity of emotional and behavioral problems—substance use, sexual abuse, sexual functioning, and social network.

**Table 25-1. Severity of suicidal ideation**

| Ideation | Severity |
|---|---|
| Vague thoughts of: "I'd be better off dead" | Least severe |
| Thoughts of killing oneself in abstract | |
| The presence of a plan for suicide | |
| The lethality of the plan | |
| The feasibility of the plan | |
| Recent suicide attempt | Most severe |

II. **Suicide.** Suicide is the third most common cause of death in adolescence. Although suicide is rare in young children, suicidal ideation is as common in young children as in teenagers. In the emergency room, suicide often presents as trauma, drug ingestion, or coma (secondary to drug ingestion).

  A. **Types of suicide**

  1. **Parasuicide.** Parasuicide is self-inflicted harm intended to be nonlethal, although death may occur due to miscalculation. It is much more common than true suicide. In many cases, parasuicide is not related to overt psychiatric illness but may be the effect of dysphoria, personality disorder, or attention-seeking in adolescents with personal or family problems. Female parasuicides outnumber males by 3 : 1.

  2. **Suicide.** Completed or attempted suicide is usually the result of medical or emotional problems or a reaction to social isolation or stress in the patient's environment. Males outnumber females by 3 : 1.

  B. **Diagnosis and assessment.** Routinely ask patients about suicidal thoughts. Judging the seriousness of suicidal ideation is critical. For a ranking of severity of suicidal ideation, see Table 25-1. Other risk factors for determining suicide potential include:

  1. Family disruption.
  2. Family history of suicide or depression.
  3. Past suicide attempts.
  4. Social isolation.
  5. Male sex.
  6. Presence of depression, especially with antisocial features.
  7. Psychosis.
  8. Recent exposure to suicide in a friend or relative.
  9. Recent severe stress or illness.

  C. **Management.** All suicide attempts should be regarded as potentially lethal. Begin by stabilizing medical problems and assessing suicide risk. Look for coexisting psychiatric problems such as depression or substance abuse and arrange for treatment.

  1. **Consultation.** Consult a child psychiatrist if in

**Table 25-2. Causes of psychosis**

| Type | Example |
| --- | --- |
| Medical | Intoxication |
| | Infection |
| | Seizure |
| | Cerebral vascular abnormalities (SLE) |
| | Metabolic and endocrine disorders: Reye's syndrome, Wilson's disease, hypoglycemia, thyrotoxicosis |
| | Cerebral hypoxia |
| | Space-occupying brain lesions |
| Psychiatric | Schizophrenic-spectrum illness |
| | Major affective disorder (depression) |
| | Reactive psychosis |
| | Personality disorders |
| | Manic phase of bipolar disorders |

doubt about the severity of the suicide attempt or to advise on treatment of depression or psychosis.

2. **Supervision.** Inform parents or guardians of the seriousness of the situation. Parents or guardians should be prepared to provide 24-hour 1 : 1 supervision to prevent suicide. If uncertain of parents' ability or motivation to do this, patient should be admitted for 1 : 1 nursing supervision. All dangerous objects should be removed from the room, and the patient should be dressed in hospital pyjamas to discourage elopement.

## III. Psychosis and delirium

A. **Psychosis.** Psychosis is defined as a gross impairment in reality testing. The presence of delusions or hallucinations, grossly disorganized behavior, and markedly bizarre or incoherent speech are evidence of underlying psychosis. The first priority is to establish the cause of psychosis (Table 25-2).

B. **Delirium.** Delirium is a psychotic state characterized by inability to maintain attention to external stimuli. It is **always** a symptom of underlying organic disease. Delirium is due to extracranial disease in 80% of cases—usually substance ingestion or metabolic derangement. Symptoms tend to wax and wane and include disorganized thinking, reduced level of consciousness, perceptual disturbance, disturbance of the sleep-wake cycle, increased or decreased psychomotor activity, disorientation, and memory impairment. Treatment of the underlying disorder will ultimately resolve the delirium.

C. **Investigation.** In all children and adolescents who present with psychosis or delirium, obtain blood specimens for complete blood count (CBC), measurement of glucose and electrolytes, and toxic screen, and urine for urinalysis and toxic screen. Patients with delirium or psychosis should undergo additional tests depending on

**Table 25-3. Dosage of medications for control of psychosis or delirium**

| Age | Dose of haloperidol every 30 minutes (PO, IV,* IM) | Dose of lorazepam every 30 minutes (PO, IV,* IM, SL) |
|---|---|---|
| > 15 years | 5 mg | 2 mg |
| 12–15 years | 3 mg | 1 mg |
| 8–14 years | 1 mg | 0.5 mg |

*Give lorazepam over 2 minutes IV. Give haloperidol over 5 minutes IV.

the differential diagnosis being considered (see Table 25-2).

  **D. Management of psychosis or delirium.** Most psychotic states are extremely unpleasant for the patient. Medications are used to relieve symptoms and distress, to allow further investigations, and to protect the patient and staff from harm. All children presenting in a psychotic or delirious state should be assessed by a child psychiatrist when possible.

    **1. Children over age 8.** In children over the age of 8 use haloperidol to normalize psychotic thinking and lorazepam to control disruptive behavior. Both drugs can be given IV, IM, or PO, but if an intravenous line is in place, this is the preferred route of administration. Cooperative patients without intravenous access can take the medication orally. Physical restraint may be required in uncooperative, dangerous, or agitated patients (one staff member for each limb and one or two to give the medication). Repeat the administration of medications every 30 minutes until target symptoms are controlled (see Table 25-3).

    **2. Children under age 8.** For treating psychosis in children less than 8 years old, thioridazine, a sedating phenothiazine, is recommended. Doses of up to 3.0 mg/kg/day PO can be used.

    **3. Side effects.** Side effects of antipsychotic drugs include sedation (haloperidol, lorazepam, thioridazine), respiratory depression (lorazepam), and orthostatic hypotension (thioridazine). Haloperidol and thioridazine administration may result in acute dystonia characterized by torticollis, oculogyric crisis, and opisthotonus. This is particularly common in teenage males. Treat acute dystonia with diphenhydramine, 2 mg/kg (maximum 50 mg) IV or IM, or benztropine mesylate (Cogentin), 0.5–2.0 mg IV or IM. Prophylactic use of PO benztropine may be considered to avoid acute dystonia in teenagers.

**IV. Depression.** Situational unhappiness is commonly found in children and adolescents, and does not always require medical therapy. Depression is a profound unremitting low mood usually accompanied by vegetative disturbance. The clinical presentation is thought to be similar in adults, teenagers, and children.

**A. Diagnosis and assessment**

    **1. Definition.** The most recent definitions of depression are contained in the DSM 111-R manual. Major depression is defined as the presence of at least five of the following nine criteria every day for a 2-week period:

        **a.** Depressed or irritable mood.

        **b.** Loss of interest or pleasure.

        **c.** Weight change or failure to gain weight.

        **d.** Insomnia or hypersomnia.

        **e.** Psychomotor agitation or retardation.

        **f.** Fatigue or loss of energy.

        **g.** Feelings of worthlessness.

        **h.** Diminished ability to think or concentrate.

        **i.** Recurrent thoughts of death or suicide.

    **2. Clinical presentation.** On most measures of clinical depression, there is no significant difference between adults, adolescents, and children. Specific differences are as follows:

        **a. Children.** Children tend to look more depressed, have more somatic complaints, psychomotor agitation, separation anxiety, phobias, and a higher incidence of hallucinations.

        **b. Adolescents.** There is more expression of hopelessness and anhedonia, hypersomnia, weight changes, and a higher lethality of suicide attempts.

**B. Management.** Determine if there is suicidal intent or psychosis—see secs. **I.C** and **II.D** for management. Most depression, even major depression, can be treated on an outpatient basis; arrange for follow-up with the family practitioner, a pediatrician, or a psychiatrist. Addressing problems at home and at school is essential. Individual or family psychotherapy is helpful. Tricyclic antidepressant therapy may be indicated.

**V. Behavior Disorders.** This group of disorders comprises the majority of psychiatric problems in the pediatrics age group.

**A. Eating disorders.** Currently in North America, there is an epidemic of eating disorders in adolescents and children, affecting 5–10% of females. Females outnumber males 10 : 1. There are two major categories: restrictors and binge-purgers.

    **1. Management.** All patients require referral to a comprehensive treatment program involving medical, nutritional, and psychiatric intervention. Patients should be admitted if there is:

        **a.** Severe acute or unremitting weight loss of greater than 30%.

        **b.** Hypotension, bradycardia, or hypothermia.

        **c.** Electrolyte imbalance, especially hypokalemia.

        **d.** Infection in a cachectic patient.

  **e.** Severe psychosocial disorganization with lack of a clear treatment plan.

**B. Conduct disturbance—delinquent behavior.** Exasperated families, social agencies, or police may arrive in the emergency room with a teenager who has a longstanding conduct problem complicated by delinquent behavior. The child often has a history of academic failure or difficulties at school. Families in particular tend to have high expectations that the child has an underlying medical problem that the doctor can remedy, thus "curing" the behavior.

  **1. Management.** Refer the child to outpatient psychiatric assessment to rule out such problems as attention deficit hyperactivity disorder, anxiety, or depression. Long-term solutions usually lie with social agencies rather than with psychiatric intervention.

**C. Family problems.** Families may present with complicated social problems in the emergency room, usually a conflict between the adolescent and the parents. There may be substance, physical, or sexual abuse within the family.

  **1. Management.** An emergency room social worker can greatly assist in assessing the problem. Hospitalization or apprehension of the child into legal custody may be necessary to protect him or her from a rejecting or disintegrating family situation. Generally, the family can be referred to a psychiatrist, psychologist, or social agency for follow-up.

**VI. Emotional problems presenting with somatic complaints.** Some patients and their families are uncomfortable with emotional issues and present with somatic complaints. Common complaints include abdominal or limb pain, headache, and nausea. In other families, emotional stress may precipitate or exaggerate physical illness. A small minority of patients meet their emotional needs by repeated contact with physicians or hospitals.

 Conversion reactions may present with a myriad of signs or symptoms including seizures and loss of motor or visual function. The classic description of "belle indifference" is not always present and does not help in making the diagnosis. Most cases are transient and resolve spontaneously. In many instances the child has real underlying disease. Conversion reaction should never be diagnosed or treated in the emergency department; admit the patient and consult a psychiatrist if this entity is suspected. In all other cases of somatic complaints, referral for outpatient psychiatric or medical assessment may be preferable to a continuing series of unproductive and expensive physical investigations.

**VII. Disposition.** The following children should be admitted: serious suicide risks, those in whom abuse or neglect is strongly suspected or confirmed, the psychotic child, those with acute intoxication or withdrawal, or those in whom there is doubt or uncertainty about the diagnosis and management. In most jurisdictions, children and adolescents can be certified and held against their will, although this is rarely necessary. Many areas have social agencies that provide emergency housing for children who do not require hospitalization on medical grounds.

**VIII. Key points**

 **A.** The best single source of psychiatric data is the child or adolescent patient.

 **B.** All children or adolescents with serious suicidal ideation require 24-hour, 1 : 1 supervision.

 **C.** Child and adolescent depression closely resembles that of adults.

 **D.** Rule out organic causes in children who present with psychosis.

 **E.** Judicious use of haloperidol and lorazepam can be helpful in symptomatic management of psychosis and delirium.

**Bibliography**

Clinton, J. E., Sterner, S., Stelmachers, Z., et al. Haloperidol for sedation of disruptive emergency patients. *Ann. Emerg. Med.* 16:3, 1987.

Dubin, W. R., Weiss, K. J., and Dorn, J. M. Pharmacotherapy of psychiatric emergencies. *J. Clin. Psychopharmacol.* 6:210, 1986.

Ellison, J. M., and Jacobs, D. Emergency psychopharmacology: A review and update. *Ann. Emerg. Med.* 15:8, 1986.

Garfinkel, B. D. Major Affective Disorders in Children and Adolescents. In G. Winkour, and P. Clayton *The Medical Basis of Psychiatry.* Philadelphia: Saunders, 1986.

Herzog, D. B., and Copeland, P. M. Eating disorders. *N. Engl. J. Med.* 313:295, 1985.

Hodgman, C. H. Recent findings in adolescent depression and suicide. *J. Develop. Behav. Pediatr.* 6:162, 1985.

Joffe, R. T., and Offord, D. R. Suicidal behavior in childhood. *Can. J. Psychiat.* 28:57, 1983.

Kazdin, A. E. Conduct disorders in childhood and adolescence. In *Developmental and Clinical Psychology and Psychiatry.* Vol. 9. Newbury Park: Sage Publication, 1985.

Ryan, N. D., Puig-Antich, J., Ambosini, P., et al. The clinical picture of major depression in children and adolescents. *Arch. Gen. Psychiat.* 44:854, 1987.

Weissman, M. M., Wickramaratne, P., Warner, V., et al. Assessing psychiatric disorders in children: Discrepancies between mothers' and children's reports. *Arch. Gen. Psychiat.* 44:102, 1987.

Vandereycken, W. *Anorexia Nervosa: A Clinician's Guide to Treatment.* Berlin: deGruyter, 1984.

---

# Sudden Unexpected Death
Andrew J. Macnab

---

Sudden, unexpected death is a traumatic event for all those concerned. Emergency room physicians rarely know the patient or the family, and this compounds the difficulty in dealing with grief. In the first hours of bereavement, family and friends may exhibit denial, anger, and guilt. Careful, sympathetic communication is of utmost importance—do not delegate this responsibility to junior staff. Effective initial intervention will reduce subsequent depression and allow earlier acceptance and recovery.

I. **Initial contact.** When possible, parents should be notified of the death of their child in person. If a telephone call is necessary, begin by identifying yourself and the hospital, and state the purpose of your call. The question "Can you come to the hospital?" is a useful introduction. Advise parents of where their child is and what has happened. Ask how long it will take for them to get to the hospital, and tell them where you will meet them. Suggest that they be accompanied by a friend or relative. News of death need not be communicated at this time, but do not deny it if a relative asks. At the end of the call repeat your name, the name of the hospital, and the address and telephone number.

II. **Arrival in the emergency room.** Emergency room staff should be told that the child has died and when and where the parents will arrive. Parents should be provided with a quiet room near the child. Make early contact. If they are met prior to the death, they may be forewarned of the seriousness of the illness and the likelihood of the child's death. If resuscitation is in progress, then you must delegate the task of communicating with parents, ensuring that someone continues to see them every 10–15 minutes. Parents are often comforted if they know that their child has been told that they are nearby. When death is imminent, allow them to be with their child.

III. **Notification of death.** Parents should be notified of the death as soon as possible. Organize your thoughts before speaking with them, and ask other family members and friends to leave the room. Relay the events in chronological order using simple and compassionate language. Touch and eye contact improve communication when dealing with the bereaved. Parents are comforted to know that their child was not in pain at the time of death. Tell them any helpful personal details, including the last wishes or words spoken. Be prepared to repeat information to allow full comprehension. Once the parents have been notified, give them time to be alone, but arrange to return shortly. When the immediate family knows the child is dead, this information should be shared with other relatives and friends—this is an important aspect of care for the grieving group as a whole.

IV. **The grief response.** Individuals express grief in a variety of ways determined by age, upbringing, culture, and experience. There is no right or wrong method. Be a good listener, and reassure the bereaved that their feelings and emotions are normal and acceptable. Do not take emotional outbursts and expressions of anger personally. It is important to address parental feelings of guilt. "If only . . ." is a common statement under such circumstances; whenever possible, explain to parents that they are not to blame for their child's illness or injury, and that everything that could have been done was done. Nursing and medical staff also need to experience grief when a child dies; take time to discuss the event with staff and address their emotional concerns.

V. **Viewing the body.** If parents are willing, they should be encouraged to see their child and say good-bye. Refer to the child by name and not as "it" or "the body." Prepare the parents by explaining how the child looks prior to the visit. The child should be made to look as clean and tidy as possible; parents find blood and vomitus particularly upsetting.

VI. **Arrangements.** Parents should be notified of plans for autopsy and other matters that require documentation. Tell them how to contact a funeral home. Arrangements should be made with their family doctor or pediatrician for a follow-up appointment within 48 hours. Explain that they should expect symptoms of grief such as anger, depression, sleep disturbance, tearfulness, loss of concentration, and poor appetite. If the parent is alone, arrange for someone to drive them home, and provide them with the hospital telephone number and your name as a contact for further questions. If there are other children in the family, help parents make plans for discussion of the death with them.

VII. **Key points**

A. Do not overlook the psychological needs of the survivors following sudden death in the emergency room.

B. Careful, empathetic intervention helps parents make a normal transition through the stages of grief.

### Bibliography

Albrizio, M. The Client Who Is Bereaved. In J. G. Gordon, and R. Partridge (eds.), *Practise and Management of Psychiatry Emergency Care* St. Louis: Mosby, 1982.

Dubin, W. R., and Sarnoff, J. R. Sudden unexpected death: Intervention with survivors. *Ann. Emerg. Med.* 15:54, 1986.

Jones, W. H. Emergency room sudden death: What can be done for survivors? *Death Education* 2:231, 1978.

Kubler-Ross, E. *On Death and Dying.* Toronto: Macmillan, 1974.

Robinson, M. A. Informing the family of sudden death. *Am. Fam. Physician* 23:115, 1981.

# Environmental
# Emergencies

# 26

# Burns and Smoke Inhalation

Gregory A. Baldwin

Burns are a devastating cause of morbidity and mortality in children. Patients with significant injury should receive care in a burn unit as soon as they have been stabilized.

## I. Diagnosis and assessment

### A. History.
Following resuscitation, inquire about past history, allergies, medications, and the mechanism of injury. Scalds, the most common type of childhood burn, are a major cause of morbidity and mortality. Suspect nonaccidental injury when histories from different sources conflict, or when the history and physical findings do not correlate.

### B. Evaluation of injury

1. **Surface area.** Body surface area (BSA) should be calculated using Lund and Browder's modified rule of nines (Fig. 26-1). As a guide, the surface area of the hand of the child is roughly equal to 1% BSA.

2. **Burn thickness**

   a. **Full-thickness burns (third-degree).** Full-thickness burns are often due to prolonged contact with a heat source, flame, or electricity. They are generally dark, hard in texture, and painless to touch, although this latter quality may be difficult to assess in an anxious child.

   b. **Partial-thickness burns (second-degree).** Partial-thickness burns may be superficial or deep. They usually follow scalds or brief contact with hot objects. They are extremely tender and sensitive.

      (1) Superficial partial-thickness burns are red and moist, with blisters.

      (2) Deep partial-thickness burns are mottled, with discrete areas of pale skin.

   c. **Superficial burns (first-degree).** Superficial burns follow minor injury. They are characterized by erythema, local pain, and tenderness but no blistering (see sec. **VI** below for treatment).

3. **Pattern of injury.** The child who has been subjected to an explosive burn should be carefully assessed for multiple system trauma. Look for clues to **nonaccidental injury:** Be suspicious of circumferential burns, scalds without splash marks, and burns that manifest the shape of the burning instrument, such as a cigarette or a curling iron (see Chap. 39).

4. **Assessment of severity. Major burns** are defined by the following criteria:

   a. Partial-thickness burns of more than 10% BSA.

   b. Full-thickness burns of more than 2% BSA.

   c. Burns of eyes, ears, face, hands, feet, or perineum.

   d. High-voltage electrical injury or electrical burns of the mouth.

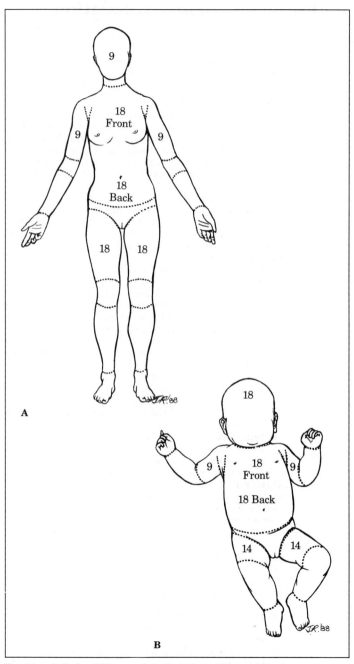

**Fig. 26-1. A. Rule of Nines, adult. B. Rules of Nines, infant.**

## II. Management of the child with major burn

**A. Airway.** The upper airway, including the larynx, may be subject to acute edema and obstruction following contact with hot air or gases. **If any of the following direct or indirect signs of injury are present in the burned child, endotracheal intubation and ventilation with 100% oxygen should be performed immediately, before complete obstruction occurs:**

1. **Direct signs.** Direct signs of airway injury include stridor, wheezing, indrawing, and cyanosis.

2. **Indirect signs**

   a. Direct burn of the face, singed nasal hair, or eyebrows.

   b. Evidence of an oropharyngeal burn, including carbonaceous sputum or a red edematous mouth or throat.

   c. Decreased level of consciousness—assume that there is significant airway or pulmonary injury.

**B. Breathing**

1. **Inhalation injury.** Smoke injury to the lower respiratory tract is due to exposure to the toxic products of combustion such as aldehydes, phosgene, and chlorine. It frequently occurs in the absence of a significant burn. Progression to respiratory failure may result and can be fatal—the result of laryngospasm, pulmonary edema, and decreased ciliary activity with obstruction of bronchioles. These effects may not be apparent clinically for up to 48 hours after injury. Suspect inhalation injury and treat with intubation and positive pressure ventilation with 100% oxygen in the following cases:

   a. When direct or indirect signs of airway injury are present (see sec. **II.A** above).

   b. When there is altered mental status (hypoxia, carbon monoxide toxicity), chest pain, or dyspnea (pneumonitis), or signs of respiratory compromise on examination or blood gas analysis.

2. **Bronchospasm.** Bronchospasm can be treated with nebulized bronchodilators such as albuterol (salbutamol), intravenous aminophylline, and if severe, ventilation (see Chap. 7).

3. **Carbon monoxide.** Carbon monoxide (CO) poisoning should be suspected in any child who is flame burned or exposed to smoke or hot gases in a contained environment. Give 100% oxygen and determine the carboxyhemoglobin level (heparinized blood sample)—see sec. **II.E** below. Carbon monoxide poisoning may present with seizures, an altered level of consciousness, and other neurologic findings. Victims of significant carbon monoxide poisoning (serum level > 20%) require 100% oxygen and may need to be intubated and ventilated. These patients may benefit from treatment in a hyperbaric chamber.

4. **Circumferential burns.** A patient with respiratory

distress associated with a circumferential burn to the chest may require an immediate escharotomy—consult a surgeon.

C. **Stop the burning process.** Burn victims may suffer ongoing injury from contact with hot, smoldering clothes or garments; remove all burning clothes and materials and apply cold soaks for a maximum of 5 minutes. Do not use ice or cold soaks for prolonged periods for pain relief—they can aggravate shock and cause cold thermal injury. In the case of a tar burn, do not try to strip the tar from the skin—the skin will come with it. Remove the tar by applying mineral oil, allow it to dissolve the tar, then wipe clean with a towel.

D. **Circulation.** Establish a large-bore-intravenous catheter if there is a burn of more than 15% body surface area (BSA) or if there is airway injury or smoke inhalation. Many children can be resuscitated with oral fluids. Evidence of shock in the first 30 minutes following injury should prompt a search for occult hemorrhage (see Chap. 32).

1. **Initial therapy.** In children in whom burns cover more than 15% of BSA, give a bolus of 400–500 ml/$m^2$ (15–20 ml/kg) of normal saline or Ringer's lactate and repeat prn to maintain a minimum urine output of 1 ml/kg/hour (normally 2–4 ml/kg/hour).

2. **Ongoing therapy.** Subsequent fluid volume should be calculated according to burn size. Do not add potassium to the fluid in the initial resuscitation. Give a total of 2000 ml/$m^2$ of maintenance fluid plus 5000 ml/$m^2$ of burned area in the first 24 hours. If surface area cannot be calculated, give 4 ml/kg/% burn area plus maintenance fluids (see Chap. 23, Fluids and Electrolytes) over the first 24 hours. Administer one-half of this total over 8 hours and the remaining half over the next 16 hours. Central venous hemodynamic monitoring (see Chap. 4) may be necessary for accurate fluid management. Aim to maintain a urine output of 1 ml/kg body weight/hour.

E. **Stabilization and monitoring**

1. **Extremities.** Examine the extremities and remove any constricting clothing or objects. In patients with circumferential burns, assess the adequacy of the distal circulation, and if compromised, consult a surgeon for escharotomy. Signs and symptoms of vascular compromise include tingling, reduced sensation, muscle weakness, and delayed capillary refill.

2. **Catheters.** Paralytic ileus and acute gastric distention are common in the severely burned child; insert a nasogastric tube if more than 15% BSA is burned or if there is gastric distention or vomiting. Place a Foley catheter to monitor urine output and guide fluid management in the severely injured child (see Table 17-1 for sizes).

3. **Pain control.** Intravenous morphine may be used for pain relief. Narcotics and sedatives should be

used with extreme caution in the nonventilated patient, especially the infant who is prone to apnea. If the child is distressed or agitated, be sure the cause is not hypoxia, shock, or carbon monoxide poisoning.

4. **Investigations.** Blood should be obtained for complete blood count (CBC), cross-matching, BUN, and measurement of carboxyhemoglobin level (heparinized tube), glucose, electrolytes, and arterial blood gas. Perform a throat culture for *Streptococcus*. If smoke inhalation is suspected, order a chest x ray as a baseline and take repeat films in 24 hours. Obtain a urine specimen for urinalysis including determinations for myoglobin, hemoglobin, and specific gravity and osmolality.

5. **Tetanus.** Administer tetanus prophylaxis to those at risk (see Appendix I).

6. **Antibiotics.** Dress wounds with 1% silver sulfadiazene cream and cover with a bulky sterile gauze dressing. Prophylactic systemic antibiotics are not required.

7. **Eyes.** If there is any evidence of damage to the eyes (including singed lashes or burns to the lids) apply sulfacetamide sodium (Sodium Sulamyd) ointment and a patch and consult an ophthalmologist immediately.

III. **Minor burns.** Initially, apply cool, sterile, saline-soaked gauze to minor partial- and full-thickness burns (limit to 20% of body surface area) for a maximum of 10 minutes to decrease tissue injury. Debride broken blisters and loose skin and clean with a weak antiseptic solution (0.5% chlorhexidine). Leave unbroken blisters intact. Give tetanus booster immunization to the child at risk (see Appendix I). Codeine phosphate, 0.5–1.0 mg/kg PO or IM, may be used for pain relief. Dress full wounds with silver sulfadiazene cream and cover with bulky dressings of sterile gauze. The face can be treated with Neosporin or Polysporin ointment and left exposed. If immediate referral is unnecessary, arrange for follow-up in 24 hours for a dressing change. For management of superficial burns, see sec. **VI** below.

IV. **Electrical burns**

A. **Low-voltage injury.** These injuries usually result from contact with wall sockets or electrical appliances. A low-voltage burn generally causes damage at the site of contact only and can be managed like a minor thermal burn. An exception is the child with an electrical burn of the mouth; this injury is fraught with complications, including late-onset scarring and heavy bleeding at 5–10 days, and surgical referral is mandatory.

B. **High-voltage injury.** High-voltage injuries are rare, occurring most often in older children involved in mishaps with power stations, live electrical rails, or live wires. Maximal tissue damage occurs at sites of entry and exit of current, and the degree of injury is usually more extensive than is apparent. Related injuries are common and include dislocations, fractures, deep visceral injury, surface arc burns across the joints, dysrhythmia, CNS injury, and renal failure secondary to hemoglobinuria or myoglobinuria.

1. **Management**

a. Assess problems in the airway, breathing, and circulation. Children with severe contact electrical burns are prone to dysrhythmias and cardiac arrest. Give oxygen by mask, start an intravenous line, and obtain blood for blood gas measurement, CBC, cross-matching, and measurement of electrolytes, BUN, and cardiac enzymes. Place the child on an electrocardiogram (ECG) monitor and insert a nasogastric tube and a Foley catheter.

b. Dipstick the first urine sample. Oliguria, anuria, dipstick-positive (myoglobin) or dark urine implies severe injury and impending renal failure from acute tubular necrosis; if this is present, give an intravenous fluid challenge with 10 ml/kg of normal saline, followed by a second challenge if the urine output does not increase in 30 minutes. Alkalinize the urine, keeping the pH above 7 by administering IV $NaHCO_3$, 50–100 mEq/liter of Ringer's lactate or normal saline. Urine output should be maintained at a minimum of 2 ml/kg/hour. Do not add potassium to the intravenous fluids in the first 24 hours. If renal function is compromised, consult a nephrologist.

c. Look for entry and exit wounds as sites of maximal tissue damage and refer to a surgeon for debridement and further therapy.

V. **Chemical burns.** Alkali burns induce liquefactive necrosis, resulting in more extensive tissue damage than the coagulative necrosis caused by acid burns. External burns should be irrigated with tap water or normal saline for a minimum of 15 minutes. Alkali burns of the eye require continuous irrigation with sterile normal saline for a minimum of 20 minutes and consultation with an ophthalmologist. For diagnosis and management of caustic ingestions, see Chap. 27.

VI. **Sunburn.** Sunburn is caused by prolonged exposure to ultraviolet B light. Erythema and discomfort are common; extreme exposure can result in heat stroke (see Chap. 29, sec. **III**).

A. **Management.** Treat mild sunburn with topical chilled emollient cream (Nivea) applied prn, and acetylsalicylic acid, 10 mg/kg/dose PO given every 4–6 hours. Cool compresses made from sheets soaked in cool water can be draped over the child to relieve pain in cases of moderate or severe sunburn. Steroids and topical anesthetic agents should not be used.

VII. **Disposition.** All children with major burns (see sec. **I.B.4** above), carbon monoxide poisoning, or inhalational injury and those in whom there is suspicion of abuse or neglect should be admitted to hospital, if possible to a burn unit.

## VIII. Key points

**A.** Follow the ABCs of resuscitation in the initial assessment and treatment of the burned child. Signs of airway or ventilatory compromise should lead to early intubation and ventilation.

**B.** If circumferential burns are compromising the limb circulation or respiratory function, an escharotomy should be performed.

**C.** Measure carboxyhemoglobin levels in the child who is flame-burned or exposed to heated gases in a contained environment.

**D.** Use cool sterile saline soaks to decrease tissue injury.

### Bibliography

Charnock, E. L., and Meehan, J. J. Postburn respiratory injuries in children. *Pediatr. Clin. North Am.* 27:661, 1980.

Herndon, D. N., Thompson, P. B., Desai, M. H., et al. Treatment of burns in children. *Pediatr. Clin. North Am.* 32:1311, 1985.

O'Neill, J. A. Evaluation and treatment of the burned child. *Pediatr. Clin. North Am.* 22:407, 1975.

Warden, G. D. Outpatient care of thermal injuries. *Surg. Clin. North Am.* 67:147, 1987.

# Toxicology

Gregory A. Baldwin

Poisoning is the third most common pediatric injury treated in emergency departments. In most cases the child is under the age of 5, and only one poison has been ingested. Morbidity in these children is usually low, and hospitalization is seldom necessary. Poisoning should also be considered in any child with unexplained coma, seizures, or affective disorder. Common ingestions are plants, household products, salicylates, acetaminophen, petroleum distillates, tranquilizers, iron, "over-the-counter" medications, and, in the adolescent, substances of abuse (see Table 27-1). Priorities in management following initial resuscitation are (1) Utilize the history, physical examination, and laboratory analysis to determine the type and severity of ingestion; (2) prevent further toxicity by removing the toxin or decreasing its absorption; (3) enhance elimination of the drug and its metabolites; (4) continue assessment of vital signs; (5) administer an antidote if possible (see Table 27-2); (6) rule out attempted suicide or child abuse.

## I. Resuscitation

**A. General principles.** The first priority in the treatment of poisoned children is to maintain the airway, breathing, and circulation. Repeated clinical assessment should include frequent monitoring of vital signs.

**B. The comatose victim.** The child with a decreased level of consciousness deserves special attention:

1. Assess the adequacy of the airway and ventilation. If there are signs of airway compromise or respiratory failure, intubate the patient with a cuffed endotracheal tube and ventilate. Determine the depth of coma and the child's response to specific stimuli (see Chap. 22, Coma).

2. Start an intravenous line, draw blood for glucose measurement, and give an IV bolus of dextrose: 2.5 ml/kg of 10% D/W in the newborn, or 1 ml/kg of 25% D/W in the child. If this is effective, follow with a dextrose infusion (see Chap. 13, Hypoglycemia).

3. Naloxone, 0.01 mg/kg IV (see Table 27-3) should be administered following the bolus of glucose; if this is ineffective, repeat with 0.1 mg/kg IV.

4. Poor perfusion or circulatory compromise should be treated with an intravenous infusion of 10 ml/kg of normal saline or Ringer's lactate (see Chap. 4), repeated prn until the patient's condition is stable.

5. Place the child on a cardiac monitor and check a rhythm strip for dysrhythmia.

6. Send samples of urine, blood, and initial gastric aspirate for toxicologic analysis and obtain blood for measurement of blood gases, serum electrolytes, glucose, ammonia, and liver function tests.

## II. Diagnosis and assessment

**A. History.** Determine the past history, current medications, allergies, the type and time of intoxication, and the maximum possible quantity of toxin ingested. When the toxin is unknown, ask about medications in the household. Obtain the empty bottle or a sample of the poison for identification. In children **over age 6,** accidental ingestion of poisons is unusual. Suspect child abuse in these cases. Poisoning in the **adolescent** usually involves a suicide attempt with multiple drug ingestion, often including acetaminophen. The history is notoriously unreliable in determining substances ingested in adolescents. Consider other possible causes of coma (see Chap. 22, Coma) in the **unconscious child** including trauma, central nervous system infection, hypoxic-ischemic injury, seizure, and Reye's syndrome.

**B. Examination.** Perform a complete physical examination and try to fit the clinical findings to a particular intoxication. Common causes of various toxic signs and symptoms are listed below; (however, this is not an inclusive list).

1. **Neurologic examination**
   a. Coma: narcotics, sedative hypnotics, barbiturates, alcohols, carbon monoxide, cyclic antidepressants, and anticholinergics.
   b. Ataxia: Dilantin, benzodiazepines, organic solvents, ethanol, and barbiturates.
   c. Seizures: theophylline, cyclic antidepressants, amphetamines, phencyclidine (PCP), camphor, ammonia, isoniazid, phenothiazines, halogenated hydrocarbons, parathion, lithium, phenol, and cocaine.
   d. Dystonic reaction (oculogyric crisis): phenothiazines, metoclopramide, and haloperidol.

2. **Eyes**
   a. Miosis: opiates, barbiturates, phenothiazines, and organophosphates.
   b. Mydriasis: amphetamines, cocaine, and anticholinergics.
   c. Nystagmus: phenyclidine and Dilantin.

3. **Vital signs**
   a. Tachycardia: alcohol, amphetamines, cocaine, theophylline, and anticholinergics.
   b. Bradycardia: cyclic antidepressants, narcotics, digitalis, barbiturates, and cholinergics.
   c. Tachypnea: amphetamines, carbon monoxide, and salicylates.
   d. Slow respirations: ethanol, barbiturates, and narcotics.
   e. Apnea: botulism, organophosphates, and any cause of slow respirations (see sec. **II.B.d** above).
   f. Wheezing: organophosphates and hydrocarbons.
   g. Hyperthermia: salicylates, hydrocarbons, amphetamines, phencyclidine, theophylline, anticholinergics, and dinitrophenols.
   h. Hypothermia: barbiturates, phenothiazines, narcotics, and ethanol.

**Table 27-1. Frequently ingested products that are usually nontoxic**

Abrasives

Adhesives

Antacids

Antibiotics

Baby product cosmetics

Ballpoint pen inks

Bathtub floating toys

Battery (conventional flashlight if bitten)

Bath oil (castor oil and perfume)

Bleach (<5% sodium hypochlorite)

Body conditioners

Bubble bath soaps (detergents)

Calamine lotion

Candles (beeswax or paraffin)

Caps, toy pistol (potassium chlorate)

Chalk (calcium carbonate)

Clay (modeling)

Colognes

Contraceptive pills

Corticosteroids

Crayons (marked A.P.,C.P.,C.S. 130-46)

Dehumidifying packets (silica, charcoal)

Detergents (phosphate-type, anionic)

Deodorants

Deodorizers (spray and refrigerator)

Elmer's glue

Etch-a-sketch

Eye make-up

Fabric softeners

Fertilizer (if no caution label)

Fish bowl additives

Fluoride, caries preventative

Glues and pastes

Golf ball (core may cause mechanical injury)

Grease

Hair products (dyes, sprays, tones)

Hand lotions and creams

Hydrogen peroxide (medicinal 3%)

Indelible markers

Ink (black, blue)

Iodophor disinfectant

Laxatives

Lipstick

Lubricant

Lubricating oils

Lysol brand disinfectant (not toilet bowl cleaner)

Magic markers

Make-up (eye, liquid facial)

Matches

Mineral oil

Newspaper

Paint, indoor latex acrylic

Perfumes (depends on alcohol content)

Petroleum jelly

Plaster patching (no lead)

Play-Doh

Pencil (lead-graphite, coloring)

Porous-tip ink marking pens

Prussian blue (ferric ferrocyanide)

Putty (< 2 oz)

Rouge

Rubber cement

Sachets (essential oils, powder)

Shampoos (liquid)

Shaving creams and lotions

Soaps and soap products

Spackles

Suntan preparations

Sweetening agents (saccharin, cyclamates, Nutrasweet)

Teething rings

Thermometers (mercury)

Toilet water

**Table 27-1.** (continued)

| | |
|---|---|
| Toothpaste | Water colors |
| Vaseline | Zinc oxide |
| Vitamins | Zirconium |

Note: An ingestion is considered nontoxic only if:
1. There is absolute identification of the product.
2. There is absolute assurance that only one product was ingested.
3. There is assurance that there is no signal word (i.e., caution, warning, danger-poison) on the container.
4. A good approximation of the amount ingested can be made.
5. There is assurance that the victim is free of symptoms.
6. The physician has the ability to call the patient back at intervals to determine that no symptoms have developed.
Source: Adapted from H. C. Mofenson, J. Greensher, and T. R. Caraccio. Ingestions considered nontoxic. *Emerg. Med. Clin. North Am.* 2:159, 1984.

> **i.** Hypertension: amphetamines, cocaine, anticholinergics, theophylline, and phencyclidine.
> **j.** Hypotension: narcotics, phenothiazines, diazepam, and other CNS depressants.

**4. Skin**
>   **a.** Hot dry skin: anticholinergics.
>   **b.** Diaphoresis: organophosphates, amphetamines, mushrooms, salicylates, and cocaine.
>   **c.** Cyanosis: methemoglobinemia, hypoxia, and carbon monoxide.
>   **d.** Flushing: anticholinergics, borate, and amphetamines.

**5. Gastrointestinal tract**
>   **a.** Ileus: anticholinergics and narcotics.
>   **b.** Violent emesis: theophylline, caustics, fluoride, salicylates, iron, and food poisoning.
>   **c.** Urinary retention: anticholinergics.

**6. Breath odor**
>   **a.** Acetone: acetone, methyl and isopropyl alcohols, and salicylates.
>   **b.** Alcohol: ethanol.
>   **c.** Bitter almonds: cyanide.
>   **d.** Coal gas: carbon monoxide.
>   **e.** Garlic: arsenic, phosphorus, and organophosphates.
>   **f.** Oil of wintergreen: methyl salicylate.
>   **g.** Fruitlike: amyl nitrate, methanol, and isopropyl alcohol.
>   **h.** Peanuts: rodenticides (Vacor).
>   **i.** Violets: turpentine.

**C. X rays.** In the child with signs of respiratory distress, order a chest x ray to look for evidence of aspiration pneumonitis or pulmonary edema. The following toxins are radiopaque and may be visible on abdominal x rays: chloral hydrate, some iron preparations, lead, phenothi-

**Table 27-2. Antidotes**

| Poison | Antidote | Dose |
| --- | --- | --- |
| Acetaminophen | N-acetylcysteine | Intravenous:<br>　Load: 150 mg/kg in 200 ml<br>　　5% D/W over 15 minutes<br>　Then: 50 mg/kg in 500 ml<br>　　5% D/W over 4 hours<br>　Then: 100 mg/kg in 1000 ml<br>　　5% D/W over 16 hours<br>　Note: Fluid volumes may be decreased in young children<br>Oral:<br>　Load: 140 mg/kg PO<br>　Then: 70 mg/kg PO q4h for 17 doses |
| Cholinergics | Atropine | 0.05 mg/kg IV prn |
| Major tranquilizers (extrapyramidal effects) | Diphenhydramine | 1–2 mg/kg IV q6h prn |
| Iron | Deferoxamine | If patient is normotensive and in mild poisoning: 50 mg IM q4h<br>If patient is hypotensive, comatose, or acidotic, or in severe poisoning: 15 mg/kg/hr IV for 4 hours, then decrease to 2–5 mg/kg/hr |

| | | |
|---|---|---|
| Narcotics | Naloxone | Maximum daily dose is 120 mg/kg or 6 gm, whichever is less<br>0.01 mg/kg IV; if no response give 0.1 mg/kg IV and repeat prn if effective |
| Methanol and ethylene glycol | Ethanol | 1 ml/kg of absolute ethanol in loading dose IV/PO; 1.4 ml/kg/hour of 10% solution IV/PO in maintenance dose if patient not being dialyzed. Maintain serum levels at 100–150 mg/dl. |
| Cyanide | Amyl nitrite<br>Sodium nitrite (3%) | Inhale for 30 seconds of each minute until sodium nitrite is given<br>If patient weighs over 25 kg: dose is 300 mg. Give at a rate of 2.5–5 ml/min IV. Stop if BP is < 80 mm Hg systolic.<br>If patient weighs under 25 kg: dose is 0.27 ml/kg. Administer IV slowly. Follow with sodium thiosulfate after 15 to 20 minutes. |
| | Sodium thiosulfate (25%) | Adult: 12.5 gm IV at 2–5 ml/min<br>Child: 1.65 ml/kg IV slowly (3–5 ml/min) |
| Organophosphate | Atropine—continue q3–5 minutes until drying of pulmonary secretions occurs | 0.05 mg/kg/dose IV q5 min prn after a test dose of 0.01 mg/kg IV. Follow with pralidoxime |
| | Pralidoxime—useful within 30 hours of exposure | 25–50 mg/kg/dose (max. 2 gm) IV slowly. May repeat in 30 min if no improvement and then at 2 hours and q8–12h prn |

azines, cyclic antidepressants, arsenic, iodides, enteric-coated medications, sodium, and potassium.

**D. Other investigations**

1. Send samples of blood, vomitus, lavage return, and urine for toxic screening. Order an electrocardiogram (ECG) on all children with significant poisoning.

2. If a particular poison is identified by the history or screening, check a serum level of the substance when possible. In teenage suicide attempts, acetaminophen is commonly ingested, and levels of this should therefore be determined. In serious poisonings, obtain blood for CBC, prothrombin time, and measurement of electrolytes, BUN, glucose, and blood gases.

3. Blood gas analysis can help to determine the poison involved. Children with salicylate toxicity often have respiratory alkalosis and metabolic acidosis. **Metabolic acidosis** with an increased anion gap occurs in a set of disorders known by the mnemonic MUD-PIES: methanol, uremia, diabetic ketoacidosis, paraldehyde, iron, isoniazid, ethanol, ethylene glycol, and salicylates. See Chap. 23, Acid-Base Metabolism.

4. The diagnosis of poisoning by ethylene glycol or the alcohols (methyl, ethyl, isopropyl) is supported by finding a positive **serum osmolar gap.** This is calculated by subtracting the measured serum osmolality from the calculated osmolality ($2 \times Na$ + glucose/18 + BUN/3 in old units, or $2 \times Na$ + BUN + glucose in SI units). A calculated difference of greater than 10 mmol/liter is significant.

5. When the poison ingested is unknown, save 30–50 ml of urine for toxic screening. The ferric chloride screening test is performed by mixing 0.5 ml of 10% FeC1 with 2.0 ml of freshly voided urine: salicylates turn purple, phenothiazines turn blue, isoniazid turns gray or green.

**III. Management.** Once the toxic substance has been identified, the local poison control authorities should be consulted regarding therapy.

**A. Gastrointestinal decontamination**

1. **Ipecac syrup.** In most instances, ipecac induces vomiting within 20 minutes. It can be safely repeated once in children who are over 1 year of age. Appropriate doses are:

| | |
|---|---|
| 6–9 months | 5 ml PO |
| 9–12 months | 10 ml PO |
| 1–12 years | 15 ml PO |
| over 12 years | 30 ml PO |

Administration of ipecac should be followed by 5 ml/kg of fluid orally to a maximum of 300 ml. Ipecac is contraindicated in the child under 6 months of age, in the child who has a depressed or decreasing level of consciousness, in the seizing child, and in the child who has ingested cyclic antidepressants, hydrocarbons, or caustic materials.

2. **Gastric lavage.** Gastric lavage should be performed in the child with massive ingestion, in patients who are obtunded, uncooperative, or comatose, or if emesis is not successfully induced. Do not perform lavage in children who have ingested a corrosive substance (see sec. **IV.D**). In the child who is comatose, convulsing, or unable to protect the airway (absent cough, gag, swallow), the airway must be secured with a cuffed endotracheal tube before lavage is performed.

   a. **Method**
      (1) Restrain the patient with a mummy wrap or papoose board (see Appendix III) and place on the left side with the head hanging over the edge of the bed.
      (2) Use a large orogastric tube—20 gauge in a toddler or infant, 30–36 gauge in 2–10 year old, and 36 gauge in the adolescent. If a cuffed endotracheal tube is in place, momentarily deflate the cuff while passing the tube; failure to do this could result in esophageal injury.
      (3) Attach a funnel to the orogastric hose. Pour in warm normal saline, 15 ml/kg/cycle (maximum 300 ml). Empty the stomach by lowering the funnel and draining the gastric contents into a container on the floor. Continue lavage until several returns are clear. Leave activated charcoal and cathartic in the stomach, and pinch the tube prior to removal to prevent aspiration.

3. **Activated charcoal.** Charcoal decreases the metabolism of the poison by an absorptive action. It is usually given in a premixed slurry of 250 ml diluent/50 gm charcoal. The dosage is 15–30 gm in children under 5 years, and 30–100 gm in older children. The preferred diluent is 35% sorbitol. Charcoal is ineffective against mineral acids, alkali, cyanide, ferrous sulfate, lithium, electrolytes, and ethyl, methyl, or isopropyl alcohol. It should not be given concurrently with or immediately prior to giving ipecac or oral $N$ acetyl cysteine (NAC) because it will cause their adsorption and inactivation. If emesis has been induced with ipecac, give charcoal 30–60 minutes later. With certain ingestions (Table 27-3), repeated activated charcoal may be given in a dose of 5–10 gm q2–4h orally or via nasogastric tube to increase clearance of the drug; this effect probably occurs by interfering with the enterohepatic circulation of the toxin. In general, cathartics should be mixed with the first dose only.

4. **Cathartics.** These are believed to increase the intestinal transit time of the toxin. The first choice is

**Table 27-3. Poisonings in which repeated activated charcoal is effective**

| | | |
|---|---|---|
| Carbamazepine | Chlordecone | Dextropropoxyphene |
| Cyclic antidepressants | Dapsone | Digoxin |
| Nadolol | Phenobarbital | Salicylates |
| Theophylline | Sotalol | Meprobamate |

35% sorbitol, which can be mixed with activated charcoal (4 ml/gm). Alternatives to sorbitol are:

    **a.** Magnesium citrate, 4 ml/kg (maximum dose 300 ml)

    **b.** Magnesium sulfate, 250 mg/kg

  **5. Increased excretion.** Forced diuresis with furosemide (Lasix) has been used to increase elimination in salicylate, bromide, phencyclidine, lithium, amphetamine, and barbiturate overdose. Forced diuresis can be hazardous; when possible it should be reconsidered in favor of hemodialysis or hemoperfusion. Alkalinization with intravenous sodium bicarbonate is effective in decreasing toxicity due to barbiturates, salicylate, and cyclic antidepressants. During alkalinization, monitor blood gases frequently.

**B. Elimination.** Although rarely indicated in the treatment of childhood ingestions, hemodialysis or hemoperfusion may be used in the following clinical situations:

  **1.** Progressive deterioration despite intensive therapy.

  **2.** Severe intoxication with hypoventilation, hypothermia, or hypotension that is not responsive to supportive therapy.

  **3.** Impairment of drug excretion due to hepatic, cardiac, or renal insufficiency.

  **4.** Hemodialysis or hemoperfusion is suitable for drug overdose with acetaminophen, aminophylline, lithium, theophylline, barbiturates, salicylates, and ethyl, methyl, or isopropyl alcohol.

**C. Surface decontamination.** Surface decontamination is required in all patients who have been exposed to organophosphates, carbamates, mace, gasoline, or caustics. Staff should wear gown and gloves, remove all articles of the child's clothing, and wash the patient's skin twice with soap and water. If the eye has been exposed, irrigate with 1–2 liters of freely running room temperature normal saline for a minimum of 15–20 minutes (see Chap. 15).

**IV. Specific poisons**

  **A. Acetaminophen**

    **1. Toxic dose.** The toxic dose is greater than 140 mg/kg. Note: the risk of toxicity is increased in children who have co-ingested barbiturates and in those with preexisting hepatic dysfunction.

2. **Toxic effects.** Four stages of acetaminophen overdose have been identified. Stage 1 occurs in the first 24 hours—in young children, in the first several hours after ingestion—and may be characterized by diaphoresis, anorexia, nausea, and vomiting. Stage 2 is a latent phase that occurs 24–48 hours after ingestion, during which gastrointestinal symptoms improve. Absence of symptoms at this time is not predictive of outcome. The target organ of acetaminophen toxicity is the liver. Hepatic necrosis, with elevation of serum transaminases (SGOT/AST > 1000 IU/liter), prothrombin time (PT), and bilirubin concentration peaks during stage 3, at 72–96 hours after ingestion. With severe toxicity there may be oliguria, jaundice, and encephalopathy leading to coma and death. Stage 4 is the recovery phase and occurs at 7–8 days.

3. **Management**

   a. If there is an accurate history of ingesting less than 140 mg/kg, the child may be treated conservatively. Ipecac, charcoal, and a cathartic should be given.

   b. If the history is unclear or more than 140 mg/kg has been ingested, give charcoal and obtain a serum acetaminophen level. Use the Rumack-Matthew nomogram (Fig. 27-1) to predict toxicity. Serum levels are predictive only when they are obtained at least 4 hours after ingestion.

   c. The child who has or is suspected of having hepatotoxic levels within 24 hours of ingestion should be treated with NAC.

      (1) Oral therapy. Prepare a 5% NAC solution by diluting one part of 20% NAC with three parts of orange or grapefruit juice. Administer this solution orally in a loading dose of 140 mg/kg and then continue with 70 mg/kg every 4 hours for 17 doses. Children who present more than 24 hours after ingestion should be given only a single loading dose of NAC until serum levels have been measured.

      (2) IV therapy. Intravenous NAC is currently not licensed for general use in the United States, but it is expected that it will soon be available. The loading dose is 150 mg/kg in 200 ml 5% D/W, given over 15 minutes. This is followed by 50 mg/kg in 500 ml 5% D/W given over 4 hours, then 100 mg/kg in 1000 ml 5% D/W given over 16 hours. The fluid volume may be decreased for young children. Intravenous use has occasionally been associated with skin rash and anaphylaxis (have diphenhydramine and epinephrine available).

      (3) During treatment with NAC, monitor liver function tests (AST, ALT, PT, bilirubin), concentrations of electrolytes, glucose, BUN, cre-

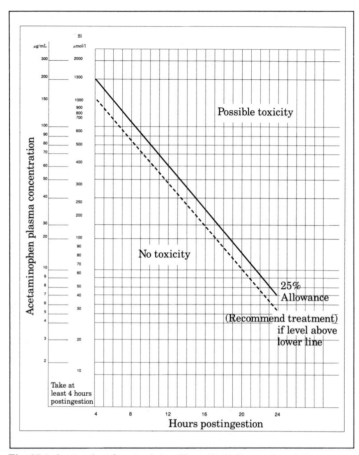

**Fig. 27-1. Acetaminophen toxicity. (From B. H. Rumack and H. Mathew, Acetaminophen poisoning and toxicity. Reproduced by permission of *Pediatrics*. 55:871. Copyright 1975.)**

atinine, and amylase, CBC, platelet count, and urinalysis.

**B. Caustic substances.** Commonly ingested alkaline substances are lyes, strong bleaches, dishwasher and laundry powders, drain and oven cleaners, and Clinitest tablets. Household hypochlorite bleach (< 5%) is considered an irritant and rarely produces significant gastrointestinal injury. Acid compounds found in the home include toilet bowl cleaners, soldering flux, and swimming pool cleaners.

**1. Toxic effect.** Drooling, vomiting, stridor, respiratory distress, and abdominal pain are signs of severe toxicity. Examination of the mouth and throat may reveal edema and ulceration of the mucosa or a white membrane that is friable and bleeds easily. **However, the absence of oropharyngeal injury does not rule out significant esophageal damage.** Severe esophageal injury results in perforation causing mediastinitis and shock (see Chap. 33). Scarring and stricture may occur up to 8 weeks after ingestion. Aspiration of a caustic substance may result in laryngeal injury and severe pneumonitis.

2. **Management**

   a. All children who ingest caustic substances should be considered to have suffered damage to the gastrointestinal tract, even if there are no burns of the oropharynx.

   b. Children with a history of ingestion of a strong acid or alkaline substance or with oropharyngeal burns, drooling, or dysphagia following alkali ingestion require prompt attention. Give oxygen by mask, start an intravenous line, and order a chest x ray, CBC, and cross-matching. Refer the child to a gastroenterologist or other endoscopist for examination within 24 hours to determine if there is gastric or esophageal injury. Endoscopy is contraindicated in the patient with acute upper airway obstruction or shock. **Do not perform lavage or administer fluids, charcoal, or ipecac to children with caustic ingestion.** Decontaminate the skin and eyes if necessary (see sec. **III.C** above).

   c. For treatment of button battery ingestion, see Chap. 16.

   d. Prophylactic antibiotics and steroids have not been proved effective.

C. **Cyclic antidepressants**

1. **Toxic effects.** Anticholinergic effects are common and include flushing, dry skin and mouth, dilated pupils, and urinary retention. Common CNS effects are sedation, confusion, and agitation. In severe poisoning, seizures, coma, and marked CNS depression with respiratory failure may be seen. The cardiovascular effects of cyclic antidepressants are hypotension, supraventricular and ventricular tachyarrhythmias, and bradyarrhythmias. A widened QRS complex ($> 0.10$ seconds) on the electrocardiogram may be associated with a poor outcome.

2. **Management**

   a. All children with suspected or proved cyclic antidepressant ingestion should be admitted and placed on a cardiac monitor. Start an intravenous line. Order the following: blood gas measurements, measurements of urine and serum for cyclic antidepressants, cyclic antidepressant levels, and an ECG.

**b.** Intubate and ventilate the comatose patient. Maintain a mild alkalemia (pH 7.40–7.50) by hyperventilation or bicarbonate infusion of 0.5–1.0 mEq/kg prn to decrease toxicity.

**c.** Treat hypotension with an intravenous infusion of 10 ml/kg of normal saline and repeat prn. If this is ineffective, infuse pressors such as phenylephrine or norepinephrine. Children with ventricular tachyarrhythmias should be started on an intravenous lidocaine infusion at 10–50 μg/kg/minute. Children with severe bradyarrhythmias require cardiac pacing. See Chap. 9.

**d.** Use intravenous diazepam or phenytoin to control seizures (see Chap. 22, Seizures).

**e.** Repeated activated charcoal administration increases clearance of cyclic antidepressants and should be administered every 2–4 hours by nasogastric tube. **Do not induce emesis.** If the child is comatose, see sec. **1.B** above.

## D. Hydrocarbons

**1. Toxic dose.** In general, hydrocarbons are toxic when **aspirated or inhaled.** Toluene, xylene, benzene, styrene, halogenated hydrocarbons, and heavy metals can cause serious systemic toxicity if more than 1 ml/kg is **ingested.**

**2. Toxic effect.** Most of the toxicity of hydrocarbons is due to pulmonary aspiration or inhalation of vapors. Volatile hydrocarbons with low viscosity (petroleum ether, turpentine, naphtha, gasoline, mineral spirits, and kerosene) are more likely to be aspirated. Early signs of aspiration are choking and gasping, followed by tachycardia and tachypnea. Nausea, vomiting, and abdominal pain are common after exposure. Signs of lower airway involvement such as grunting, nasal flaring, retractions, and wheezing often occur within 6 hours of aspiration and become worse during the subsequent 24–48 hours. Hypoxemia generally accompanies severe chest disease.

Chest x rays are frequently positive (60%) in the absence of chest symptoms and show alveolar infiltrates and atelectasis in the lower lobes. Pneumatoceles, pneumomediastinum, and pneumothorax are rare complications.

Central nervous system toxicity is usually limited to dizziness, headache, and somnolence. Seizures, coma, and other severe central nervous system effects are more likely to occur following ingestion of aromatic (toluene, benzene, styrene, xylene) or halogenated varieties.

Fever and leukocytosis with a left shift are frequent. Pulmonary edema and dysrhythmia may also occur.

**3. Management**

**a.** Obtain a chest x ray and blood gas measurements in any child suspected of hydrocarbon ingestion. When there are no radiographic or clinical signs of toxicity, observe the child for a minimum of 4 hours. If a repeat chest x ray at 4 hours is normal, the child may be discharged and the parents instructed to return if there are further problems. Admit all children with aromatic or halogenated hydrocarbon ingestion, CNS depression, respiratory symptoms, or an abnormal chest x ray.

   **b.** In children with evidence of ingestion or aspiration obtain serum electrolyte measurements, liver function tests, a complete blood count, and an ECG. In general, do not perform gastrointestinal decontamination with ipecac, gastric lavage, charcoal, or cathartics. In children who have ingested > 1 ml/kg of **neurotoxic hydrocarbons** (benzene, toluene, styrene, xylene, halogenated hydrocarbons), controlled gastric lavage may be undertaken after the patient has been intubated with a cuffed endotracheal tube.

   **c.** Give oxygen to all children with signs of chest disease. Children with severe chest pathology require admission to an intensive care unit for ventilation and monitoring. Treat bronchospasm with nebulized bronchodilators such as albuterol (salbutamol—see Chap. 7). Most children who have fever, x-ray evidence of consolidation, and leukocytosis with a left shift are not infected. Use antimicrobials in children with severe pneumonia with increasing fever or white blood cell count and in debilitated children (undernourished, preexisting chest disease, immune deficient).

**E. Iron**
   **1. Toxic dose**
      **a.** Mild to moderate: 20–60 mg/kg elemental iron
      **b.** Severe: more than 60 mg/kg elemental iron
      **c.** Ferrous sulfate = 20% elemental iron; ferrous gluconate = 12% elemental iron; ferrous fumarate = 33% elemental iron.
   **2. Toxic effect.** Most of the toxic effect of iron is exerted on the gastrointestinal and cardiovascular systems. Gastrointestinal symptoms usually occur in the first few hours (stage 1, 0.5–6 hours) after ingestion with vomiting, diarrhea, abdominal pain, and gastrointestinal bleeding. This is followed by a latent stage (stage 2), 6–24 hours after ingestion. The presence of gastrointestinal or hypovolemic symptoms during this phase suggests severe poisoning. In the third stage of iron overdose (12–30 hours after ingestion), the child deteriorates into shock. There may be fever, hyperglycemia, and severe bleeding. These patients require aggressive resuscitation and monitoring and should be managed in an intensive care unit. Stage 4 (48–96 hours) is characterized by coma, seizures, and hepatic failure. Rarely, there is progression to stage 5 at 2–5 weeks, associated with gastric outlet obstruction secondary to scarring.

**3. Management**

    **a.** Do not give charcoal. A child who appears well following ingestion of 20–60 mg/kg of elemental iron should be lavaged or given ipecac and admitted for observation.

    **b.** If the dose is greater than 60 mg/kg or if the victim is an adolescent, give ipecac and perform gastric lavage.

    **c.** When severe iron poisoning results in shock, massive fluid replacement with central venous pressure monitoring is necessary. A raised hematocrit is often indicative of incipient shock.

    **d.** When a toxic ingestion is suspected, obtain blood specimens for measuring serum iron, total iron-binding capacity (TIBC), liver function, CBC, cross-match, blood gases, glucose, electrolytes, and calcium. Obtain an abdominal x ray to determine if a large number of tablets have yet to be absorbed and require removal. Not all iron tablets are radiopaque.

    **e.** Chelation therapy:

        **(1)** If there is any doubt about serious toxicity or if the serum iron concentration is greater than 90 μmol/liter (500 μg/dl), begin treatment with deferoxamine.

        **(2)** If the level is between 55 μmol/liter (300 μg/dl) and 90 μmol/liter (500 μg/dl), begin chelation therapy if:

            **(a)** The serum iron level exceeds the TIBC.

            **(b)** The child is symptomatic.

            **(c)** The white blood cell count is greater than 15,000 or the serum glucose concentration is greater than 8.5 mmol/liter (150 mg/dl).

        **(3)** If the patient is normotensive and stable, give deferoxamine, 50 mg IM q4h. If the ingestion is severe or the patient is hypotensive, acidotic, or comatose, give an intravenous infusion of deferoxamine; start slowly and increase over 30 minutes to a rate of 15 mg/kg/hour. Infuse at 15 mg/kg/hour for 4 hours, then reduce the rate to 2–5 mg/kg/hour. The maximum daily dose is 120 mg/kg/day or 6 gm, whichever is less. Deferoxamine may cause hypotension if it is infused too rapidly.

        **(4)** The decision as to whether or not chelation therapy is continued should be based on the status of the patient and the serum iron level. Although a change in urine color to pink has traditionally been considered a sign that chelation is effective and should continue, this sign is not always reliable. Continue therapy until 24 hours after the urine has cleared or until the serum iron level has fallen below 50 μmol/liter (300 μg/dl).

**F. Salicylates**
   **1. Toxic dose**
      **a.** Mild to moderate: 150–300 mg/kg
      **b.** Potentially severe: greater than 300 mg/kg
   **2. Toxic effects.** Ingestion of child and adult aspirin or oil of wintergreen syrup is the most common cause of severe salicylate toxicity. The signs of salicylate toxicity resemble those of diabetic ketoacidosis, with deep, driven respirations and a decreased level of consciousness. Severe central nervous system effects can occur, resulting in coma, convulsions, and death. Dehydration is common secondary to vomiting, increased renal losses, and increased insensible losses from the lungs. Noncardiogenic pulmonary edema has occurred following salicylate ingestion. There may be bleeding and hepatic dysfunction in some cases. The biochemical effects of **acute** salicylate toxicity vary with age. In young infants, metabolic acidosis may be the only abnormality of acid-base status. In older children, an initial respiratory alkalosis evolves to combined respiratory alkalosis and metabolic acidosis. Hypokalemia is common, and serum glucose concentration may be elevated or decreased. **Chronic** salicylate toxicity results in prominent CNS signs and symptoms; acid-base abnormalities are rare.
   **3. Management**
      **a.** Begin with gastrointestinal tract decontamination, using ipecac and activated charcoal or gastric lavage, and activated charcoal. Patients with severe toxicity may benefit from repeated activated charcoal administration.
      **b.** Draw blood to obtain a serum salicylate level. Admit and treat patients with levels greater than 50 gm/dl and obtain measurements of blood gases, electrolytes, ketones and glucose, a complete blood count; and coagulation studies. In selected cases, the Done nomogram (Fig. 27-2) may be helpful in determining severity when levels are drawn 6 hours after acute ingestion (not helpful in chronic ingestion).
      **c.** Circulating fluid volume must be restored.
         **(1)** Use an intravenous solution containing 75 mEq NaCl and 88 mEq $HCO_3$ (2 ampules) per liter of 5% dextrose; this solution is given at a rate of 10–15 ml/kg/hour in the first 2 hours. Maintain a urine output of 3–6 ml/kg/hour. If acidosis is severe, an extra 1–2 mEq/kg of $NaHCO_3$ may be added to increase urinary pH above 7 to improve salicylate excretion.
         **(2)** After the first 2 hours, 35 mEq/liter of KCl should be added to the intravenous fluid (ex-

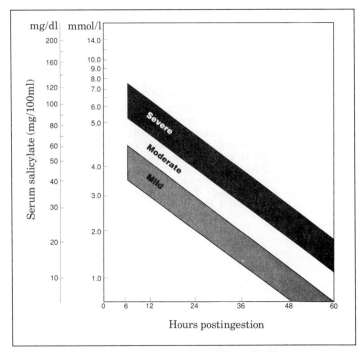

**Fig. 27-2.** Salicylate nomogram. (From A. K. Done, Salicylate intoxication. Reproduced by permission of *Pediatrics*. **26**:805. Copyright 1960.)

cept in patients with renal failure) and the infusion rate decreased to 5 ml/kg/hour, until the serum salicylate level is therapeutic at 0.7–1.4 mmol/liter (10–20 mg/dl).

(3) Treat hyperthermia with a cooling blanket, seizures with intravenous diazepam, and bleeding with vitamin K, 2–5 mg IM.

d. Hemodialysis should be considered in cases of severe toxicity associated with renal failure, noncardiogenic pulmonary edema, seizures, or severe acidosis, and in patients with salicylate levels of more than 9.5 mmol/liter (130 mg/dl).

G. **Theophylline**
1. **Toxic effect.** Theophylline toxicity may be acute, chronic, or acute-on-chronic. The latter state often occurs in children with decreased theophylline clearance due to viral illness, fever, pneumonia, hepatic dysfunction, congestive heart failure, or hypoalbuminemia. Medications that may decrease clearance include erythromycin, cimetidine, and propranolol.

a. In mild to moderate toxicity (drug level < 280 μmol/liter or 50 μg/ml), vomiting, sinus tachycardia, tremor, agitation, and abdominal pain are common.

**b.** Obtundation, dysrhythmia, and seizures may occur in children with drug levels of greater than 280 μmol/liter (50 μg/ml). Seizures with acute toxicity are a poor prognostic sign and are often refractory to treatment. Other abnormalities include hyperthermia, metabolic acidosis, hypoglycemia, hyperglycemia, hypokalemia, and gastrointestinal bleeding.

**c.** Children with chronic toxicity are more likely to present with seizures.

**2. Management**

**a.** Admit all children who are symptomatic or have drug levels greater than 165 μmol/liter (30 μg/ml). Start an intravenous line and draw blood for toxicology screening, theophylline level, CBC, differential count, platelet count, prothrombin time (PT), partial thromboplastin time (PTT), and measurement of electrolytes, BUN, creatinine, phosphate, magnesium, glucose, and blood gases. Give intravenous fluid, 5% D/W with 15 mEq KCl and 15 mEq KPO$_4$/liter, at the maintenance rate. Place the child on a cardiac monitor.

**b.** Empty the gastrointestinal tract by means of emesis or lavage, and give charcoal. Children with significant toxicity should be treated with repeated administration of activated charcoal q2h.

**c.** If seizures occur, intravenous diazepam and phenytoin is the initial treatment of choice (see Chap. 22, Seizures).

**d.** Consider hemoperfusion in children with high drug levels—greater than 440 μmol/liter (80 μg/ml) in acute intoxication, or greater than 330 μmol/liter (60 μg/ml) in chronic intoxication—who do not respond to supportive care.

**H. Substances of abuse**

**1. Phencyclidine** (PCP, angel dust). Phencyclidine produces a dissociative state resulting in an altered sensation of pain and self-injurious activity. Patients may exhibit violent behavior, making restraint difficult. Moderate or severe toxicity results in sustained muscle contractions and causes hyperthermia, rhabdomyolysis, and renal failure. Other effects include hypertension, a depressed level of consciousness, seizures, and psychosis.

**a. Management**

**(1)** Patients who are medically stable should be placed in a quiet dark room to decrease sensory stimulation. If necessary, use soft restraints to prevent injury.

**(2)** Patients who are agitated may be treated with intravenous diazepam. Reduce fever with a cooling blanket and tepid sponging.

**2. LSD and mescaline.** These drugs distort the user's

perception of the environment, and panic may result from disordered thought processes. Severe side effects are coma, convulsions, and respiratory arrest.

    **a. Management.** Psychologic support will suffice in most cases. Severe panic reactions can be treated with intravenous diazepam. In general, avoid gastrointestinal decontamination in the intoxicated patient.

**3. Mushrooms.** Psilocybin-containing mushrooms cause hallucinations similar to those that occur with LSD and mescaline. Mushrooms of the *Amanita* class may contain varying amounts of cholinergic and anticholinergic substances. The most common lethal mushroom ingestions are due to *Amanita phalloides* and *A. virosa*. These result in gastrointestinal symptoms followed by renal and liver failure. Signs of poisoning that occur within 2–3 hours of ingestion are unlikely to be due to a deadly variety of mushroom.

    **a. Management**

        **(1)** Start by emptying the stomach with ipecac and charcoal or gastric lavage. When hallucinogenic effects are severe, treat with intravenous diazepam.

        **(2)** Anticholinergic signs (hot dry skin, fever, tachycardia, mydriasis, decreased bowel sounds, urinary retention) do not require treatment.

        **(3)** Cholinergic signs (salivation, lacrimation, urination, defecation, emesis) can be treated with atropine, 0.05 mg/kg intravenously.

**4. Stimulants** (amphetamines, caffeine, phenylpropanolamine). Overdose with this group of drugs produces acute paranoid psychosis, often with pallor, flushing, hypertension, mydriasis, and hyperthermia. Central nervous system effects include agitation, hallucinations, and seizures. Dysrhythmias may also occur.

    **a. Management**

        **(1)** Following gastrointestinal decontamination (see sec. **III.A** above), treat agitated and convulsing children with intravenous diazepam and reduce fever if present. If seizures are refractory to therapy with diazepam, consult the anesthesia department about the possibility of paralysis and intubation (see Chap. 22, Status Epilepticus).

        **(2)** Treat ventricular dysrhythmias with phenytoin; cardioversion may be necessary (see Chap. 9). Hypertension may respond to a change of position—place the child in a reverse Trendelenburg position. Diazoxide or nitroprusside should be given if hypertension is severe (see Chap. 23, Hypertension).

**5. Cocaine and crack.** Cocaine toxicity resembles toxicity due to phencyclidine and stimulants, with excessive sympathetic stimulation. Nausea, vomiting, flushing, dysrhythmias, hyperthermia, paranoid delusions, convulsions, and cardiorespiratory arrest may occur.

  **a. Management.** Seizures and dysrhythmias are life-threatening complications. Treatment is similar to that used for amphetamine overdose (see sec. **IV.H.4.a** above).

**6. Ethyl alcohol.** Severe intoxication with alcohol may result in autonomic overactivity, hallucinations, seizures, hypoglycemia, and hypothermia.

  **a. Management.** Start an intravenous line and administer a bolus of IV dextrose to alcohol-intoxicated children who have an altered sensorium. Treat hypothermia aggressively (see Chap. 29). Examine the child carefully for signs of trauma, and draw blood for measurement of electrolytes, BUN, ethanol level, and hematocrit.

**7. Narcotics and barbiturates.** The classic triad of signs in narcotic overdose are CNS depression, respiratory depression, and miotic pupils. Parenteral use may result in noncardiogenic pulmonary edema. Hypotension occurs in severe cases. The signs of barbiturate overdose resemble those of narcotic overdose except for the presence of miosis, which is variable. Seizures may result following pentobarbital or secobarbital intoxication.

  **a. Management.** Naloxone is the antidote for narcotic overdose. Initially give 0.01 mg/kg; if there is no response, increase this dose by a factor of 10 to 0.1 mg/kg. If naloxone is effective, repeat the dose every 5–10 minutes prn. In general, treat barbiturate overdose with gastric emptying and supportive measures. Alkalinization or dialysis may be effective in treating overdose due to phenobarbital (for method, see sec. **IV.F** above).

**V. Disposition.** Admit all patients with serious poisoning (see specific sections above), or when suicide or child abuse is suspected.

**VI. Key points**

  **A.** Early gastric decontamination, followed by antidotal therapy when available, is the treatment of choice in most cases.

  **B.** Seizing or comatose children must have their airway secured prior to gastric lavage.

  **C.** When possible, consult local poison control authorities before commencing treatment.

**Bibliography**

Baker, M. D. Theophylline toxicity in children. *J. Pediatr.* 109:538, 1986.

Goldfrank, L. R. *Toxicologic Emergencies* (3rd ed.). Norwalk, CT: Appleton-Century-Crofts, 1986.

Mofenson, H. C. Gastrointestinal dialysis with activated charcoal in the treatment of adolescent intoxications. *Toxicology* 24:678, 1985.

Mofenson, H. C., and Greensher, J. The unknown poison. *Pediatrics* 54:336, 1974.

Pediatric toxicology. *Pediatr. Clin. North Am.* 33:April, 1986.

Symposium on medical toxicology. *Emerg. Clin. North Am.* 2(1), Feb., 1984.

Truemper, E., De La Rocha, S. R., and Atkinson, S. D. Clinical characteristics, pathophysiology, and management of hydrocarbon ingestion: Case report and review of the literature. *Pediatr. Emerg. Care* 3:187, 1987.

Victoria, M. S., and Nangia, B. S. Hydrocarbon poisoning: A review. *Pediatr. Emerg. Care* 3:184, 1987.

# 28

# Drowning and Near-Drowning

Andrew J. Macnab

In North America, drowning is the third most common cause of death in children aged 1–14 years. *Drowning* refers to those children who die within 24 hours of submersion injury. *Near-drowning* means survival, at least temporarily, following asphyxia due to submersion. Most victims are males and either toddlers or adolescents. Over 85% of incidents occur in swimming pools or bodies of water near the child's home. The lung is the target organ. Aspiration of water depletes surfactant, causing atelectasis and alveolar collapse. Lung compliance is decreased, and pulmonary edema develops. Brain injury may result from respiratory insufficiency, hypoxia, hypercapnia, and acidosis.

I. **Diagnosis and assessment**
   A. **History.** Water temperature, the duration of submersion, and the time of onset and type of resuscitation are important prognostic factors in the history. A child with a seizure disorder is more likely to have suffered prolonged submersion with massive aspiration, whereas near-drowning following diving injury may be associated with cervical spine and head injury.
   B. **Examination.** Assess problems in the airway, breathing, and circulation. Noncardiogenic pulmonary edema may lead to respiratory failure. Milder cases present with dyspnea, chest pain, and tachycardia. Hypotension may be severe. Assess neurologic status; an altered level of consciousness is usually due to hypoxic or anoxic brain injury. Seizures may result from hypoxia, anoxia, or electrolyte imbalance. Hypothermia may be severe and can be fatal; measure the core (rectal) temperature of all near-drowning victims with a low-reading thermometer.

II. **Management.** Management begins at the scene of the accident with cardiopulmonary resuscitation. Mouth-to-mouth breathing can be initiated in the water. Specific management of near-drowning victims depends on respiratory function, core temperature, and the level of consciousness on arrival.
   A. **Airway and cervical spine.** In the apneic victim begin mouth-to-mouth or bag-mask ventilation immediately. Do not try to drain fluid from the lungs. If the chest does not move when ventilation is attempted, use the standard procedure to position and clear the airway (see Chap. 1). In victims of diving accidents or unwitnessed near-drowning, stabilize the cervical spine with a semirigid collar or tape and sandbags until x rays can be performed.
   B. **Breathing.** Treat all near-drowning victims with 100% oxygen. Intubate and ventilate children with cyanosis, apnea, or other evidence of respiratory failure (see Chapter 1). Pulmonary edema may develop up to 12 hours after submersion, often requiring ventilation with

continuous positive airway pressure (CPAP) or positive end-expiratory pressure (PEEP).

**C. Circulation and warming.** Start an intravenous line. Administer cardiopulmonary resuscitation when there is inadequate cardiac output. Vigorously resuscitate the child with fluid infusion to achieve normovolemia; after salt-water drowning, large volumes (30–40 ml/kg) may be required. Hypothermic children with dysrhythmia are special cases (see sec. **III** and Chap. 29, sec. **I**).

**D. Central nervous system.** If the patient is comatose or if the level of consciousness has decreased since submersion (see Table 28-1), hypoxic brain injury is likely. Full brain resuscitation should be undertaken in these children. This includes controlled elective intubation, hyperventilation, fluid restriction to 50% of maintenance, sedation, temperature control, correct positioning, and aggressive treatment of seizures (see Chap. 22, Seizures and Chap. 22, Increased Intracranial Pressure). There is no evidence that dexamethasone, phenobarbital, or sustained hypothermia are useful in controlling the cerebral edema associated with near-drowning. Acute cerebral edema requires aggressive hyperventilation and diuresis.

**E. Temperature.** Submersion, even in relatively warm water, can result in severe hypothermia. Check the rectal temperature and warm the child if the body temperature is less than 35°C (see sec. **IV** below and Chap. 29, sec. **I**). Avoid a rebound rise of core temperature above 36.5°C.

**F. Stabilization.** Insert a Foley catheter in all children who require resuscitation. A nasogastric tube should usually be placed. However, if there is severe hypothermia (core temperature under 30°C) delay nasogastric tube placement, as passage may contribute to dysrhythmia.

**Table 28-1. Near-drowning classification: Emergency room assessment 1 hour postrescue**

| Category | Description |
|---|---|
| A (awake) | Alert, fully conscious |
| B (blunted) | Obtunded, stuporous, but arousable<br>Purposeful response to pain<br>Normal respiration |
| C (comatose) | Unrousable<br>Abnormal response to pain<br>Abnormal respiration |
| C-1 (decorticate) | Pain response—flexor |
| C-2 (decerebrate) | Pain response—extensor |
| C-3 (flaccid) | Pain response—none |
| C-4 (dead?) | Resuscitation unsuccessful within 1 hour but cardiac rhythm and blood pressure obtained subsequently |

G. **Laboratory and x-ray studies.** Check arterial blood gas measurements to determine acid-base status and ventilation. Electrolyte imbalance and hemolysis may occur in the drowning victim owing to changes in serum osmolality. Obtain and follow measurements of serum electrolytes, BUN, creatinine, and hemoglobin. A chest x ray should be performed to rule out pulmonary edema, and cervical spine films should be ordered when indicated (see sec. **I.A** above).

H. **Antibiotics.** Children who drown in warm water (hot tubs, spa pool) or contaminated water have an increased risk of pneumonia and sepsis. Hot tub or spa pool near-drowning victims should receive intravenous ceftazidime, 100 mg/kg/day divided q8h, to anticipate infection with *Pseudomonas aeruginosa.* Other cases of near-drowning should be treated expectantly, with twice daily Gram's stain and cultures of tracheal aspirates, and chest x rays and cultures of blood as appropriate.

III. **Disposition.** All children with a history of submersion should be admitted to an intensive care unit for observation. Those who require resuscitation and those who have abnormal blood gas measurements or chest x ray, or a decreased level of consciousness (level B or C) are at high risk for complications (see Table 28-1).

IV. **Cold water drowning.** Hypothermia has a protective action on the brain of the near-drowned child. Cold water that is aspirated or swallowed on contact will drop the core temperature rapidly. Hypothermia prior to anoxia reduces cerebral injury. Children have survived intact following submersions of greater than 60 minutes in water below 10°C. Victims of cold water submersion injury may appear to be dead at the scene or on arrival in the emergency room. There may be apnea, impalpable pulses, and fixed, dilated pupils. Do not give up. Full resuscitation efforts with cardiopulmonary resuscitation and rewarming may result in a complete recovery. (For specific therapy of hypothermia see Chap. 29, sec. **I**).

V. **Key points**

A. Prompt, effective cardiopulmonary resuscitation significantly improves prognosis and outcome in near-drowning victims.

B. Near-drowning victims who are pulseless, apneic, and cold should receive full resuscitation with rewarming.

C. Near-drowning victims with an altered level of consciousness should be electively intubated, ventilated, and sedated.

D. With prolonged submersion, children who drown in cold water have the best prognosis.

**Bibliography**

Bohn, D. J., et al. Influence of hypothermia, barbiturate therapy, and intracranial pressure monitoring on morbidity and mortality after near-drowning. *Crit. Care Med.* 14:529, 1986.

Conn, A. W., et al. Near drowning in cold fresh water: Current treatment regimen. *Can. Anaesth. Soc. J.* 25:229, 1978.

Frewin, T. C., Sumabat, W. O., Han, V. K., et al. Cerebral resuscitation therapy in pediatric near drowning. *J. Pediatr.* 106:615, 1985.

Macnab, A. J., et al. Near drowning in British Columbia. *Br. C. Med. J.* 30:339, 1988.

Modell, J. H. Treatment of near drowning: Is there a role for HYPER therapy? *Crit. Care Med.* 14:593, 1986.

Orlowski, J. P. Drowning, near-drowning, and ice water submersions. *Pediatr. Clin. North Am.* 34:75, 1987.

# Hypothermia, Frostbite, and Heat Stress

Gregory A. Baldwin

**I. Hypothermia.** When a child's core temperature drops below 35°C, significant effects on the cardiovascular, respiratory, and nervous systems result. Hypothermia in children is commonly seen following near-drowning, trauma, or prolonged outdoor exposure in winter months.

**A. Assessment.** Hypothermia is often overlooked; only low reading or digital thermometers are capable of detecting it. Physical findings in the **hypothermic infant** are often vague and variable—the only signs may be irritability and poor feeding. In **older children and adolescents,** manifestations vary with the core temperature.

**1. Mild hypothermia** (core temperature 32–35°C). Children with mild hypothermia may have slurred speech, poor coordination, and decreased cognitive function. Shivering is usually evident.

**2. Moderate hypothermia** (core temperature 29.5–32°C). The level of consciousness is further decreased—most children with a temperature of less than 29.5°C will be unconscious. The skin may be cyanotic and edematous. There is muscle rigidity instead of shivering, and respiratory drive and cardiac output are decreased. Rarely, ventricular fibrillation and bradyarrhythmias occur.

**3. Severe hypothermia** (core temperature less than 29.5°C). At this temperature, children are comatose. The pupils are fixed and dilated, and there is areflexia. Ventricular dysrhythmias and respiratory arrest are likely. Metabolic abnormalities, gastrointestinal bleeding, renal failure, thrombosis, and coagulopathy may occur.

**B. Management**

**1. Stabilization.** Ideally, treatment of hypothermia begins in the field by removing wet garments and surrounding the child with heat from warmed blankets or the body of the rescuer. Attach an electrocardiographic (ECG) monitor and start an intravenous line; there may be hypovolemia secondary to increased losses and decreased intake.

**2. Initial resuscitation.** Begin cardiopulmonary resuscitation if no pulse or respirations are obtainable. Although stimulation of the airway may cause ventricular dysrhythmias in the severely hypothermic patient, airway management and ventilation must take precedence over all else; do not hesitate to intubate and ventilate the apneic child.

**3. Ongoing resuscitation**

**a.** On arrival in the emergency room, maintain the airway, breathing, and circulation and measure the core (rectal) temperature.

**b.** Children with severe hypothermia may appear to be dead, but do not assume that any child is dead until the core temperature is above 32°C. Even children with severe bradycardia or asystole can recover without sequelae.

**c.** If there is ventricular fibrillation and the core temperature is below 29.5°C, direct current (DC) shock cardioversion or medications are unlikely to be helpful. Continue cardiopulmonary resuscitation and administer rapid rewarming measures (see sec. **I.B.4** below) until the temperature is above 29.5°C.

**d.** If ventricular fibrillation occurs at a core temperature of 29.5–32°C, make one attempt at DC shock defibrillation with 2 joules/kg in *nonsynchronized* mode. If this fails, continue warming until the temperature is above 32°C.

**e.** Obtain an electrocardiogram (ECG), urinalysis, and blood specimens for measurement of electrolytes, glucose, amylase, renal and liver function, coagulation studies, and blood gases in all hypothermic children.

**f.** In severe cases, insert a Foley catheter to enable monitoring of urine output. Nasogastric tube insertion may lead to ventricular dysrhythmia and should generally not be performed until the core temperature is above 30°C.

**4. Rewarming**

**a.** Patients with **mild hypothermia** who have stable cardiovascular function can be rewarmed slowly with warming blankets or with immersion in a tub of warm (32–41°C) water. The immersion method is dangerous except in mild cases in healthy children because resuscitation and monitoring are difficult.

**b.** In children with **moderate hypothermia,** slow deliberate rewarming is achieved by increasing the ambient room temperature, giving warmed IV fluids via a blood warmer, using a warming blanket, and giving heated, humidified oxygen by mask.

**c.** Those with **severe hypothermia** are at high risk for ventricular fibrillation and require rapid rewarming. Methods for rapid rewarming include warming blankets, administration of warmed IV fluids via a blood warmer, colonic lavage with warmed (40–45°C) fluid, and peritoneal dialysis with warmed (40–45°C) fluid. The child with a heartbeat and respiratory rate, no matter how slow, must be treated gently to avoid precipitating ventricular dysrhythmia. In refractory cases where there is ventricular fibrillation, heroic measures such as thoracotomy with mediastinal lavage and open chest cardiac massage, or partial cardiopulmonary bypass with a heat exchanger, can be considered.

C. **Disposition.** Admit all patients with a core temperature below 35°C. Children with a core temperature below 32°C, or those who have complications or who have required resuscitation should be admitted to an intensive care unit.

D. **Key points**
   1. Do not assume that a hypothermic child is dead until the core temperature is above 32°C.
   2. Defibrillation is unlikely to be effective in children with a core temperature below 29.5°C.

II. **Frostbite.** Cold tissue injury occurs most commonly in the ears, nose, fingers, toes, hands, and feet. Early signs of frostbite include blanching of the skin, followed by numbness, pallor, mottling, and a hard wooden or waxy texture. Assessment of tissue viability in the first hours following injury is often inaccurate.

   A. **Management**
   1. Remove wet, cold, and constricting garments and cover injured areas with warm, dry, padded gauze. Do not rub or expose areas of frostbite to dry heat.
   2. In children presenting within 24 hours of injury, rewarm the frozen areas by immersing them in water at 40–42°C for 20–40 minutes or until the distal tip is completely thawed—a flush is visible when this occurs. This process is usually painful, and analgesia with codeine or IV morphine is required. Do not rewarm if the area has thawed. Never begin rewarming if there is any possibility of refreezing (i.e., in the field) because this will lead to increased tissue damage.
   3. Using strict aseptic technique, debride white (nonhemorrhagic) blisters and leave red (hemorrhagic) blisters intact.
   4. Elevate and splint the involved part if necessary and cover it with a loose, padded dressing.
   5. Give a tetanus booster immunization to those at risk and consult a plastic surgeon.

   B. **Disposition.** All children with frostbite injury should be admitted to a plastic surgical or burn unit.

   C. **Key points**
   1. Warm areas of frostbite injury by immersing them in warm water and transfer the patient to a burn unit.

III. **Heat stress.** Heat stress may present as heat cramps, heat exhaustion, or heat stroke. **Exertional heat stroke** is usually seen in athletic adolescents who engage in strenuous activity. Infants and young children may suffer **nonexertional heat stroke,** often as a result of overdressing during fever or being locked in unventilated vehicles on hot sunny days. Heat stress is more likely to occur in dehydrated children, newborns, children with cystic fibrosis, children with a congenital abnormality of sweating (ectodermal dysplasia), poorly conditioned adolescents, and children taking amphetamines, tricyclic antidepressants, phenothiazine, or other medications that prevent sweating.

   A. **Diagnosis**
   1. **Heat cramps.** The mildest form of heat stress is

heat cramps; these occur in the leg and abdomen following exertion in hot weather. There is no associated morbidity.

**2. Heat exhaustion.** Heat exhaustion presents with dehydration, nausea, vomiting, headache, and occasionally syncope. Core temperature may be mildly elevated; serious complications are rare.

**3. Heat stroke.** Heat stroke is a medical emergency with a significant risk of mortality. It occurs during heat waves and can affect any age group. Victims have rectal temperatures of over 40°C and often over 42°C. The child with heat stroke has red, hot, dry skin. Restlessness, drowsiness, and coma are common secondary to cerebral edema. There may be loss of brain stem reflexes with pupillary constriction. Headache, ataxia, areflexia, seizures, and cardiovascular collapse due to hypovolemia are also seen. Rare complications include adult respiratory distress syndrome (ARDS), disseminated intravascular coagulation, and acute hepatic and renal failure.

**B. Management**

**1. Heat cramps.** Patients with heat cramps can be treated with rest and oral fluids.

**2. Heat exhaustion.** Children with heat exhaustion should be placed in a cool room. Administer normal saline or Ringer's lactate, 10 ml/kg intravenously as a bolus infusion, and treat dehydration subsequently as outlined in Chap. 23, Fluids and Electrolytes.

**3. Heat stroke**

**a.** The child with heat stroke needs to be cooled rapidly. This is best achieved by the evaporative method. The child is placed in a room at the lowest possible temperature, covered with a gauze or light cotton sheet, and continuously sprayed with tepid tap water while electric fans (at least three) blow air onto him.

**b.** Start an intravenous line; if there are signs of hypovolemia (see Chap. 4), give 10 ml/kg of Ringer's lactate or normal saline and repeat as necessary. Children with respiratory distress usually require intubation and ventilation. A Foley catheter and nasogastric tube should be inserted.

**c.** Check measurements of serum electrolytes, blood gases (correct for temperature), glucose concentration, liver and renal function tests, and amylase level, and obtain a CBC. Obtain coagulation studies when indicated.

**d.** Treat seizures with intravenous diazepam.

**e.** Any child with hyperpyrexia and signs and symptoms of heat stroke should be evaluated for possible sepsis and meningitis.

**C. Disposition.** Children with heat stroke should be admitted to an intensive care unit for observation.

**D. Key points**

**1.** Heat stroke is a medical emergency; victims must be

rapidly cooled by the evaporative method and admitted to an intensive care unit for observation.

## Bibliography

Leads from the MMWR—illness and death due to environmental heat—Georgia and St. Louis, 1983. *J.A.M.A.* 252:20, 1984.

McCauley, R. L., et al. Frostbite injuries: A rational approach based on the pathophysiology. *J. Trauma* 23:143, 1983.

Robinson, M., and Seward, P. N. Environmental hypothermia in children. *Pediatr. Emerg. Care* 2:254, 1986.

Treatment of hypothermia. *Med. Lett.* 123–124, 1985.

Yaqub, B. A., et al. Heat stroke at the Mekkah pilgrimage: Clinical characteristics and course of 30 patients. *Q. J. Med.* 59:523, 1986.

# Allergic Emergencies

John M. Dean

I. **Anaphylaxis.** The anaphylaxis syndrome is a potentially life-threatening systemic response to foreign matter. The etiology may be allergic (*anaphylactic reaction*—IgE-mediated) or nonallergic (*anaphylactoid reaction*—not IgE-mediated). Commonly, anaphylaxis occurs following exposure (by ingestion, inhalation, or injection) to penicillins or other drugs, insect stings (hymenoptera), foods (nuts, peanuts, seafood, eggs, milk, berries), immunotherapeutic agents, hormones (insulin, adrenocorticotropic hormone [ACTH]), or radiocontrast media. Target organs include the circulatory system, respiratory tract, alimentary tract, genitourinary tract, and skin. Most fatalities occur within 1 hour and are due to laryngeal edema.

A. **Diagnosis and assessment.** In most cases, there is a history of exposure to the provocative substance, followed by a rapid (usually in minutes, seldom hours) onset of symptoms and clinical deterioration. In general, severe attacks occur immediately after exposure. Any combination of symptoms can occur; the same combination tends to recur in each individual. Increasing severity of episodes (particularly if there are cardiac or respiratory symptoms) on repeated exposure is a malignant sign. The differential diagnosis includes isolated urticaria and angioedema, hereditary angioneurotic edema (see sec. **II** below), epiglottitis (see Chap. 6), vasovagal reactions, hysteria, and other causes of coma, shock, and respiratory distress.

1. **Skin.** The common skin reactions are generalized pruritus and urticaria, often most intense at the site of antigen access. Angioedema is less common and rarely leads to airway compromise from external pressure. Skin reactions tend to be self-limited and subside within 48 hours (see Chap. 12).

2. **Respiratory symptoms.** Mild upper airway symptoms include tingling, pruritus, and a sense of fullness in the mouth. There may be nasal congestion, sneezing, and general itchiness of the mouth, throat, eyes, and ears. Laryngeal and supraglottic edema causes upper airway obstruction characterized by hoarseness, stridor, dyspnea, and finally, respiratory arrest. Bronchospasm may occur, with signs ranging from mild wheeziness and coughing to severe dyspnea, cyanosis, and respiratory failure.

3. **Cardiovascular symptoms.** The cardiovascular effects of anaphylaxis are hypotension, shock, and cardiac dysrhythmia. These are probably secondary to distributive changes (venous pooling, transudation of fluid) rather than any primary effect on the heart. Patients often feel flushed and warm and have a sense of impending doom. Syncope and palpitations are common.

4. **Other symptoms.** Gastrointestinal symptoms— mouth and throat swelling, diarrhea, vomiting, and cramping—are more likely to occur when the antigen has been ingested. There may also be urinary urgency and uterine cramping.

B. **Management.** Rapid assessment and action are vital. In all cases, control of airway, breathing, and circulation is the first priority. Children with anaphylaxis who are also on beta-blocker therapy often require prolonged intensive support.

1. **Airway.** The airway must be maintained. Give oxygen by mask or nasal prongs and place the child on a cardiac monitor. Intubation should be performed if laryngeal edema results in upper airway obstruction.

2. **Epinephrine.** Administer epinephrine, *0.01 ml/kg of a 1 : 1000 concentration (maximum 0.3 ml) subcutaneously* and repeat every 15–20 minutes as necessary. If anaphylaxis is the consequence of a sting or intramuscular injection, give a further 0.1 ml of epinephrine at the site to slow antigen absorption. If the site is on a limb, apply a proximal tourniquet and loosen it every 5 minutes for 1 minute.

3. **Antihistamines.** Antihistamines should be given, but they are not a substitute for epinephrine. Give diphenhydramine (Benadryl), 1–2 mg/kg (maximum 50 mg) IV, IM, or PO, and continue q8h for 48 hours.

4. **Monitoring.** Determine vital signs every 5–15 minutes.

5. **Vascular access.** If the patient presents with more than just urticaria or if there is no improvement with the above measures, start two large-bore intravenous lines.

6. **Shock** (see Chap. 4). The child with hypotension or shock should be placed in the Trendelenburg position. Rapidly administer 10 ml/kg aliquots of intravenous normal saline; most patients will require 30 ml/kg given over 20–30 minutes. Continue fluid administration until the child's condition is stable. If the response to fluid and subcutaneous epinephrine is unsatisfactory, start an infusion of dopamine (see Chap. 4). *Epinephrine, 0.1 ml/kg (maximum 3.0 ml) of 1 : 10,000 solution, can be given slowly intravenously over 5 minutes* while the dopamine infusion is being prepared.

7. **Bronchospasm.** In the child with bronchospasm, obtain measurements of blood gases and treat the patient with a nebulized bronchodilator such as salbutamol (albuterol), 0.02 ml/kg in 2–3 ml of normal saline via oxygen-powered nebulizer mask. Repeat up to q15minutes prn. In addition, intravenous aminophylline, 6 mg/kg as a bolus over 30 minutes in normal saline, should be given to the patient who is not currently taking theophylline medication. If the patient is taking theophylline, a bolus of up to 3 mg/

kg can be given depending on the time of the last dose. Follow the bolus with a maintenance infusion of 1 mg/kg/hour, subsequently adjusted according to blood levels (see Chap. 7).

8. **Corticosteroids.** Corticosteroids prevent the late phase of the allergic response. If symptoms are mild, give prednisone, initially 2 mg/kg/day (maximum 40 mg) PO divided q12h, then taper the dose over 4–5 days. For more severe symptoms, hydrocortisone, 5 mg/kg q8h, should be administered intravenously.

9. **Stabilization.** Treatment should be continued until the need for therapeutic support ceases. This generally takes less than 24 hours, although laryngeal edema may persist for a week.

10. **Prevention.** Every attempt should be made to identify the provoking agent or event and to indoctrinate the patient in means of avoiding future exposure. A bracelet (Medic-alert) stating the problem should be worn. When avoidance is not always feasible, such as with allergies to insect stings, the child should carry a first-aid kit containing epinephrine and antihistamine injections.

C. **Key points**
   1. The management of anaphylaxis can be summarized by the familiar ABCs: airway, breathing, and circulation.
   2. Prevention by AVOIDANCE is the ultimate goal.
   3. Most cases of fatal anaphylaxis occur within 1 hour of exposure and are the result of laryngeal edema.

II. **Hereditary angioneurotic edema.** This rare autosomal dominant inherited disorder is caused by an absolute or functional deficiency of C1 esterase inhibitor. It rarely presents before puberty. The common symptoms are cramping abdominal pain and nonpitting, nonpruritic, nonerythematous edema of the cutaneous and subcutaneous tissues. Life-threatening laryngeal edema is a rare complication.

A. **Management of laryngeal edema.** About 50% of patients will improve on the following protocol. The rest will require definitive airway management by intubation or tracheostomy.
   1. Give epinephrine, *0.01 ml/kg of a 1 : 1000 solution* subcutaneously (maximum dose 0.3 ml), and hydrocortisone, 5 mg/kg q6h intravenously. Full histamine receptor blockade ($H_1$ and $H_2$) is achieved by giving intravenous Benadryl, 5 mg/kg/day divided q8h, and intravenous cimetidine, 20–40 mg/kg/day divided q8h. In adolescents, aminocaproic acid (Amicar) can also be given in a dose of 3 gm IV q3h (maximum dose 12 gm/day) until the attack subsides.
   2. Refer all cases to a surgeon immediately. Avoid trauma to the neck because this may increase the edema.

B. **Disposition.** Admit all patients with laryngeal edema and consult an ENT surgeon immediately.

C. **Key points**
   1. Treat children with laryngeal edema secondary

to hereditary angioneurotic edema with epinephrine, hydrocortisone, and histamine blockers. Avoid trauma or manipulation of the neck.

## BIBLIOGRAPHY

Fauci, L. (ed.). *Immunology and Rheumatology*. St. Louis: Mosby, 1985.

Lawlor, G. J., and Fischer, T. J. (eds.). *Manual of Allergy and Immunology*. Boston: Little Brown, 1981.

Middleton, E., Reed, C. E., and Ellis, E. F. (eds.). *Allergy: Principles and Practice*. St. Louis: Mosby, 1978.

Patterson, R. (ed.). *Allergic Diseases* (third ed.). Philadelphia: Lippincott, 1985.

# Bites and Stings

Loretta Fiorillo and Gregory A. Baldwin

I. **Hymenoptera (bees, wasps, hornets).** Hymenoptera is a large order of insects containing about 100,000 species, many of which have evolved poison glands and modified the ovidepositor for stinging. Their bites cause more than 30 deaths per year in the United States—more than any other venomous animal—and are responsible for many painful and near-fatal reactions.

A. **Diagnosis and assessment.** The sting produces immediate burning pain, often severe, followed by local erythema and edema. Antigenic substances in the venom may cause immediate (less than 30 minutes) allergic hypersensitivity, ranging in severity from an intense local reaction to anaphylaxis. Severe or fatal reactions tend to occur immediately after exposure. Stings on the face or mucous membranes are the most dangerous.

B. **Management**

1. **Resuscitation.** If systemic symptoms of anaphylaxis are present, treat the patient with epinephrine and other medications (see Chap. 30, sec. **I**).

2. **0–2 Hours after bite**

a. Cleanse the area with soap and water.

b. Remove the bee stinger by gently scraping the area with the dull edge of a No. 10 scalpel blade.

c. Follow with cold compresses composed of a 1 : 20 dilution of Burow's solution or tap water for 20 minutes. Topical application of an antiperspirant containing aluminum hydroxide usually provides adequate pain relief.

d. Patients with local reactions only can be discharged with instructions to reapply antiperspirant every 4–6 hours. Advise parents to return for follow-up if the swelling persists or increases after 24 hours.

3. **24–72 Hours after bite.** Increased tenderness, deepening erythema, and pus at the site of the sting suggest bacterial infection. Obtain a swab of the area for Gram's stain and culture and begin treatment with cephalexin, 50 mg/kg/day PO divided q6h, or cloxacillin, 50 mg/kg/day PO divided q6h. If secondary infection is excluded, persistent local reactions can be treated with topical 1% hydrocortisone cream or lotion qid, and diphenhydramine (Benadryl), 1 mg/kg PO q6h.

II. **Spider bite.** Two varieties of spider are particularly dangerous: the black widow spider (*Latrodectus mactans*) and the brown recluse spider (*Loxosceles reclusa*). Both are commonly found in warm climates.

A. **Diagnosis and assessment**

1. **Black widow spider.** There may be momentary pain at the time of the bite, but more commonly the bite is unnoticed, leaving two tiny red marks at the

entry site of the fangs. Within 10 minutes to an hour a dull cramping pain and numbness start to spread from the inoculation site toward the torso. The abdomen may become excruciatingly painful and rigid. Pain usually peaks in 2–3 hours but may last up to 2 days. There may be nausea and vomiting, dizziness, headache, seizures, shock, coma, and death.

   2. **Brown recluse spider.** Pain develops within 2–8 hours of most bites, although onset may be delayed for 24 hours. The initial lesion is a vesicle that evolves into a purplish plaque with tissue necrosis in severe cases. Systemic signs and symptoms are more common with large lesions and appear within 72 hours. They include fever, malaise, urticaria, arthralgia, myalgia, headache, seizures, hemolysis, disseminated intravascular coagulation (DIC), jaundice, hematuria, hemoglobinuria, and proteinuria. Systemic loxoscelism can result in shock, coma, and death.

B. **Management**
   1. **Black widow**
      a. **Immediate.** Apply ice packs to the affected area and give analgesia (acetaminophen, codeine) as required. Morphine may be necessary for severe pain.
      b. **Subsequent.** Administration of antivenin (Lyovac), 2.5 ml intravenously or by IM injection, is sufficient to relieve most of the symptoms within 1–2 hours.
   2. **Brown recluse**
      a. **Immediate.** Apply an ice pack to the area for immediate pain relief; then replace it with a sterile dressing. Splint the involved limb if the reaction is severe and give a tetanus booster immunization to those at risk (see Appendix I).
      b. **Subsequent.** Acetaminophen or acetylsalicylic acid (ASA) may be given for analgesia when pain is mild. Prescribe antibiotics when secondary bacterial infection is suspected, after obtaining a swab of the involved area for Gram's stain and culture. Bites with necrotic centers greater than 2 cm in diameter should be treated with prednisone, 1 mg/kg/day PO divided q12h for 5 days. Plastic surgery may be necessary at a later date to cover large skin defects. Early surgical excision is not recommended.

III. **Tick bites.** Although tick bites are usually benign, they are associated with tick paralysis, Rocky Mountain spotted fever, tularemia, relapsing fever, and Lyme arthritis.

   A. **Management.** Ticks should be removed in toto, without leaving the mouth parts embedded in the skin. This is accomplished by gently and steadily pulling on the exposed portion of the body with a pair of curved forceps. It takes roughly 2–3 minutes to remove the tick in this manner. If the mouth parts remain embedded, a 2-mm punch skin biopsy will suffice to remove them. Application of chloroform, local heat, Vaseline, or other substances is not effective.

IV. **Human bites.** True bites or injuries incurred by direct trauma with the mouth (punching injury) are at high risk for infection and should be treated with prophylactic phenoxymethyl penicillin, 50 mg/kg/day PO divided q6h, and cloxacillin, 50 mg/kg/day PO divided q6h (clindamycin is an alternative). After careful irrigation and debridement, dress the wound. All lacerations should be treated by delayed closure in 3–4 days (see Chap. 35). If there is any suspicion of bony injury or penetration of a joint, obtain x rays and consult an orthopedic or hand surgeon. If infection has developed, take a swab of the wound for Gram's stain and culture, admit the patient and treat with intravenous cefuroxime *or* ampicillin, 100 mg/kg/day divided q6h, and cloxacillin or oxacillin, 100 mg/kg/day divided q6h (or other suitable antistaphylococcal drug), and consult a surgeon. Administer tetanus booster immunization to those at risk (see Appendix I).

V. **Animal bites.** All injuries other than superficial scratches are prone to infection from a multitude of organisms including *Pasteurella, Staphylococcus aureus,* streptococci, and aerobic and anaerobic mouth flora. Although only 5% of dog and 15% of cat bites become infected, it is probably wise to treat patients with large wounds, wounds that involve the face, and wounds more than 4 hours old with phenoxymethyl penicillin, 50 mg/kg/day PO divided q6h, or cephalexin, 25–50 mg/kg/day PO divided q6h for 5 days. Established infection in **serious or deep bites** should be treated with intravenous ampicillin, 100–200 mg/kg/day divided q6h, or cefuroxime, 75–100 mg/kg/day divided q8h. **Minor** infections can be treated with clavulanic acid and amoxicillin (Augmentin), 40 mg/kg/day as amoxicillin component PO divided q8h, or oral doxycycline (in children over age 8). Penicillin-allergic patients can be treated with clindamycin, 20–40 mg/kg/day PO or IV, divided q6–8h. Administer tetanus booster immunization to those at risk (see Appendix I).

VI. **Rabies prophylaxis.** Rabies virus can infect any mammal. Cats, dogs, bats, raccoons, skunks, foxes, and farm livestock are most likely to be affected. Animals vaccinated in North America are unlikely to cause disease. Determine the behavior of the animal and whether the attack was provoked or not—petting and feeding an animal are considered provocations. Bites or contamination of scratches, open wounds, abrasions, or mucous membranes with body fluids or tissue from a rabid animal constitute significant exposure. Rabies infection presents with sensory changes (hypoesthesia, paresthesia) at the site of the inoculation followed by rapid progression to hydrophobia, seizures, and death.

A. **Management.** Begin with thorough local debridement, cleaning with soap, and administration of tetanus booster immunization as necessary (see Appendix I). In

**Table 31-1. Postexposure rabies prophylaxis guide**

| Details of animal | Nature of exposure | Management of child |
|---|---|---|
| Rabid, **OR** Suspected rabid, **OR** Wild animal in an endemic area, **OR** Escaped dog or cat in endemic area*—animal should be killed and tested immediately | No skin or mucosal contact with animal or casual contact<br><br>Bite or contamination of scratch, abrasion, open wound or mucous membrane with saliva, body fluids, or tissue | No treatment<br>1. Local wound toilet<br>2. RIG (local and IM)<br>3. Full course of HDCV |
| Apparently healthy domestic dog or cat that is confined for 10 days | Bite or contamination of scratch, abrasion, open wound or mucous membrane with saliva, body fluids or tissue | 1. Local wound toilet<br>2. At first sign of rabies in animal give RIG (local and IM) and start full course of HDCV |

Key: RIG = Rabies immune globulin, human; HDCV = human diploid cell vaccine
*Consult local public health authorities.
Source: Reprinted from Advisory Committee on Immunization, Government of Canada. *A Guide to Immunizations for Canadians*. Ottawa: Government of Canada, Dept. of Health and Welfare, 1981.

areas where rabies occurs, domestic healthy animals should be confined for 10 days of observation; if rabies is suspected the animal must be killed and the head examined for rabies at an appropriate laboratory. Strays and wild animals that are caught should similarly be sacrificed for examination. Other animals (livestock, rodents, etc.) should be considered individually; follow local public health recommendations. For management of previously rabies-immunized persons also consult local public health authorities.

**VI. Disposition.** Admit all children with anaphylaxis after hymenoptera stings, those with black widow or brown recluse spider bites who have systemic symptoms, children with a human bite associated with fracture or joint penetration, and children exposed to rabies.

**VII. Key points**
   **A.** Treat all human and most animal bites with systemic antibiotics and delayed wound closure.
   **B.** Remove ticks with steady pressure, using curved forceps.

## Bibliography

Advisory Committee on Immunization, Government of Canada. *A Guide to Immunizations for Canadians.* Ottawa: Government of Canada Dept. of Health and Welfare, 1981.

Fitzpatrick, T. B. (ed.). *Dermatology in General Medicine* (3rd ed.). New York: McGraw Hill, 1987.

Kingston, L. E. Spider bites. *Arch. Dermatol.* 123:41, 1987.

# Trauma

# Multiple Trauma

Geoffrey K. Blair

Trauma is the most common cause of death in children over 1 year of age. Most injuries are blunt in nature and are sustained by passengers or pedestrians in motor vehicle accidents. Multiple trauma can also occur in victims of child abuse.

I. **Principles of trauma management.** Death usually results from central nervous system (CNS) injury; in most cases the CNS injury cannot be ameliorated. Morbidity and mortality can be reduced when they are secondary to hypovolemia or metabolic, respiratory, or infectious complications. The cardinal rules for management of the traumatized child are:

   A. Do not waste time—a child who appears well may be marginally compensated.

   B. Be suspicious of occult injury. A stable outward appearance often belies serious internal damage.

   C. Consider the unique aspects of the child trauma victim including anatomy, physiology, drug metabolism, and emotional response to injury.

   D. Use a systematic approach. Get help from qualified specialists. When possible, a "trauma team" should be available, consisting of general and subspecialist surgeons, emergency physicians, anesthetists, nurses, and paramedical personnel. Have appropriate equipment ready in a "trauma cart"; for a sample list of equipment see Table 32-1.

II. **Rapid initial assessment**

   A. **Airway**

      1. **Assessment.** Never assume that the airway is clear. Inspiratory stridor or a tracheal "tug" may indicate upper airway compromise. Infants up to 6 months of age are often obligate nasal breathers, and obstruction of the nose by blood or swelling can lead to respiratory failure.

      2. **Initial management.** Initial airway management includes a jaw thrust or chin lift (see Chap. 1). An oropharyngeal airway can be inserted immediately, and a suction catheter may be passed through it to clear secretions, blood, and other debris.

      3. **Intubation.** If endotracheal intubation is required, it may be done orally or nasally; nasal intubation is contraindicated in patients with suspected basilar skull fracture. Maintain in-line traction on the neck if cervical spine injury is suspected. Auscultate both sides of the chest to ensure correct tube position (see Chap. 1).

      4. **Oxygen.** Give maximal oxygen by mask to all multiple trauma victims.

      5. **Cricothyroidotomy.** Surgical cricothyroidotomy is rarely necessary in childhood trauma. Needle cricothyroidotomy, with a 14- or 12-gauge intravenous

**Table 32-1. Emergency room pediatric trauma equipment**

| Category | Equipment |
|---|---|
| Airway | High-flow oxygen masks |
| | Endotracheal tubes (see Chap. 1) |
| | 10–14-gauge catheter-over-needle IV sets for needle cricothyroidotomy |
| | Oxygen administration and ventilation equipment (see Chap. 1) |
| | Semirigid cervical collars and sandbags |
| | Suction equipment |
| Breathing | 14-gauge catheter-over-needle IV (thoracostomy) |
| | 10–28 F chest tubes, two of each |
| | Two chest tube insertion trays and a thoracotomy equipment pan |
| Circulation | 14–25-gauge IV cannulae and tourniquets |
| | Central venous catheters, Seldinger sets |
| | Two IV cutdown trays |
| | IV and blood administration sets with pumps and warmers, IV solutions (Ringer's, normal saline, 5% albumin, 50% dextrose) |
| | Pericardiocentesis tray |
| | ECG monitor |
| Other | NG tubes—10–18 F, with catheter tip 50-ml syringes |
| | Suture tray with variety of suture types and sizes—silk is most versatile in acute trauma |
| | One general surgical equipment tray with peritoneal dialysis catheter |
| | Electrocautery unit |
| | Operative light source |
| | Heat lamps, warm blanket |
| | Foley catheters 8–16 F |
| | Orthopedic splinting and casting materials |
| | Spine board |

catheter inserted downward at a 45-degree angle through the cricothyroid membrane, is an appropriate temporizing measure if intubation attempts fail. Pneumothorax may occur in children ventilated by high pressure jet insufflation via needle cricothyroidotomy.

6. **Spine stabilization.** All children with significant injury above the level of the clavicles, and trauma victims who are comatose should be assumed to have cervical spine injury. **Trauma to the spine can produce spinal cord injury with or without a fracture.** When injury is suspected, fix the spine with a semirigid collar or by taping the forehead down to the bed with sandbags placed at each side of the head. Order a lateral cervical spine x ray in all cases, ensuring that all seven vertebrae are visible

on the film. See Chap. 24, sec. **V.B,** for specific diagnosis and management.

**B. Breathing**

**1. Assessment.** Initially, respiratory impairment is a clinical diagnosis. Signs of respiratory impairment include restlessness, tachypnea (>45 breaths/minute in an infant or toddler, >30 breaths/minute in a child) grunting respirations, cyanosis, and intercostal indrawing. Inspect the chest, front and back, for signs of injury. Palpate the trachea for deviation and auscultate for presence and symmetry of breath sounds.

**2. Management.** If there are signs of respiratory impairment in a multiple trauma victim, immediate intubation and ventilation with 100% oxygen is indicated. For diagnosis and management of specific chest injuries, see Chap. 33.

**C. Circulation.** Traumatic shock in children is usually secondary to blood loss from the extremities or concealed hemorrhage into the chest or abdomen.

**1. Assessment.** Early signs of shock include tachycardia, mottled skin, cool extremities, and delayed capillary refill (normally 2 seconds at the thenar eminence). Hypotension is a very late sign. Hypovolemic children whose condition decompensates into shock are often very difficult to treat.

**2. Stop hemorrhage.** Control external hemorrhage using direct pressure. Rarely, MAST pants may be required in the older child or adolescent. Contraindications to MAST pants include pregnancy, congestive heart failure, pulmonary edema, and abdominal evisceration or impalement injury.

**3. Intravenous access and blood work.** Start two large-bore intravenous lines. If the child is "flat," with unobtainable vital signs, gain intravenous access in the groin by using a cutdown or Seldinger technique (see Chap. 2). Obtain blood samples for cross-match, complete blood count (CBC), platelet count, measurement of electrolytes, blood glucose, and amylase, BUN, prothrombin time (PT), partial thromboplastin time (PTT), and liver function tests.

**4. Fluids.** Inadequate intravenous fluid administration is a common error in trauma management. Treat hypovolemia initially with Ringer's lactate, 10 ml/kg given as a bolus infusion and repeated prn. Frequently reassess the patient's volume status including heart rate, capillary filling, warmth of the extremities, and blood pressure. Warmed whole blood, 10 ml/kg given prn, or packed red cells, 5 ml/kg given prn, may be administered if the child remains unstable. Uncross-matched group O, Rh-negative blood may be used if type-specific blood is not available, although this situation is very rarely encountered in a modern hospital setting. In patients requiring massive transfusions, use a blood warmer, monitor the patient frequently for coagulopathy or thrombocytopenia, and give platelet concentrate, fresh frozen plasma, or cryoprecipitate as needed (see Chap. 19).

**D. Neurologic status**

1. **Assessment.** Determine and record the level of consciousness, pupil size and symmetry, and the Glasgow Coma Scale score (see Chap. 41).

2. **Management.** Inadequate treatment of hypoxia, hypovolemia, or hypercapnia may worsen existing brain injury. Reduction of cerebral edema by fluid restriction should be instituted only after hemodynamic stabilization has been achieved. See Chap. 41.

**E. Detailed assessment, support, and disposal**

1. **Expose the patient.** Remove all clothing. Core rectal temperature should be measured on all trauma victims and appropriate warming procedures undertaken if necessary (see Chap. 29, I).

2. **Examination.** Examine the child in a systematic fashion from head to toe. For more detailed descriptions of the diagnosis and management of individual injuries, see appropriate chapters.

   a. Head and neck. Carefully inspect and palpate the head for evidence of trauma. Examine the ears, eyes (pupils, fundi, visual acuity), nose, mouth (including teeth), throat, and scalp. Rule out maxillofacial trauma. Without moving the neck, carefully palpate the cervical spine for tenderness. Perform a complete neurologic examination, including power, tone, reflexes, sensation, and cranial nerves, and recheck the Glasgow Coma Scale score.

   b. Chest. Inspect for serious injuries such as open pneumothorax or flail segments. Palpate the entire chest to search for crepitus and tenderness. Percuss and auscultate the chest. Log roll the patient while maintaining alignment of the spine to view the back and test for tenderness and crepitus over the thoracolumbar spine.

   c. Abdomen. Inspect for distention or bruising, percuss for dullness (fluid) or tympany (gas), and palpate for tenderness or rigidity. Apply pressure on the pelvis at the anterior superior iliac spines and the symphysis pubis.

   d. Rectum. Look for blood and feel for a boggy or high-riding prostate or pelvic fracture; assess the anal tone. Guaiac test the stool.

   e. Genitourinary system. Inspect for blood at the urethral meatus and bleeding or trauma to the vulva, hymen, penis, or scrotum.

   f. Extremities. Look for bruising, swelling, and obvious deformity. Assess the peripheral pulses, capillary filling, and temperature. Test the range of motion and palpate for crepitus and tenderness.

3. **Monitoring and stabilizing**

   a. Place the child on a cardiac monitor and frequently measure the vital signs. If available, use an automatic sphygmomanometer (Doppler) for continuous monitoring of blood pressure and pulse.

**b.** Place a nasogastric tube (orogastric when basal skull fracture is suspected) and a Foley catheter (use caution when there is blood at the meatus, a high-riding prostate, scrotal hematoma, or other suspicion of urethral injury—see Chap. 17). Perform a gross and microscopic urinalysis to search for signs of bleeding. Give fluids to maintain a minimum urine output of 1 ml/kg/hour (ideally, 2–4 ml/kg/hour). Give a tetanus booster immunization to those at risk (see Appendix I).

**c.** Assign a team member to record information on a trauma flow sheet including vital signs, medications, laboratory investigations, x rays, and procedures performed.

**4. Investigations.** Order blood work (see sec. **II.C.3** above) and a urinalysis. Using a portable x-ray machine, obtain x rays of the spine, chest, and abdomen. CT scans, nuclear medicine scans, and angiographic studies are often useful in evaluation of specific injuries in the multiple trauma victim.

**5. History.** Determine details of the accident (mechanism of injury, other people injured, seatbelts, damage to vehicle) and preceding events as well as information on the patient's allergies, medications, and past health. Ambulance attendants and accident witnesses are often helpful historians. Contradictory histories from different caretakers or a history that doesn't "fit" the physical findings should arouse suspicion of child abuse (see Chap. 39).

**6. Ongoing assessment and treatment.** If the child remains unstable and requires transfer to the operating room or another hospital, ensure the following:

**a.** If possible, warn anesthetists, operating room staff, and other personnel well in advance.

**b.** Transfer should be speedy and smooth without sacrificing control of airway or vital functions. Monitoring and resuscitation equipment must accompany the child during transport.

**c.** Take adequate time for consultation and transfer arrangements. Copy all records, laboratory results, and x rays and send them with the child.

**7. Preexisting disease or congenital defects.** Existing diseases or congenital anomalies (i.e., cardiac or renal abnormalities) can "tip the scales" against an injured child, making management more difficult.

**a.** These anomalies may be revealed for the first time by the injury.

**b.** Seemingly minor trauma may cause significant impairment in the child with an underlying disorder or congenital defect.

**III. Disposition.** Admit all multiple trauma victims.

## IV. Key points
   **A.** Airway control and cervical spine stabilization are the first steps in management of children with multiple trauma.
   **B.** A team approach, including early consultation with surgeons and anesthesiologists, is advised, preferably before the child arrives in the emergency department.

### Bibliography

American College of Surgeons. *Student Manual, Advanced Trauma Life Support Course.* Chicago: A.C.O.S., 1984.

Hurst, J. M. (ed.). *Common Problems in Trauma.* Chicago: Year Book Medical Publishers, 1987.

King, D. Trauma in infancy and childhood: Initial evaluation and management. *Pediatr. Clin. North Am.* 32:1299, 1985.

Proceedings of the first national conference on pediatric trauma. *Pediatr. Emerg. Care* 2:113, 1986.

Zuidema, G. D. (ed.). *The Management of Trauma* (4th ed.). Philadelphia: Saunders, 1985.

# Chest Trauma

Geoffrey K. Blair

The chest encloses not only the lungs and lower airways but also the heart, great vessels, esophagus, and thoracic spine. **An initial rapid assessment** (see Chap. 32) should detect signs of severe life-threatening injuries. In the **subsequent detailed assessment,** search for subtle signs of traumatic injury.

I. **Diagnosis and assessment**
   A. **Examination**
      1. **Inspection.** If there are signs of respiratory failure such as cyanosis, tracheal tug, or indrawing following chest trauma, immediate intubation and ventilation are indicated. Look for open or sucking wounds, flail segments, asymmetry of movement (hemothorax, pneumothorax), and fullness of the chest. Though difficult to detect in the young child, an elevated jugular venous pressure may indicate cardiac tamponade or tension pneumothorax. Bruising or swelling of the chest wall may be indirect signs of internal injury.
      2. **Palpation.** Feel the position of the trachea (deviated in tension pneumothorax) and palpate the chest wall for asymmetry (hemothorax, pneumothorax), flail segments, and crepitus (pneumothorax).
      3. **Percussion.** Percuss the position and excursion of the diaphragm (rupture) and note the presence of hyperresonance (pneumothorax) or dullness (hemothorax, traumatic diaphragmatic hernia).
      4. **Auscultation.** Evaluate the equality of air entry—this is especially important after endotracheal intubation to ensure tube position is correct. In general, coarse sounds come from the large airways, whereas fine crepitations suggest alveolar disease. Listen for rubs, "crunches," bronchial breathing, intrathoracic bowel sounds, and the loudness and character of the heart sounds.
   B. **Investigation**
      1. **Chest x ray.** X rays should never delay therapy of life-threatening injury. Six-foot upright anteroposterior and lateral films are preferred. If this is impossible because of suspected spinal or other injuries, a supine portable film will suffice. See Table 33-1 for a summary of findings.
      2. **Arterial blood gases.** Arterial blood gas measurements should be obtained as soon as possible and are usually taken from the femoral artery. Arterial catheter placement should be deferred until resuscitation is completed. If available, pulse oximetry can be an excellent method for continuously monitoring oxygen saturation. Capillary blood gas measurements are unreliable for determining oxygenation and

**405**

**Table 33-1. X-ray findings in chest trauma**

| Examination | Findings |
| --- | --- |
| Bones | Vertebral fractures or misalignment, rib fractures (greenstick fractures, old fractures, and especially first or second rib fractures), clavicular fractures, scapular fractures, shoulder dislocations or fractures |
| Lungs and pleural space | Contusion, atelectasis, consolidation, hemothorax, apical capping; note the position of any chest drains that have been inserted |
| Airways | Shifts in position, foreign bodies (teeth); note position of the endotracheal tube |
| Mediastinum | Shift to one side (tension pneumothorax), widening (aortic trauma—may be hard to assess in the young child with a large thymus), pneumomediastinum, pneumopericardium; note the size and shape of the heart, the shape and position of the aortic arch |
| Diaphragm | Rupture, traumatic herniation of abdominal viscera, elevation, paralysis |
| Soft tissues | Swelling, subcutaneous air, foreign bodies |

should not be relied on for assessment of the trauma victim.

3. **Electrocardiographic (ECG) monitoring.** Immediately place the child on a cardiac monitor. A 12-lead ECG may be necessary during the detailed assessment.

II. **Common chest injuries.** Contusion and pneumothorax account for the great majority of chest injuries in children. In all cases, give oxygen by mask or nasal prongs and be prepared to intubate and ventilate the child.

A. **Lung contusion.** Severe contusion results in lung edema, arteriovenous shunting, and hypoxia. It may occur in the absence of rib fractures or other injury and may present in a slow and insidious fashion, hours after trauma.

1. **Diagnosis.** The child is dyspneic, and examination reveals tachypnea, with fine crepitations on auscultation. Cyanosis and marked hypoxemia occur in severe cases. Initially, the chest x ray may be normal,

but eventually it shows patchy infiltrates or consolidation.

2. **Management.** Treatment is supportive and includes oxygen, monitoring, and, if necessary, intubation and mechanical ventilation, often with positive end-expiratory pressure (PEEP) or continuous positive airway pressure (CPAP). Avoid fluid overload that can worsen lung edema; excessive administration of crystalloid fluid is especially hazardous. In most cases the contusion resolves in 2–3 days.

B. **Pneumothorax.** Pneumothorax is a consequence of a tear of the lung, bronchus, or trachea, resulting in a collection of air in the pleural space. It can occur following blunt or penetrating trauma. Open and tension pneumothorax are surgical emergencies (see sec. **III.A** and **B** below). Nontraumatic pneumothorax can occur in children with lower airway obstruction (asthma, foreign body aspiration, cystic fibrosis), in newborns, and spontaneously in otherwise healthy children and adults.

1. **Diagnosis.** The child with pneumothorax usually has pleuritic chest pain. A large pneumothorax presents with decreased breath sounds, hyperresonance to percussion, and signs of respiratory distress or failure. Tachypnea may be the only sign of a small pneumothorax. The diagnosis is confirmed by x ray. Associated signs may include subcutaneous emphysema on palpation and pneumomediastinum on x ray.

2. **Management.** All children with pneumothorax should be admitted for observation and given maximum oxygen therapy by mask. Start an intravenous line and proceed with chest tube insertion if more than 10% of the lung surface area is collapsed (estimate the amount from the chest x ray), if there has been trauma, or if there are signs of hypovolemia or respiratory distress. Pneumothorax in patients with cystic fibrosis may require surgical treatment.

III. **Other chest injuries**

A. **Tension pneumothorax.** This injury often occurs secondary to penetration by a fractured rib (although it may occur in the absence of rib fracture). Untreated, it can be rapidly fatal.

1. **Diagnosis and assessment.** The presentation is similar to that of simple pneumothorax (see sec. **II.B** above), although respiratory distress is more severe. The child is often restless and cyanosed, and the trachea may be deviated to the contralateral side; also, there may be a raised jugular venous pressure (usually not visible in young children).

2. **Management**

a. **Immediate treatment.** Decompress the pneumothorax with a 14- or 16-gauge intravenous catheter. This is placed in the midclavicular line at the second intercostal space anteriorly, aimed directly posterior, and pushed to the hilt. The stylet is then removed and the catheter is left in place. A rush of air is usually heard or felt when the pneumothorax is drained.

  **b.** Chest tube. Following catheter decompression, insert a chest tube at the midaxillary line at nipple level (see sec. **IV.A** below). Suction may be applied up to $-10$ to $-20$ cm of water. If there is a massive air leak, one or more tubes may be inserted and attached to a suction device. In all cases, follow the procedure with an x ray to check tube position and confirm drainage of the pneumothorax. Do not clamp the chest tube because this may result in rapid reaccumulation of air. Thoracotomy is indicated when there are major bronchial or tracheal tears, as suggested by a continued large air leak.

**B. Open pneumothorax.** This is caused by a penetrating injury. Open pneumothorax causes a to-and-fro movement of the mediastinum, resulting in inadequate ventilation.

  **1. Diagnosis.** The child complains of pain and dyspnea. On examination, there may be tachypnea, restlessness, or cyanosis. There is a sucking chest wound and poor air entry bilaterally.

  **2. Management.** Immediately apply an occlusive dressing to the wound and tape it down on three of four sides. Insert an ipsilateral chest tube at a site remote from the wound. Most children will require definitive surgical debridement and repair in the operating room.

**C. Hemothorax.** Intrathoracic bleeding usually originates from the intercostal vessels or the lung and is self-limited. Fatal hemorrhage may follow penetrating injury to the heart or great vessels or, rarely, deceleration injury to the arch of the aorta (see sec. **III.K**). Pneumothorax and lung contusion are commonly associated injuries.

  **1. Diagnosis.** The major complaints are pain and dyspnea. On examination there may be restlessness, cyanosis, or shock. Decreased air entry and dullness to percussion over the hemothorax are usually found. Severe hemothorax may result in mediastinal shift with tracheal deviation to the contralateral side.

  **2. Management.** These children require rapid intravenous volume replacement and insertion of a chest tube. Thoracotomy may be necessary if the bleeding continues or is severe.

**D. Cardiac tamponade.** This rare complication may be the result of penetrating or blunt trauma. Rapid accumulation of as little as 30–40 ml of blood in the pericardial cavity may be fatal. Tamponade may also occur in children with inflammatory or infectious pericarditis; the presentation in these patients is generally more benign.

  **1. Diagnosis.** The child may have dyspnea or air hunger. On examination, there are usually a pulsus paradoxus (inspiratory blood pressure is at least 10 mm

Hg higher than expiratory blood pressure) and poor peripheral perfusion. Although it is not always present, look for Beck's triad: decreased arterial pressure, elevated jugular venous pressure, and muffled heart sounds. In the stable patient with a nontraumatic effusion, the diagnosis can be confirmed by echocardiography.

2. **Management.** Treatment is by subxiphoid pericardiocentesis during continuous ECG, blood pressure, and pulse monitoring. Withdrawal of as little as 30 ml of fluid (Fig. 33-1) may result in a dramatic clinical improvement. Pericardial blood may reaccumulate rapidly; a catheter can be left in the pericardial cavity to allow for repeated withdrawal of blood. Open pericardiotomy and repair of the myocardium may be necessary—consult a surgeon.

**E. Flail chest.** Blunt injury may produce multiple rib fractures that destabilize the chest wall and result in ineffective ventilation. This injury is uncommon in children.

1. **Diagnosis.** Chest pain and dyspnea are present with tenderness and bony crepitus over the flail segment. Observation of the breathing pattern may reveal paradoxical movement of a segment of the chest wall. On auscultation, air entry is poor, and there may be crepitations due to an underlying lung contusion.

2. **Management.** Do not externally stabilize or strap the chest wall. These children require intubation and mechanical ventilation. Analgesia can be achieved by intercostal nerve block using a solution of 0.25% bupivacaine mixed with equal portions of dextran (bupivacaine maximum dose is 2 mg/kg).

**F. Myocardial contusion.** Myocardial contusion occurs following direct blunt trauma and may result in serious dysrhythmia.

1. **Diagnosis.** The child complains of chest pain. Examination reveals chest wall tenderness or fracture of the sternum. The most common sign is tachycardia, which is disproportionate to the degree of hypovolemia. Cardiac enzymes may be increased (creatine phosphokinase, lactic dehydrogenase, aspartate aminotransferase) and ECG analysis may reveal ST-segment elevation and premature ventricular contractions.

2. **Management.** Treatment is supportive, with monitoring and antiarrhythmic therapy (see Chap. 9). Obtain measurements of cardiac enzymes and echocardiographic studies after stabilization.

**G. Penetrating chest trauma.** Children with penetrating chest trauma often appear to be surprisingly well. Most cases involve missile injuries or impalement by objects such as arrows, sticks, or fence posts.

1. **Diagnosis.** There may be signs of shock and evidence of hemothorax, pneumothorax, and cardiac or great vessel injury.

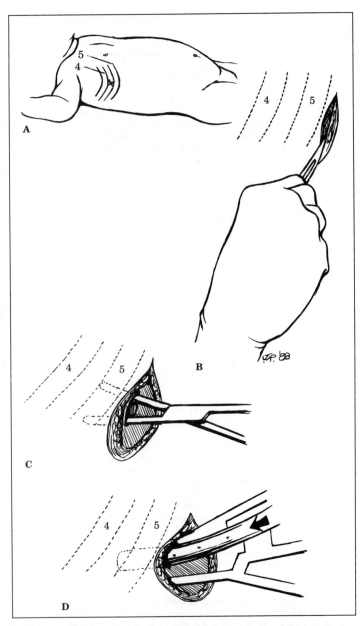

Fig. 33-1. Chest tube insertion. A. Site of chest tube insertion. B. Make incision at superior border of rib. C. Blunt dissect to border of rib with curved hemostat. Open wide to let air or fluid surge out. D. Thread tube through open jaws of hemostat toward superior pole of lung. Suture in place and attach to underwater sealed drainage.

2. **Management. In children with an impalement injury, do not remove the impaling object.** Impaling objects and missiles should be removed in the operating room during thoracotomy. Treat the accompanying chest injuries as outlined in sec. **III.A–F** above and consider arteriography to rule out great vessel trauma. In children who have a penetrating injury at or below the fifth intercostal space, rule out abdominal or diaphragmatic injury (see Chap. 34).

**H. Esophageal rupture.** Esophageal rupture may follow penetrating injury, blunt injury, or caustic or foreign body ingestion. The majority of cases are associated with severe blunt trauma to the upper abdomen.

1. **Diagnosis.** Disruption of the esophagus presents with the signs and symptoms of mediastinitis. Patients may complain of chest pain, abdominal pain, dysphagia, or nausea. On examination there may be tachypnea, fever, evidence of a pneumothorax, Hamman's sign (precordial "crunch" on auscultation), or shock that is out of proportion to the apparent severity of the injury. Diagnosis is confirmed by an upper GI series using a water-soluble contrast material such as Gastrografin.

2. **Management.** Place a chest tube or tubes for drainage and treat with intravenous antibiotics: clindamycin, 30 mg/kg/day divided q6h and chloramphenicol, 75 mg/kg/day divided q6h. Most patients require thoracotomy for esophageal repair and possible gastrostomy.

**I. Traumatic diaphragmatic hernia.** This type of hernia is usually the result of blunt trauma to the chest or abdomen and nearly always occurs on the left side. Herniation of the abdominal contents into the chest results in lung displacement and ineffective ventilation. The diagnosis is often missed on the initial examination.

1. **Diagnosis.** The child is usually dyspneic. On chest auscultation there may be decreased air entry on the ipsilateral side. Bowel sounds are only rarely heard over the chest, but when heard, they are pathognomonic. The chest x ray shows evidence of stomach (including a nasogastric tube), bowel, spleen, or liver in the chest and loss of the diaphragmatic outline. Occasionally, the diagnosis is made when abdominal viscera are seen during chest tube insertion.

2. **Management.** Insert a nasogastric tube to allow gastrointestinal decompression and rule out concomitant intraabdominal injury. Surgical repair of the diaphragm is required.

**J. Traumatic asphyxia.** Traumatic asphyxia follows acute, high-pressure compression of the chest and commonly occurs in children who are run over by a motor vehicle. Compression against a closed glottis results in a severe rise in venous pressure that is transmitted peripherally, causing the distinctive clinical presentation of traumatic asphyxia.

1. **Diagnosis.** The child complains of chest pain and

dyspnea. On examination there are petechiae and suffusion (sunburned appearance) of the head, neck, and upper torso. There are often conjunctival hemorrhages, and there may be fundal hemorrhages and exudates. Thoracic fractures do not always occur; the only signs of injury may be tire-tread marks on the chest. Lung contusion is commonly associated. Seizures and visual disorders such as diplopia and decreased acuity may result from CNS or retinal injury.

    **2. Management.** Treatment is supportive (see sec. **II.A** above). Monitor for myocardial, nervous system, and abdominal injury. A complete eye examination is mandatory prior to discharge.

**K. Aortic rupture.** Aortic rupture is extremely rare in children; the presentation includes chest and arm pain, shock, and loss of left arm or lower limb pulses. Death is common from hypovolemia. On chest x ray there may be widening of the mediastinum, apical capping, tracheal deviation to the right, and first or second rib fracture. In the young child, a large thymus can make interpretation of mediastinal widening difficult. Consult a surgeon for management, including arteriography and surgery.

## IV. Procedures
### A. Insertion of a chest tube
#### 1. Equipment
    **a.** Appropriate-sized chest tube
        **(1)** 10F in neonate
        **(2)** 15F in young child
        **(3)** 20–28F in older child
    **b.** Underwater seal vacuum set with tubing and adaptor
    **c.** Scalpel blade (No. 15) and handle
    **d.** Lidocaine 1% for elective or semielective placement
    **e.** Sutures
    **f.** Curved hemostat or Kelly clamp
    **g.** Gloves, gown, mask
    **h.** 0.5% tincture of chlorhexidine, or povidone-iodine antiseptic solution

#### 2. Method (see Fig. 33-2)
    **a.** Identify the site for tube thoracostomy, at the fourth or fifth intercostal space in the midaxillary line.
    **b.** Using aseptic technique, clean the skin with chlorhexidine and infiltrate the site with 1% lidocaine down to the periosteum of the rib.
    **c.** Make a 2–4-cm incision with the scalpel at the superior border of the rib.
    **d.** Use the curved hemostat to dissect bluntly through muscle and fascia to the superior border of the rib and puncture the intercostal muscles and pleura. Do not allow the instrument to enter more than 1 cm into the pleural cavity.
    **e.** Open the instrument wide and let air or fluid surge out. Insert the index finger to widen the tract.

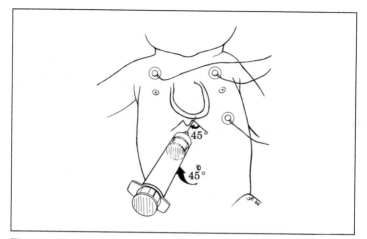

**Fig. 33-2. Pericardiocentesis.**

    **f.** Grasp the tip of the chest tube with the hemostat and advance it through the incision into the pleural cavity. Thread the tube through the open jaws of the hemostat toward the superior pole of the lung.

    **g.** Suture the tube in place and attach to an underwater seal drainage.

    **h.** Obtain a chest x ray following the procedure.

   **3. Complications**

    **a.** Injury to the chest contents—heart, lung, diaphragm, liver, spleen, or bronchus

    **b.** Bleeding

    **c.** Pneumothorax, hemothorax

    **d.** Infection

**B. Pericardiocentesis.** When possible, this procedure should be performed by a surgeon or cardiologist.

   **1. Equipment**

    **a.** 18–20-gauge cardiac needle or long central venous catheter with needle introducer

    **b.** Three-way stopcock

    **c.** 30-ml syringe

    **d.** ECG monitor

    **e.** Antiseptic chlorhexidine and alcohol or povido-iodine solution

    **f.** Gloves, gown, mask

   **2. Method**

    **a.** Assess the patient's vital signs continuously and place the child on a cardiac monitor.

    **b.** If time permits, wash the lower chest and upper abdomen with antiseptic solution.

    **c.** Identify a point one fingerbreadth inferior and to the left of the xiphichondral junction; if time permits, anesthetize the skin at this point with 1 ml of 1% plain lidocaine.

   **d.** Incise the skin with a scalpel, introduce the needle, and aim it toward the inferior tip of the left scapula. Aspirate for blood and monitor the ECG as the needle is advanced.

   **e.** Premature ventricular contractions, wide QRS complexes, or ST–T changes indicate that the needle has entered the myocardium; withdraw the needle until the ECG normalizes.

   **f.** In the child with cardiac tamponade, aspiration of pericardial fluid results in a dramatic improvement. The catheter may be left in the pericardial space and attached to the stopcock in case repeat aspiration becomes necessary.

   **g.** Obtain a chest x ray and a 12-lead ECG following the procedure.

**3. Complications**
   **a.** Pneumothorax
   **b.** Injury to myocardium or coronary vessels
   **c.** Dysrhythmias
   **d.** Mediastinal injury (to the aorta, esophagus, or vena cava)
   **e.** Iatrogenic hemopericardium

**V. Disposition.** Admit patients with evidence or suspicion of serious chest trauma, including all the examples listed in this chapter. Most cases of open pneumothorax, hemothorax, cardiac tamponade, great vessel injury, penetrating trauma, esophageal rupture, and diaphragmatic hernia require definitive treatment in the operating room.

**VI. Key points**
   **A.** Lung contusion, a common cause of mortality from chest trauma, is often asymptomatic in the early hours—maintain a high index of suspicion for this injury.
   **B.** Do not wait for measurements of blood gases or chest x rays in the trauma victim with signs of respiratory failure—intubate and ventilate the patient.
   **C.** When pneumothorax is suspected in the child with respiratory failure, immediate chest tube placement is indicated. Do not wait for the chest x ray.

**Bibliography**

Brooks, B. F. (ed.). *The Injured Child.* Austin: University of Texas Press, 1985.

Dunham, C. M., and Cowley, R. A. (eds.). *Shock Trauma/Critical Care Handbook.* Rockville, Md.: Aspen Publishers, 1986.

# 34

# Abdominal Trauma

Geoffrey K. Blair

Serious abdominal injury is usually due to blunt trauma resulting from motor vehicle accidents, child abuse, or falls. Injury to solid viscera may lead to bleeding; injury to hollow viscera can result in peritonitis. The liver and spleen are the organs most often affected.

I. **Resuscitation and initial assessment.** During the initial trauma assessment (see Chap. 32) look for abdominal distention—this may indicate intraabdominal hemorrhage. Insert a nasogastric tube (an orogastric tube in patients with suspected basilar skull fracture), aspirate the gastric contents, and look for evidence of gross or occult bleeding (Gastroccult test card). See Chap. 32.

II. **Detailed assessment**

  A. **History.** Determine the mechanism of injury, the past history including previous abdominal surgery, and the time of the last meal. Ask about pain; generalized pain is usually due to peritonitis resulting from blood or bowel contents. Consider the diagnosis of child abuse when there is a discrepancy between the history and physical findings or when histories taken from different people are conflicting.

  B. **Examination.** Inspect, percuss, palpate, and auscultate, remembering that the abdomen has six sides: anterior, posterior, two flanks, and the diaphragmatic and pelvic aspects. Interpretation of findings is often difficult, especially in the child with head injury who has an altered level of consciousness.

   1. **Inspection.** Look for distention, bruises, lacerations, abrasions, penetrating wounds, and surgical scars. Carefully log roll the patient to view the back if there is a suspicion of spinal injury. Observe the patient for splinting of the abdomen with movement or respiration as a sign of pain.

   2. **Palpation.** When feasible, ask the child to locate the pain before palpating. Note any guarding, tenderness (including costovertebral angle tenderness), masses, or organomegaly. Muscle guarding is an important finding; rigidity usually indicates peritonitis. Pain or crepitus with pressure on the symphysis pubis or anterior superior iliac spines suggests pelvic fracture.

   3. **Percussion.** Percuss all quadrants and locate the diaphragm, liver, and bladder. Percussion is particularly useful in distinguishing distention due to gas (tympanitic) from that due to blood (dull). Lack of dullness over the liver suggests pneumoperitoneum. Pain caused by percussion is a sensitive sign of rebound tenderness and peritonitis.

   4. **Auscultation.** Auscultation is generally unreliable in the evaluation of the injured abdomen, although

it can help to confirm correct nasogastric tube position.

5. **Rectal examination.** Although the prostate is not always palpable in the young child, the finding of a high-riding prostate or a boggy anterior mass on rectal examination is highly suspicious of rupture of the membranous urethra (see Chap. 17). Look for perianal signs of trauma and check the anal tone. The presence of blood in the rectum is suggestive of bowel injury. In the child with a pelvic fracture, feel for any bony fragments that may have lacerated the rectum.

C. **Laboratory investigations.** In the child with abdominal trauma, obtain blood specimens for the following tests:

1. Hemoglobin/hematocrit. These may be normal despite acute hypovolemia from blood loss.
2. A white bloood cell count is taken for a baseline study; it is unreliable in the acute phase.
3. Amylase level is often normal, even in the presence of pancreatic or bowel trauma.
4. Liver enzyme levels may be elevated in acute liver injury.
5. Electrolyte, BUN, and blood glucose concentrations.
6. Cross-match for 4–8 units of packed red blood cells and plasma if hemorrhage is suspected.

D. **X-ray and imaging studies**

1. **Abdominal x rays.** Order supine and upright or lateral decubitus views in all children with suspected abdominal injury. Although the presence of free air is pathognomonic of perforation, up to 80% of perforations are not evident on x ray. Note the vertebral alignment and the position of the nasogastric tube.
2. **Chest x ray.** Note the position and integrity of the diaphragm and look for signs of chest injury (see Table 33-1).
3. **Abdominal ultrasound examination.** Although this is a useful screening test for major solid organ damage or hemoperitoneum, it is not always reliable.
4. **Computed tomography (CT).** This is the most accurate modality for imaging the injured abdomen; it can reliably assess liver, spleen, and kidney damage. When upper bowel perforation is suspected, give 100 ml of water-soluble contrast material (Gastrografin) via nasogastric tube 20–30 minutes prior to the scan and look for leakage. CT scans are especially useful in head-injured children when examination is difficult.
5. **Liver-spleen radionuclide scanning.** Liver-spleen scanning is a reliable method of diagnosing injury of the liver or spleen.
6. **Magnetic resonance imaging** (MRI). To date, very little has been published on the use of MRI in the assessment of abdominal trauma in children.

E. **Peritoneal lavage.** The role of peritoneal lavage in the assessment of childhood abdominal injuries is controversial. It should be performed by a surgeon under direct vision and using careful dissection.

  1. **Method.** Local anesthesia is achieved by injection of 1% lidocaine with epinephrine. The incision is made in the midline subumbilically, and lavage is performed with 10 ml/kg of warm, sterile, normal saline or Ringer's solution.

  2. **Interpretation.** The presence of blood is not an indication for laparotomy. Although the presence of white blood cells, vegetable fibers, or a raised amylase concentration in the lavage returns is significant, these findings are not always present in patients requiring laparotomy. Lavage may be useful for identifying:

      **a.** The source of blood loss when there is unexplained shock in the injured child.

      **b.** The need for transport to a tertiary treatment facility—send a sample of lavage returns with the child. Always consult with a surgeon in the tertiary center before undertaking peritoneal lavage.

  F. **Laparoscopy.** Laparoscopy may be useful in the evaluation of the injured child's abdomen. It should be performed by a surgeon.

III. **Monitoring and reassessment.** Concealed injury often becomes manifest hours or days after the initial trauma. Frequent reevaluation and reexamination are therefore mandatory.

IV. **Laparotomy.** Immediate laparotomy is indicated in the following situations:

  A. Penetrating abdominal trauma.

  B. Intraabdominal hemorrhage when the child cannot be stabilized by transfusion.

  C. Pneumoperitoneum or stomach or bowel perforation.

  D. Diaphragmatic rupture.

  E. Rectal perforation.

  F. Some specific urinary tract injuries such as renovascular injury or bladder or urethral rupture.

  G. Biliary tract rupture.

  H. When the diagnosis is in doubt and there is suspicion of a serious or potentially fatal injury such as duodenal rupture.

V. **Management.** In all cases of suspected abdominal trauma, a surgeon should be consulted immediately for diagnosis and management. Give oxygen, start two large-bore intravenous lines, place a nasogastric tube, and follow guidelines for management as described in Chap. 32. **No analgesics should be administered until a surgeon has assessed the child.**

VI. **Specific injuries**

  A. **Spleen injuries.** Spleen injuries rarely require splenectomy; most can be managed nonoperatively by a surgeon with monitoring in an intensive care unit. Signs of splenic injury include left upper quadrant pain and tenderness and left shoulder tip pain (Kehr's sign). In the stable child, the diagnosis may be confirmed by nuclear medicine or CT scan.

**B. Liver injuries.** Although many liver injuries do not require operative intervention, others may result in violent intraabdominal hemorrhage. Right upper quadrant pain and signs of heavy occult bleeding should arouse suspicion of liver injury; immediately notify a surgeon, anesthesiologist, and the operating room for urgent laparotomy. In the stable child, the diagnosis may be confirmed by nuclear medicine or CT scan.

**C. Bowel perforation.** These rare injuries are often missed in the early assessment. The diagnosis is suggested by increasing signs of peritoneal irritation. Initial x rays often do not show free air; consider contrast studies (see sec. **II.C**, above). Laparotomy and repair are required.

**D. Duodenal hematoma.** Classically, these children are initially well and then develop intractable vomiting 6–18 hours later with the onset of duodenal obstruction. Upper GI contrast studies may reveal a typical "coiled-spring" pattern. Beware of underlying duodenal rupture or traumatic pancreatitis. Most duodenal hematomas can be managed nonoperatively with continuous nasogastric suction and intravenous fluids.

**E. Rectal injuries.** If a rectal injury remains undetected, the consequences are severe. When it is associated with a pelvic fracture, there is a risk of osteomyelitis. Rectal injury presents with bleeding, often in association with penetrating trauma or pelvic fracture. Patients require surgical repair with colostomy and drainage.

**F. Penetrating injury.** Children with penetrating abdominal trauma require laparotomy for exploration and repair. Do not remove impaling objects prior to laparotomy.

**G. Pancreatic injury.** Pancreatic injury is often occult in the early stages after trauma. The classic case occurs in the child who falls forward, landing on the abdomen ("handlebar" injury). There may be epigastric or periumbilical pain and vomiting. The amylase level is often raised, but it may be normal. Treatment is supportive in most cases, with intravenous fluids and continuous nasogastric suction.

**H. Stomach injuries.** Stomach perforation is suggested by the presence of fresh blood in the nasogastric tube and free air on x rays (reliably present in this injury). Surgical repair is required.

**I. Biliary tract perforation.** This is a rare injury and is difficult to diagnose on clinical grounds alone. Most such injuries are diagnosed at laparotomy following a course of progressive posttraumatic peritonitis.

**J. Retroperitoneal hemorrhage** (RPH). RPH occurs in conjunction with severe back or pelvic injuries and may lead to hypovolemic shock. There is a profound paralytic ileus that may last for days. Initial treatment is accomplished with continuous nasogastric suction, intravenous fluids, and blood transfusion. Severe hemorrhage requires angiographic embolization.

K. **Paralytic ileus.** Paralytic ileus is common after injury; the stomach is involved in most cases. Distention occurs and is increased by crying and air swallowing. Children present with abdominal pain and vomiting, signs that frequently mimic those seen with primary abdominal injury. Treat with nasogastric tube insertion and intravenous fluid administration. Most cases resolve within 12 hours.

L. **Seat belt injury.** In the classic case, the victim is wearing a lap belt but no shoulder belt and is involved in a head-on collision. The abdomen is acutely flexed over the lap belt, resulting in a triad of injuries: (1) abdominal wall contusion, often with severe tearing of the anterior muscles; (2) bowel perforation; and (3) fracture-dislocation of the lumbar spine that may result in paraplegia (Chance fracture). Maintain the child supine on a fracture board or firm mattress until spinal injury is ruled out (see Musculoskeletal Injuries). If bowel perforation is suspected, laparotomy is required.

VII. **Disposition.** Admit all children with abdominal trauma except trivial cases. Evidence of intraabdominal hemorrhage, even if it is minor and the child's condition is stable, demands continuous monitoring in an intensive care unit. For indications for emergency surgery see sec. **IV,** above.

VIII. **Key points**

A. The majority of serious abdominal trauma is due to spleen or liver injury.

B. Suspect liver injury in a child with signs of hemoperitoneum; urgent laparotomy is indicated.

### Bibliography

American College of Surgeons. *Student Manual Advanced Trauma Life Support Course.* Chicago: ACOS, 1984.

David, K. Trauma in infancy and childhood: Initial evaluation and management. *Pediatr. Clin. North Am.* 32:1299, 1985.

Proceedings of the first national conference on pediatric trauma. *Pediatr. Emerg. Care* 2:113, 1986.

Shires, G. T. *Principles of Trauma Care* (3rd ed.). New York: McGraw Hill, 1985.

# 35

# Minor Trauma

Leslie A. Scott

**I. Approach to minor trauma in the child.** Children are apprehensive about hospitals in general and painful procedures in particular; a caring, empathetic approach is important. If the child is uncooperative, restraint (Appendix III) or, in some cases, sedation or general anesthesia is necessary for examination or treatment following injury. If the child is attentive, explain the procedure carefully using appropriate language and state that everything will be done to make it as painless as possible. Explain which aspects will be uncomfortable or painful both prior to and during the procedure. Let the child watch if possible. In all cases, assess tetanus immunization status and treat those at risk (see Appendix I).

**A. Local anesthesia.** Local anesthesia can be achieved with 1% plain lidocaine using a small gauge (25 or 26) needle. The maximum dose is 4 mg/kg of plain lidocaine and 7 mg/kg of lidocaine with epinephrine (1 : 100,000). In the fingers or toes, create a digital block by infiltrating 0.5–1.0 ml of 1% plain lidocaine into the dorsal aspect of both sides of the digit at the level of the web. For wounds, infiltrate from the corners of the laceration to minimize needle pricks. An alternative to lidocaine infiltration of wounds is application of topical TAC (0.5% tetracaine, 1 : 2000 epinephrine, 11.8% cocaine), which is applied by soaking a 2-inch gauze pad or cotton pledget with 3 ml of solution and holding it on the wound for 10–15 minutes. Use of TAC and lidocaine with epinephrine is contraindicated in lacerations of the pinna, nipple, nasal bridge and alae, tarsal plate of the eye, digits, penis, or other areas of limited circulation. TAC should not be used in children less than 1 year old or on the face of young children if there is any chance of sniffing or swallowing it—fatalities can occur secondary to overdose.

**B. Abrasions.** Abrasions are friction injuries causing loss of superficial epithelium. There may be profuse bleeding from capillaries, and pain is often severe. Full-thickness abrasions should be referred to a plastic surgeon.

**1. Management.** Carefully clean the surface of all foreign material to avoid tattooing of the skin. After applying local anesthetic, scrub with a soft scrub brush and Hibitane soap until the skin is clean. If the affected area is extensive or if there are multiple injuries, general anesthesia may be necessary. Cover with an antibiotic cream such as mupirocin or Neosporin in exposed areas and a plastic film dressing in areas that will be covered by clothing.

**C. Lacerations.** Evaluate age of the injury, extent of contamination, degree of contusion and edema, and the possible presence of a foreign body. Small wounds with closely approximated edges that are not in areas under tension may be treated with Steri-Strips. Friars' Balsam should be applied to adjacent skin prior to the placement of Steri-Strips. Extensive or difficult lacerations in cosmetically important areas should be referred to a pediatric or plastic surgeon.

1. **Delayed closure.** Wounds over 24 hours old, human bites, barnyard injuries, and areas of poor vascular supply (bony shin), are at high risk for infection. They should be debrided, dressed, and closed in 3–5 days' time if they appear clean at that time. Lacerations that are infected should be allowed to close by secondary intention.

2. **Primary closure.** In general, lacerations that are less than 24 hours old, clean, or amenable to surgical cleaning may be closed primarily.

3. **Method**
   a. Restrain the child if necessary (see Appendix III).
   b. Shaving around the laceration in hair-bearing areas is usually unnecessary and should never be done in eyebrow lacerations.
   c. Achieve local anesthesia. This is unnecessary when only one or two sutures are required. In hand injuries, a full sensory-motor examination must be performed prior to using local anesthetic.
   d. Using gloves and aseptic technique, clean the wound and a generous margin of the surrounding skin with povidone-iodine or 0.5% tincture of chlorhexidine.
   e. Explore the wound to determine the depth of injury and rule out the presence of a foreign body, especially in hand lacerations. If in doubt about a fracture or foreign body, obtain an x ray.
   f. If bleeding is heavy, achieve hemostasis with a tourniquet or point pressure. Never blindly clamp areas because damage to vital structures may result.
   g. Forcefully irrigate the area with an aqueous preparation or dilute hydrogen peroxide solution, using a syringe attached to an 18-gauge needle. Excise the ragged edges and nonviable or crushed soft tissue or skin.
   h. If the wound is deep or gaping, subcutaneous tissues should be approximated with fine absorbable sutures such as 4–0 or 5–0 chromic or vicryl. Start subcutaneous sutures in the deep portion of the wound to bury the knot.
   i. Approximate the skin edges with fine nonabsorbable material such as nylon or silk using interrupted or running simple sutures. The needle should enter and exit the skin at points equidistant from the wound margin at a 90-degree angle to the skin surface. When suturing scalp lacerations use a color of suture material that contrasts with hair. Place the sutures close to the wound margins and include the dermis. Skin edges should lie together but not tightly. When suturing through a hairline or a vermilion border, accurate

**Table 35-1. Suturing guidelines**

| Site | Size | Days till removal |
|------|------|-------------------|
| Face | 5–0 or 6–0 | 4 days |
| Scalp | 3–0 or 4–0 | 5 days |
| Anterior neck | 4–0 or 5–0 | 4 days |
| Chest and abdomen | 3–0 or 4–0 | 7 days |
| Back | 3–0 or 4–0 | 10 days |
| Limbs | 4–0 or 5–0 | 10 days |
| Hands | 5–0 or 6–0 | 7 days |
| Feet | 4–0 or 5–0 | 10 days |

alignment must be achieved. A guide to suture size and length of time sutures should remain in place is given in Table 35-1.

II. **Foreign bodies.** Foreign body penetration of the skin or soft tissues is frequent in small children who have been playing or crawling on the floor. Treatment depends on the time elapsed since penetration, the type of foreign body involved, and the site. X rays will show glass, wood splinters, plastic, and metals—two perpendicular views are necessary for accurate localization. Placement of radiopaque markers such as paper clips over the area may be helpful. Transillumination of the site may be useful in the very young child.

A. **Management.** Removal is indicated for all foreign bodies made of wood and for objects embedded in the hand or foot because they may migrate. Steel or glass fragments that are deeply embedded in soft tissue and are asymptomatic can be left in place and explored at a later date if symptoms arise. Visible or palpable foreign bodies may be removed under local anesthesia in a cooperative child. In all other cases, removal should be done with fluoroscopy under sedation or general anesthesia. Removal of the visible or palpable object is accomplished by infiltrating the area with 1% plain lidocaine around the most superficial portion of the foreign body and incising along the length of the object with a No. 11 scalpel blade. Pull the object free with a small mosquito clamp, explore the wound with a gloved finger, irrigate, and close. To remove a barbed fishhook, infiltrate the area with 1% plain lidocaine, then push the barb through the skin and cut it off with a pair of wire cutters. This will enable the hook to be removed through the entrance wound.

III. **Hair tourniquet of fingers or toes.** In infants, irritability accompanied by edema of the fingers or toes may be the result of a loose hair that encircles the base of the digit, causing strangulation. There is usually a deep circular groove at the base, but the hair may be difficult to see. Use cool compresses to decrease swelling, then gently wash in warm water. If the hair does not come free, it must be carefully cut. Following removal, observe the child until the swelling has resolved.

**IV. Disposition.** Admit children with infected wounds and those who require repair under general anesthesia.

**V. Key points**

    **A.** Explaining procedures to the child will decrease anxiety and increase cooperation.

    **B.** Wounds more than 24 hours old, human bites, barnyard injuries, and areas of poor vascular supply should have delayed closure.

    **C.** Most foreign bodies should be removed with fluoroscopy under general anesthesia.

    **D.** Do not use epinephrine-containing local anesthetics in areas of potential vascular compromise.

**Bibliography**

Anderson, A. B., et al. Optimal local anesthesia in pediatric patients: Topical TAC versus lidocaine. *Pediatr. Emerg. Care* 3:283, 1987.

Fleisher, G., and Ludwig, S. (eds.). *Textbook of Pediatric Emergency Medicine*. Baltimore: Williams and Wilkins, 1984.

# Hand Injury and Infection

Leslie A. Scott and Gregory A. Baldwin

## I. Hand injury

**A. Diagnosis and assessment.** Determine capillary filling and the color of all digits prior to sensory or motor examination. If there is suspicion of a vascular injury, urgent surgical assessment is required. In flexion, all fingers should point toward the anatomic "snuffbox" if not there may be a rotational deformity.

### 1. Sensory examination

**a. Older child.** Test pinprick or two-point discrimination in all digits using a paper clip. The normal range is 3–5 mm. Compare radial and ulnar sides; any difference suggests digital nerve injury. Sensation supplied by the ulnar nerve can be tested in the little finger, and the median nerve can be tested in the index, long finger, and palmar thumb. The radial nerve can be assessed on the dorsum of the thumb.

**b. Younger child.** Avoid pinprick sensory testing in children in this age group because it frightens the child and makes further examination impossible. Absence of normal sweat beading indicates nerve injury. This may be visible under tangential light, or it may be felt by lightly stroking the digits. Alternatively, the hand may be soaked in warm water for 10 minutes—normal skin wrinkles whereas denervated skin remains smooth.

### 2. Motor examination

**a. Older child.** Test flexion, extension, and abduction of the thumb. Opposition of the thumb may be tested by asking the child to form a ring with the thumb and each finger and then attempting to break the ring. Spreading of the fingers tests the intrinsic muscles. Flexion of finger joints should be tested as follows: (1) **Profundus.** The DIP joint is flexed while the PIP is held in extension. (2) **Superficialis.** The PIP joint is flexed while all the other fingers are held in extension. Extensor tendon injuries usually present with a flexion deformity when the child is asked to hold all fingers in full extension.

**b. Younger child.** In the younger child, observe the hand in the resting position. Asymmetry may be due to tendon or motor nerve injury. If there is pain, local anesthesia may allow active movement of the hand and digits, facilitating an examination to determine if there are deficits in flexion or extension.

**B. Principles in management of hand injuries**

1. All significant hand injuries should be referred to a hand surgeon for evaluation.

2. Do not clamp bleeding areas. Elevate and apply pressure until the surgeon arrives.

3. In any laceration of the hand or wrist, a thorough assessment of function must be performed prior to infiltration with local anesthetic.

4. All injuries other than superficial lacerations should be radiographed to look for fractures or foreign bodies. If there is confusion regarding epiphyses, use a radiologic text or films of the opposite hand for comparison.

C. **Specific injuries**

1. **Fingertip injuries (incomplete amputation).** These injuries occur frequently. Fortunately, even in severe injuries, amputation is rarely complete. If there is moderate crushing and only a bridge of skin is intact, the tip will usually survive. Gently clean and place a minimal number of sutures to fix the tip in place. Immobilize the finger with a soft splint and bulky dressing, and arrange for follow-up examination in 48 hours' time.

2. **Complete amputation.** Revascularization should be attempted when amputation occurs at or proximal to the distal phalanx. The amputated portion is washed and wrapped in gauze soaked with Ringer's lactate and sealed in a plastic bag, which is placed on ice. If amputation occurs at or beyond the distal phalanx in a child, revascularization is unnecessary. Refer all cases to a hand surgeon for treatment.

3. **Fingernail injury.** Partial nail plate avulsion is treated with excision of the detached portion and reinsertion of the root after a V is cut out to allow drainage. Look for laceration of the nail matrix—this must be repaired with a fine (6–0 or 7–0) absorbable suture to avoid deformity. If the nail can be replaced, it will splint the healing matrix. In all cases, obtain x rays to check for epiphyseal fracture.

4. **Fractures and dislocations**

   a. Metacarpal fractures, and in particular, fifth metacarpal fractures, may require closed reduction if rotation or angulation is suspected. Undisplaced fractures without deformity can be treated with a splint.

   b. Phalangeal injuries

      (1) **Fractures** involving the middle or distal phalanx should be immobilized with a splint and taping to the next finger. In proximal fractures, the splint should extend over the wrist to hold it in 30 degrees of extension, with the metacarpophalangeal (MCP) joint flexed to 90 degrees and the interphalangeal (IP) joint kept at 0 degrees. Intraarticular fractures, compound fractures, and any rotational or angular deformities requires surgical management.

      (2) Most **dislocations** follow hyperextension or a blow to the fingertip. The finger is deformed and cannot be flexed. DIP dislocation should be reduced by hyperextension and

then returning the joint into position without using excessive force. After reduction, examine it for ligament laxity and obtain an x ray to rule out fracture; if none is present, buddy-tape and splint the digit for 10–14 days. All other fractures and dislocations should be referred to a surgeon. For management of suspected scaphoid or carpal injury, see Chap. 38.

(3) **Skier's thumb (gamekeeper's thumb)** follows a hyperextension injury of the MCP joint, classically occurring in the child who falls while holding a ski pole strap. Tenderness and swelling are present over the ulnar side of the first MCP joint, which is lax when stressed in a radial direction. Check an x ray to rule out fracture. Treatment is accomplished by thumb spica cast or, if laxity is severe, surgical repair.

(4) **Mallet finger** follows sudden forced flexion, typically after the tip is struck by a ball. This results in an avulsion of the extensor tendon where it inserts at the base of the distal phalanx—a Salter 1 or Salter 2 injury. In adolescents there may be an associated avulsion fracture, resulting in a Salter 3 injury. The child with a mallet finger is unable to actively extend the DIP joint. If the fragment of avulsed bone is large and involves more than one-fourth of the joint surface, open repair is required. If the fragment is small or if there is no associated fracture, treatment consists in splinting in hyperextension and referring the patient to a hand or orthopedic surgeon for follow-up.

5. **Subungual hematomas** occur after direct trauma to the nail. Drainage of the hematoma results in immediate relief of pain and is best achieved by using a hot metal wire or paper clip to perforate the nail. Alternatively, a 23- or 25-gauge needle can be used, applying pressure with a to-and-fro rotating motion until the nail is punctured.

## II. Hand infection

A. **Paronychia.** This is an infection of the skin surrounding the fingernail. The area is red and exquisitely tender. If no pus is seen under the nail, achieve drainage by elevating the skin edge over the nail with a No. 15 scalpel blade (Fig. 36-1). This procedure should be followed with daily saline soaks for a week. If pus is visible under the nail, the lateral part of the nail must be excised under digital block.

B. **Felon.** A felon is a pulp space abscess under the fingertip. Do not confuse it with whitlow, a herpetic infection characterized by a painful vesicobullous eruption, erythema, and swelling. A felon can cause necrosis of the overlying skin. Under digital nerve block, drain the le-

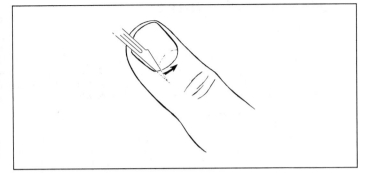

**Fig. 36-1. Treatment of paronychia. Method of elevation of skin over nail.**

sion by incising it along the skin lines over the area of necrosis or maximal tenderness.

**C. Subcutaneous abscess.** This abscess arises on the lateral surface of the finger following penetrating injury of the volar aspect. Drain it by incising directly over the fluctuant area, avoiding the neurovascular bundle.

**D. Tenosynovitis.** This is an acute infection inside the tendon sheath, usually secondary to a penetrating injury. The finger is swollen and held in slight flexion. There is tenderness along the length of the tendon with severe pain on extension. Consult a hand surgeon for admission and give intravenous cloxacillin or oxacillin, 150 mg/kg/day divided q6h, or another suitable antistaphylococcal medication. Exploration is indicated if there is no improvement in 8–12 hours.

**III. Disposition.** Admit children with tenosynovitis, vascular compromise, amputation, and fracture/dislocations requiring repair under general anesthesia.

**IV. Key points**

**A.** Perform a sensory and motor examination before giving local anesthetic in hand injuries.

**B.** Do not blindly clamp bleeding areas in the hand.

**Bibliography**

Markison, R. E., and Kilgore, E. Hand. In J. H. Davis (ed.), *Clinical Surgery*. St. Louis: C. V. Mosby, 1987. Pp. 2293–2353.

Zacher, J. B. Management of injuries of the distal phalanx. *Surg. Clin. North Am.* 64:747, 1984.

# Maxillofacial Injury

Gerald Wittenberg and Karen Wardill

Maxillofacial injuries usually follow motor vehicle accidents or falls. Mandibular trauma is common and often involves the subcondylar region. Lacerations of the chin, lips, and intraoral mucosal tears are commonly associated.

## I. Diagnosis and assessment
### A. Initial assessment
1. **Extraoral.** Inspect the face for areas of swelling, bruising, and asymmetry by observing it from the front, side, and above the head. Lacerations may be associated with underlying bony fracture. Subconjunctival ecchymosis may indicate a lateral orbital rim fracture (zygoma). Palpate the facial bones in a systematic fashion from top to bottom, comparing the sides for asymmetry. Use the index finger to circle over the orbital rims, feeling for a step-off as evidence of a fracture (particularly laterally and inferiorly). Use the index finger and thumb to palpate the nasal bones for irregularities. Press the area lateral to the nose to evaluate the anterior maxillary wall and continue across the zygomatic arch to detect any depressions or dimpling as evidence of disruption of the zygomaticotemporal suture. Now palpate the temporomandibular joints and ask the child to open, close, and "wiggle" the jaw. Pain and reduced palpability of the condyle indicate a possible subcondylar bone fracture. Deviation of the jaw toward one side can indicate unilateral muscle spasm or fracture. Palpate along the jaw line for steps or deformity.

2. **Intraoral.** Examine the inside of the mouth for lacerations, loosened or lost teeth, and bony fracture. Missing teeth with blood-filled sockets must be accounted for to determine whether they are embedded in the lips, aspirated, lost, or if fractured roots remain in the bone. Dental x rays are required. Displacement of teeth and their supporting bone is called an alveolar fracture and is usually local to a few teeth. Grasp the maxilla above the teeth with the index finger and thumb while stabilizing the head and attempt to move the maxilla. Palpate above the teeth to the back of the mouth to detect fracture of the base of the zygoma (above the first molar). Inspect the floor of the mouth for ecchymosis, which is indicative of mandibular fracture. Place one thumb on top of the molars with the index and middle fingers under the mandible and place the other hand in a similar position further forward; torque the hands in opposite directions to detect mandibular body fracture. Repeat on the other side. Subcondylar fractures result in limited opening of the jaw,

a bite that is "off," and tenderness over the preauricular area. X rays are confirmatory.

**B. Associated injuries.** Perform a complete eye examination. Enophthalmos, limited extraocular movement, and asymmetry of the eye level suggest a blowout fracture (see Chap. 15). Subconjunctival ecchymosis without a lateral limit indicates zygomatic fracture. Rule out cervical spine, head, dental, nasal, and ear injury in all cases (see appropriate chapters). Look for clear discharge from the nose or ears as evidence of cerebrospinal fluid (CSF) leakage and basal skull fracture, and test the function of the fifth cranial nerve (sensory division) and the seventh (motor) cranial nerve.

**C. X rays.** The following three x rays are usually sufficient for evaluation of facial bone fractures.

1. Waters' view—provides a good view of the orbital rims and the maxillary sinuses.
2. Posteroanterior (PA) view of the face and mandible.
3. Lateral view—when taken with the PA view will demonstrate the integrity of the mandible, sinuses, and nasal bones.
4. If a mandibular fracture is suspected, the following supplemental views may be ordered:
   a. A Townes' view shows the ascending rami and condyles.
   b. Other views include a PA view, a submentovertex view, and bilateral oblique views.
   c. If available, a panoramic view is useful.

## II. Initial management

**A.** The first priority is airway maintenance. Suctioning may be necessary to remove vomitus, blood, secretions, or foreign bodies. If the tongue is obstructing the airway and mandibular fracture prevents successful positioning or intubation, place a towel clip through the tongue and pull it forward. Rarely, tracheostomy is required.

**B.** Support the cervical spine with sandbags or a collar in children with facial fracture (other than isolated nasal fracture) or neurologic impairment until x rays have excluded injury.

**C.** Rule out associated trauma to the head, larynx, thorax, and abdomen (see Chaps. 32, 33, and 41).

**D.** In all cases, determine tetanus immunization status and treat those at risk.

## III. Specific injuries

**A. Soft tissue injury.** Severe or cosmetically disfiguring lacerations should be referred to a plastic surgeon. Consult with a surgeon prior to suturing lacerations when there is an underlying fracture. Wounds lateral to the eye and inferior to a line drawn from the tragus to the nasal tip can result in injury to the facial nerve, parotid gland, and duct. The presence of saliva in this type of wound suggests disruption of the parotid gland or duct. Lacerations through the vermilion border of the lip require careful reconstruction. Mark the border with a colored pen prior to injection of local anesthetic to aid in accurate alignment. The first suture is placed at the mucosa/skin junction. Close wounds involving the mouth and skin from "inside to outside." Mucosal lacerations more than 1 cm in length should be sutured. If debris (e.g., gravel) cannot be completely removed, leave the oral wound to heal by secondary intention. Lacerations of the eyebrows or hairline must be carefully approximated—never shave the eyebrows. Evert the edges when suturing wounds of the nasal alae to avoid notch deformity due to scar contracture. Chin lacerations also require a careful and everted skin closure.

**B. Facial bone fractures**

    **1. Nasal fractures.** See Chap. 14.

    **2. Mandibular fractures.** The most frequent mandibular fracture in children is a **subcondylar fracture,** which often results from a fall onto the chin. There is an open bite deformity with minimal displacement of the mandible and tongue. The most common signs are malocclusion and limited opening. On examination there is pain on palpation or torqueing of the mandible (see sec. **I.A.2,** above). In a **mandibular body fracture** there may be gingival mucosal tears or anesthesia of the teeth and lower lip— the latter manifestation is a sign of entrapment of the inferior alveolar nerve. A hematoma may be visible on the floor of the mouth. A malocclusion may be evident and the normal curvature of the dental arch may be distorted.

        **a. Management**

            **(1)** Treatment of a subcondylar fracture is usually conservative, consisting of immobilization and a liquid diet. Displaced subcondylar fractures should be carefully monitored for growth disturbance.

            **(2)** Children with displaced compound mandibular fractures (skin or intraoral gingival tears) should be treated with prophylactic antibiotics—penicillin is the drug of choice. Refer the patient to an oral and maxillofacial surgeon for splinting. It is very important that the surgeon be familiar with bite assessment. Mandibular fractures without mucosal tears or with minimal displacement may not need surgical therapy. The presence of unerupted or erupted teeth in the line of fracture requires assessment by a dentist for treatment and follow-up.

    **3. Midface fractures**

        **a. Maxilla proper** (including LeFort fractures). Symptoms of maxillary fracture include malocclusion (most common), numbness of the upper lip and gums, pain, and swelling. Elongation of the face is the most consistent sign. There are often coexisting significant eye injury, nasal obstruction, and a "floating maxilla." X rays often reveal opacification or air–fluid levels in the maxillary sinuses (not well seen in children under 4 years of age), and fractures often follow predictable patterns. LeFort fractures of the maxilla can occur alone or in combination and are classified as follows:

LeFort I   —A transverse fracture that separates the hard palate from the rest of the maxilla. It runs above the roots of the teeth.

LeFort II —A pyramidal fracture that separates the nose, midmaxilla, and palate (one large fragment).

LeFort III—A fracture that separates the zygomas, nose, and entire maxilla from the rest of the skull. CSF leaks can occur.

  (1) **Management.** Ensure an adequate and stable airway; start broad-spectrum prophylactic antibiotics and refer to a surgeon for reduction and fixation. Ophthalmologic evaluation is necessary with LeFort III fractures.

 b. **Zygomatic bone**—"tripod fracture." A tripod fracture is commonly seen after a motor vehicle accident and may occur in conjunction with a maxillary fracture. Characteristically, it has three detectable fracture lines—the frontozygomatic suture line, the zygomatic arch, and the orbital rim. Intraoral bony disruption at the area above the first molar is frequent. Displacement can occur at any of three sites. There may be swelling over the malar eminence with flattening; this sign is often obscured initially. A depression of the inferior orbital rim may be felt, and there may be eye injury and limitation of eye motion in an upward gaze. Anesthesia over the cheek in the distribution of the infraorbital nerve can occur. Limited mandibular opening due to blockage of the coronoid process of the mandible can occur. Referral to a surgeon is indicated.

 c. **Blowout fracture of the orbit.** See Chap. 15.

 d. Other fractures include alveolar bone fractures, frontal bone fractures, and nasofrontal fractures.

**IV. Disposition.** Children with severe facial fractures and patients with abnormal neurologic signs following facial injury require admission. Consultation with an ophthalmologist is required for fractures involving the orbital floor or when there is eye muscle entrapment. Consultation with an oral and maxillofacial surgeon is necessary when there is malocclusion or a subcondylar fracture.

**V. Key points**

 A. Rule out airway obstruction and cervical spine injury in all children with significant facial trauma.

 B. Subcondylar fracture is the most common mandibular

injury in children. It can lead to facial bone growth disturbances.

**C.** Malocclusion is the most consistent sign of maxillary fracture.

## Bibliography

Suen, J. Y., and Wetmore, S. J. *Emergencies in Otolaryngology.* New York: Churchill–Livingstone, 1986.

Fleischer, G., and Ludwig, S. *Textbook of Pediatric Emergency Medicine.* Baltimore: Williams & Wilkins, 1983.

# Musculoskeletal Injury

Richard D. Beauchamp

Musculoskeletal injuries account for up to 15% of disorders in children presenting to the emergency department. The unique features of the musculoskeletal system of the child must be kept in mind when assessing orthopedic injuries: (1) Children with open growth plates who injure the physis or epiphyseal plate may develop growth disturbances; (2) a tough, elastic periosteum tends to maintain the alignment of fractured bones; (3) in general, predictable patterns of fracture occur in each age group; (4) in the prepubertal child, ligamentous injuries rarely occur without epiphyseal plate injury. Suspect epiphyseal injury in any prepubertal child with a "sprain."

I. **Classification of fractures.** Injuries involving growth plates are classified into five groups according to Salter and Harris. In general, the risk of growth disturbance varies with the type of injury, ranging from minimal with type 1 to highest with type 5 (Fig. 38-1).

Type 1. These injuries occur through the zone of provisional calcification—the weakest area of the epiphyseal plate. A common example is distal fibular physeal injury, which mimics ankle sprain. Treatment is symptomatic unless there is displacement, in which case closed reduction may be required.

Type 2. This type of injury comprises the majority of epiphyseal plate injuries requiring treatment. Common sites are the distal radius and the tibia. The periosteal hinge is intact, facilitating closed reduction.

Type 3. This injury is an intraarticular fracture that needs anatomic reduction. Displaced fractures may require open reduction and internal fixation.

Type 4. This injury is a combination of an intraarticular and a transphyseal injury that frequently requires open reduction and internal fixation.

Type 5. This compressive injury damages the zone of resting cells. Growth disturbance is a frequent complication. These injuries are difficult to diagnose on initial radiographs: Maintain a high index of suspicion in children who have been subjected to a compressive force on bone (as in falls or motor vehicle accidents).

II. **Complicated injury**

A. **Compound fracture.** Any open wound in the vicinity of a fracture should prompt suspicion of a compound injury—the most benign-appearing open injury may become complicated by secondary infection or gas gangrene. Debridement under general anesthesia should be performed within 6 hours. Give intravenous antibiotics (penicillin and cloxacillin, or cefazolin), splint the fracture, and dress the wound. Administer tetanus booster immunization to those at risk (see Appendix I) and consult an orthopedic surgeon.

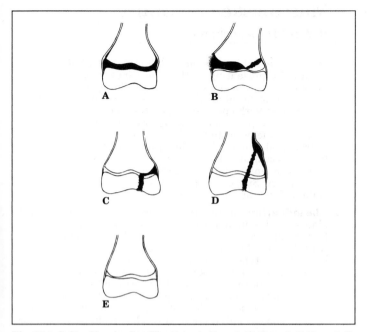

Fig. 38-1. Salter Harris classification. A. Type 1. B. Type 2. C. Type 3. D. Type 4. E. Type 5.

    **B. Compartment syndrome.** Increased intracompartmental pressure can lead to ischemic necrosis and loss of function. Typically, fractures of the tibia produce compartment syndromes in the leg, and displaced supracondylar fractures produce compartment syndromes in the forearm. Neurovascular assessment is the key to clinical diagnosis. The hallmark of this phenomenon is excessive pain in the extremity. Other signs include decreased temperature, capillary refill, or pulses, pallor, or pain on passive movement of the fingers or toes. If suspected, immediately consult a surgeon.

**III. Diagnosis and assessment of musculoskeletal injury**

    **A. History.** Determine the history of the injury, location of the pain, and past history of fractures or bone diseases such as osteogenesis imperfecta, osteopetrosis, or rickets. Young children may present with refusal to use a limb, often with little outward evidence of fracture. In the very young child with fracture of a long bone, and in any child with unusual fractures or a suspicious history of injury, consider the possibility of child abuse.

    **B. Examination.** Assess the neurovascular status (see sec. **II.B** above). Look for evidence of displacement, bony tenderness, crepitus, bruising, or swelling. In the comatose patient, contusions, abrasions, or bony crepitus on palpation may be the only signs of fracture. Look for wounds near the injury as evidence of possible compound fracture. Ligamentous injuries present with swelling around the joint or tenderness over the injured ligament. Following examination, elevate the injured limb and use ice and splints for pain relief.

C. **X rays.** Apply a radiolucent splint (e.g., fiberglass, Thomas splint for the femur) to the injured limb prior to obtaining x rays. X rays should include the joint proximal and the joint distal to the injured area. In all cases, anteroposterior (AP) and lateral films are required. When there is confusion about the epiphyseal plates or growth centers, use a textbook of normal x rays or films of the opposite limb for comparison. Stress x rays may help in diagnosis of ligamentous or Salter I injuries; these should be obtained only after consultation with a surgeon. Elbows and ankles may require oblique x rays for evaluation.

IV. **The principles of management** expressed in the mnemonic RIP should be applied to any fractured bone.

A. **R—Reduction.** Most fractures associated with clinical deformity must be reduced to allow return of function. Fractures associated with neurovascular compromise should be reduced immediately. In young children, general anesthesia is usually required; a cooperative adolescent may be treated after regional anesthesia has been achieved. Fractures close to the growth plate do not always require anatomic reduction. This is particularly true in the young child (who has considerable growth potential) when displacement is minimal (i.e., less than 10 degrees) and is in the line of movement of the adjacent joint.

B. **I—Immobilization.** In most cases, closed fractures require immobilization in a plaster of Paris cast, using three-point pressure. Immobilization must fix the joint above and below the injury, and the cast should be snug and smooth to prevent deformity or slippage. Parents should be told to keep it dry and clean, and elevate it as much as possible during the first 48 hours. Advise them to return immediately to have the cast split if there are signs of neurovascular compromise (pain, paresthesia, pallor, puffiness, pulselessness). Follow-up should be arranged in a minimum of 7 days.

C. **P—Preservation of function.** Following cast removal, mobilization and physiotherapy are necessary for a full return of power, mobility, and function. Follow-up is important to diagnose and treat any growth deformity.

V. **Specific injuries**

A. **Soft tissue**

1. **Sprains.** In the prepubertal child ligaments are stronger than the physis, and sprains are usually associated with type 1 epiphyseal plate injury. Be suspicious of ligamentous disruption in pubertal children with an injury of the knee or ankle. Test joint stability by comparing each joint with that of the

contralateral limb, or by stress x rays (consult with an orthopedic surgeon before performing these). A grade 1 injury (minor, no tear) is stable; a grade 2 injury (incomplete tear) shows increased laxity, and a grade 3 injury (complete tear) is unstable. Grade 1 injuries can be treated with ice, pressure, and elevation. Grade 2 or 3 ligamentous injuries require immobilization and referral to a surgeon for management.

2. **Meniscus injury of the knee.** This type of injury is rare before adolescence. It usually occurs following a twisting motion during weight bearing and is commonly seen in contact sports such as football. There is a joint effusion with tenderness along the joint line over the meniscus, and pain is increased with flexion. In some cases the joint may lock in a flexed position. Obtain x rays of the knee, splint the knee in extension with a long leg (Robert-Jones) bandage, and arrange outpatient follow-up with a surgeon in 24–48 hours.

B. **Cervical spine.** All children with diving injuries, hanging injuries, or significant trauma above the level of the clavicles, and trauma victims who are comatose should be assumed to have cervical spine injury. **Trauma to the spine can produce spinal cord injury with or without a fracture.** Conditions associated with an increased risk of instability of the cervical spine include congenital spinal abnormalities, Down's syndrome, skeletal dysplasias, rheumatoid arthritis, and Marfan's syndrome.

1. **Management**
   a. **Stabilize the spine.** When injury is suspected, fix the spine. Use a semirigid collar or tape the forehead down to the bed, placing sandbags at each side of the head.
   b. **X rays.** A cross-table lateral x ray should be performed, including all of the upper 7 vertebrae. If the lower vertebrae cannot be seen, obtain a swimmer's view (elevate the opposite limb, which is then shot through in a lateral x ray) or have an assistant pull down on the shoulders during the x ray. Assess the intervals between the occiput and C1, and between C1 and C2. On a lateral view, instability is suggested by a gap of more than 3–5 mm between the anterior aspect of the odontoid and the posterior aspect of the C1 arch. Look for soft tissue swelling anterior to C3 or C4—a width of more than 10 mm should arouse suspicion of injury (see Fig. 38-2). Flexion/extension views or CT scan may be required to diagnose "pseudosubluxation" of C3 on C4; these x rays or scans should be ordered only after consulting with a surgeon.
   c. **Examination.** If the x rays are normal and a collar is in place, gently remove it. Without moving the neck, palpate the cervical spine for tender-

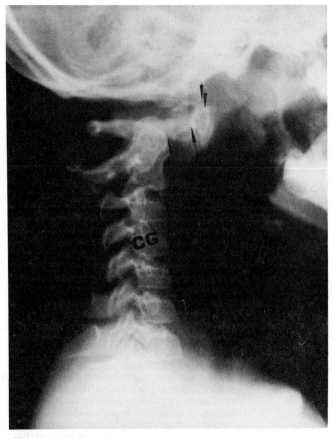

**Fig. 38-2. Cervical spine injury revealing an increased distance between C1 and C2.**

ness. Perform a full neurologic examination, noting power, sensation, and reflexes. Respiratory distress due to paralysis can occur in high cervical spine injury (above C4); intubation and mechanical ventilation may be required (see Chap. 1).

    **d. Management.** In the patient with evidence of significant cervical spine injury, give oxygen, start an intravenous line, obtain blood for complete blood count (CBC) and cross-match, and catheterize the bladder (see Chap. 32). An orthopedic surgeon should be consulted whether or not there is a neurologic deficit.

**C. Thoracolumbar spine.** When thoracolumbar spine injuries are suspected, the child should be splinted by strapping and taping him or her to a fracture board. Examine the spine by carefully log-rolling the child; look for ecchymoses or swelling and palpate for tenderness. Seat-belt or Chance fractures of the lumbar spine occur in children who are involved in motor vehicle accidents while wearing lap belts but no shoulder belts—there may be contusions in the shape of the belt over the anterior abdominal wall. Assume that such injuries are unstable until proved otherwise: Give oxygen, start an intravenous line, obtain blood for cross-match and CBC, and catheterize the bladder. In all cases of suspected injury, consult an orthopedic surgeon.

**D. Pelvis.** Children with high-energy axial skeleton injuries should be assessed for a fractured pelvis, particularly when there is hypovolemia or shock. Pain or crepitus on compression of the anterior or superior iliac spines or the symphysis pubis suggests pelvic fracture. Associated visceral injuries include bladder rupture (signs of peritonitis), urethral disruption (blood at the urethral meatus, boggy anterior mass, or a high-riding prostate on rectal examination in males), and laceration of the bowel by a bony fragment (blood or palpable bony fragment on rectal examination)—see Chaps. 17 and 32. Compound fractures into the vagina are particularly hazardous. Blood loss can be considerable; give oxygen by mask, start two large-bore intravenous lines, and obtain blood for CBC and cross-match. Pelvic fractures require assessment by orthopedic and general surgeons. A urologist or gynecologist should be consulted immediately if urologic or pelvic injury is suspected.

**E. Upper extremities**

**1. Shoulder and humerus**

  **a.** Fractures of the upper humerus are common after direct trauma or a fall. Although there may be significant displacement, very little anatomic reduction is required. Most displacements can be treated with a collar and cuff or a Vietnam Velpeau sling (see Fig. 38-3). Always rule out axillary and radial nerve injury by testing sensation over the deltoid area and the dorsum of the thumb.

  **b.** Proximal epiphyseal injury, usually Salter 2 in type, also occurs after direct trauma or a fall. Minor angulation of less than 40 degrees without rotation can be treated with a collar and cuff or a Vietnam Velpeau sling (Fig. 38-3). Injury with angulation of more than 40 degrees, and rotated or comminuted fractures may require admission to hospital—consult an orthopedic surgeon.

  **c.** Anterior dislocation of the shoulder occurs after direct trauma or a fall onto an externally rotated abducted arm. This type of injury rarely occurs before adolescence. Examination reveals a flattened deltoid muscle, with the arm held in internal rotation and adduction. Abduction and external rotation are limited. In the common anterior dislocation, x rays reveal inferior displacement of

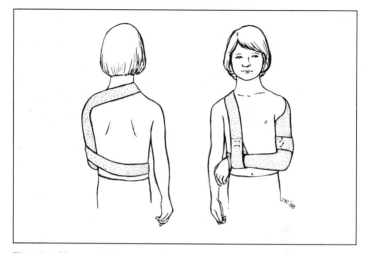

**Fig. 38-3. Vietnam Velpeau sling.**

the humeral head. Always rule out an associated fracture. This injury is managed with closed reduction after intravenous sedation with Demerol and Valium. Reduction may be achieved by having the child lie prone with the shoulder and arm hanging over the edge of the bed, then attaching a weight to the hand of approximately one-tenth body weight. If this maneuver is ineffective, consult an orthopedic surgeon for reduction. After reduction, place the child in a Vietnam Velpeau sling and arrange for a follow-up visit with a surgeon within 1 week.

   **d.** Fracture of the clavicle usually follows a fall onto the shoulder or outstretched arm or a direct compression injury. Patients can be placed in a figure-of-eight bandage and sling for comfort (Fig. 38-4).

   **e.** Acromioclavicular injuries are benign in children and rarely need treatment. Children with complete acromioclavicular joint separation may develop a "bump" that causes cosmetic deformity. Treat with a regular or Velpeau sling (see sec. **V.E.1.d** above).

**2. Elbow.** The elbow is the most common area of major orthopedic trauma in children. X rays may be difficult to interpret, and comparison with films of the contralateral elbow or a radiologic textbook is advised.

   **a. Supracondylar fractures.** These injuries usually follow a fall onto an outstretched hand or, rarely, onto a flexed elbow. Children present with

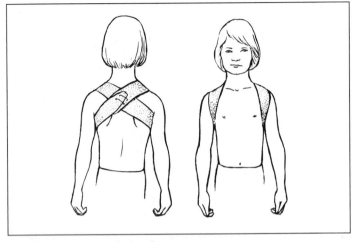

**Fig. 38-4. Figure-of-eight bandage.**

pain on elbow flexion and tenderness of the distal humerus. Assess neurovascular function, splint, and consult a surgeon about reduction and immobilization.

  (1) Displaced fractures present with deformity and gross swelling. There is x-ray evidence of posterior displacement. Neurovascular compromise can occur (see sec. **II.B,** above).

  (2) In undisplaced fractures there is swelling but no deformity; the only radiologic sign may be displacement of the posterior fat pad above the olecranon.

**b. Lateral condylar fractures** are common in children between 4 and 10 years of age. The mechanism of injury is similar to that causing supracondylar fracture. The child presents with tenderness and swelling, which is maximal over the lateral aspect of the elbow. This is a Salter 4 injury, and orthopedic referral for anatomic reduction is required.

**c. Posterior elbow dislocation** may be associated with a small avulsion of the medial epicondyle or coronoid process. Neurovascular compromise can occur, especially median nerve injury, which causes decreased sensation over the index and long fingers. X rays may reveal an associated fracture and posterior fat pad displacement (see sec. **V.E.2.a,** above). Reduction and immobilization under general anesthesia may be required.

**d. "Pulled elbow,"** or "nursemaid's elbow," is often misdiagnosed. Patients are usually infants or toddlers who have been picked up by the arms.

They are unwilling to supinate or pronate the extended elbow. In general, x rays are not required. Obtain x rays if the mode of injury is atypical, if there is tenderness over the distal humerus, or if reduction with symptomatic relief is not easily achieved. Reduce the injury by placing pressure over the radial head with the thumb, fully pronating, supinating, then flexing the elbow—a "click" may be heard or felt when reduction is achieved. When the injury has been present for more than 3–4 hours, reduction can be difficult; if these children are treated with a posterior slab overnight, the pain will resolve, and the range of motion will return to normal in a few days.

3. **Radial head.** Fracture of the radial head follows a fall onto an outstretched hand. Evidence of angulation of more than 30 degrees on either the anteroposterior or lateral x ray requires closed reduction under general anesthesia. Minor displacement is treated with immobilization in a posterior slab for 7–10 days.

4. **Forearm.** These fractures are usually due to a fall on the hand or direct trauma to the forearm.

   a. Single bone fractures are often associated with injury of the proximal or distal radioulnar joints—x rays of adjacent joints are therefore mandatory in forearm injuries. A line drawn proximally through the long axis of the radius should pass through the capitellum in all views; if it does not, there is radial subluxation or dislocation. Angulation of more than 10 degrees or a rotational deformity requires reduction. Other minor injuries (buckle, greenstick fracture) can be treated with a well-molded forearm cast.

      (1) An isolated fracture of the ulna with displacement implies dislocation of the radius proximally (Monteggia fracture-dislocation). Closed reduction under general anesthesia is required.

      (2) Fracture of the radius alone implies displacement of the ulna distally (Galeazzi fracture-dislocation). Closed reduction under general anesthesia is required.

   b. Fractures of both bones usually require reduction and application of a long arm cast under general anesthesia. Adolescents are best treated with open reduction and internal fixation.

5. **Wrist.** Injuries to the wrist are common in children. Many are metaphyseal fractures, and most epiphyseal injuries are Salter 2. If deformity is apparent clinically, closed reduction and application of a long arm cast under general anesthesia are required.

   Carpal injuries are rare in children. Scaphoid fractures often follow a fall onto an outstretched hand; they are uncommon in children under the age of 10. Older children and adolescents with tenderness in the anatomic snuffbox should be assumed to have a fractured scaphoid even if the x ray is normal. Treatment is accomplished by immobilization in a thumb spica cast for 10–14 days, followed by a repeat x ray of the wrist out of the cast.

**F. Lower extremity**

1. **Hip fracture.** A hip fracture is associated with high-velocity trauma. On examination, there is shortening and external rotation of the leg. Open reduction and internal fixation are frequently required.

2. **Femoral shaft fracture.** Femoral shaft fracture usually follows a fall or motor vehicle trauma, typically when a child pedestrian is struck by the bumper of a car. Immobilize the limb with a Thomas splint or external rigid apparatus prior to taking an x ray. Adolescents may require open reduction.

3. **Distal femur/tibial plateau.** These fractures present with effusion and pain following varus or valgus stress or direct trauma to the area. They are frequently Salter 2, but there may be an associated Salter 5 injury resulting in growth disturbance. Refer all cases to an orthopedic surgeon; any displacement requires anatomic reduction.

4. **Patellar dislocation.** Patellar dislocation is common in adolescent girls who present with a frankly dislocated patella and a flexed knee. Simple extension of the knee usually achieves reduction. Following reduction anteroposterior, lateral, tunnel, and skyline x rays should be obtained to rule out osteochondral fracture; this requires orthopedic assessment to determine the need for possible internal fixation. Simple patellar dislocations require immobilization in a cylinder cast for 6 weeks followed by physiotherapy.

5. **Swelling of the knee.** Swelling of the knee is common after injury. Always order x rays to rule out bony injury.

   a. In any child with swelling of the knee and fever, all causes of monoarthritis must be considered, including septic arthritis (see Chap. 24, Acute Arthritis).

   b. Serous effusion is usually caused by trauma to the synovium or a strain of the ligaments or capsule. It forms slowly over 24 hours or more and usually does not become tense. Treat with elevation and immobilization in a Robert-Jones bandage (long leg bandage in full extension) or extension splint and provide outpatient orthopedic referral.

   c. Hemarthrosis tends to form during a period of a few hours after injury and is often tense and painful. All cases of significant hemarthrosis should be evaluated by a surgeon. In the **adolescent,** hemarthrosis is often associated with dislocation of the patella. In addition, be suspicious of possible anterior cruciate ligament rupture with joint instability (positive anterior drawer sign). This commonly occurs after lateral trauma to the knee in sports such as football. Jumping injuries can cause avulsion of the tibial spine and anterior cruciate instability. Treatment of significant hemarthrosis is accomplished by needle aspiration (see Chap. 24, Acute Arthritis) and immobilization in a Robert-Jones bandage, extension splint, or cylinder cast. Patients with unstable injuries (grade 3) should be referred for outpatient orthopedic assessment (see sec. **V.A** above).

6. **Fracture of the tibia.** A frequent injury in children is a rotational spiral fracture of the tibia with an intact fibula. These children present with a rotated foot, usually externally rotated. When the rotation is clinically apparent, treatment consists of closed reduction and immobilization in a long leg cast.

7. **Valgus injuries, fractured proximal tibia.** This injury is most commonly seen in children aged 2–6 years. The medial cortex of the metaphysis is disrupted by an almost undisplaced fracture, but the fibula is intact. Marked growth disturbance and valgus deformity may result. The injury is managed by anatomic reduction under general anesthesia and immobilization in a long leg cast with the knee extended.

8. **Ankle injury**
   a. Fracture. Epiphyseal plate injuries are frequent in the growing ankle. **Tillaux** fractures occur in adolescents and involve the distal growth plate with avulsion of the lateral aspect of the tibia; they are Salter 3 injuries that require open reduction and internal fixation. **Bimalleolar** fractures are common and may require open reduction. **Posterior Salter 2** injuries of the distal tibia may be diagnosed by lateral x ray; when the tibia is minimally displaced, treatment is achieved by immobilization in a long leg cast with the foot in dorsiflexion.
   b. Sprain. Assume the presence of an associated Salter 1 epiphyseal injury in the prepubertal child with a sprain. Perform an x ray to rule out bony injury. Minor sprains without laxity (grade 1) can be treated with ice, elevation, and a tensor bandage for pressure. Unstable sprains (grade 2 or 3) require referral to an orthopedic surgeon for immobilization or repair.

9. **Foot injury.** Fractures of the metatarsals (particularly the fifth metatarsal) are common. Treatment is symptomatic; a below knee cast may be required for pain relief. A Lisfranc fracture-dislocation should be suspected when there is significant soft tissue swelling over the second metatarsal; open reduction may be required.

VI. **Disposition.** All significant injuries should be referred to an orthopedic surgeon for management. Exceptions to this rule include minor sprains, some undisplaced buckle fractures, pulled elbow, acromioclavicular joint injury, uncomplicated fracture of the clavicle, minor soft tissue injury of the knee, and uncomplicated fractures of the metatarsals; follow-up should be arranged in all cases. Admission is required for fractures associated with multiple trauma, compound fractures, all injuries of the femur, pelvis, or spine, fractures with neurovascular compromise, and those requiring reduction under general anesthesia.

**VII. Key points**

    **A.** Assess neurovascular function in all cases. Beware of compartment syndrome in injuries of the elbow, forearm, or tibia.

    **B.** Follow the pneumonic RIP for the management of musculoskeletal injury. Order a minimum of two views of each fracture and include the joint above and below the injury.

    **C.** Assume the presence of epiphyseal injury in prepubertal children with ankle sprains.

    **D.** In children with significant head trauma, stabilize the cervical spine until injury can be ruled out.

**Bibliography**

Houghton, G. R., and Thompson, G. H. *Problematic Musculoskeletal Injuries in Children*. London: Butterworth, 1983.

Ogden, J. A. *Skeletal Injury in the Child*. Philadelphia: Lea & Febiger, 1982.

Rangm, M. *Children's Fractures* (2nd ed.). Philadelphia: J. B. Lippincott, 1983.

Salter, R. B. *Textbook of Disorders and Injuries of the Musculoskeletal System* (2nd ed.). Baltimore: Williams & Wilkins, 1983.

Salter, R. B., and Harris, W. R. Injuries involving the epiphyseal plate. *J. Bone Joint Surg.* 45A:587, 1963.

# Child Abuse

Jean Hlady

About 1 million children are abused or neglected each year in the United States, and about 2 thousand die from non-accidental injury. Child abuse is more likely to occur in the younger child—40% of victims are under 5 years of age. It is more common than appendicitis, and the mortality is many times higher.

I. **Physical abuse.** Physical abuse accounts for 60–65% of reported cases. The abused child is a victim of his family; an appreciation of the family situation is important for prompt diagnosis and treatment.

  A. **The situation**

    1. **The parent.** Abusive parents are often poorly prepared for child rearing. They have unrealistic expectations of the child, are frequently impulsive, and tend to use corporal punishment. Many were abused themselves as children and have poor role models. These parents usually have little social support and often misuse drugs and alcohol.

    2. **The child.** One child is often singled out in a family. Frequently, these children have had a difficult neonatal period, are handicapped, or are developmentally delayed.

    3. **The trigger.** A specific event often triggers the abuse. This may be the loss of a job, an illness, or a death in the family. Crowded housing also plays a role. No social class is immune.

  B. **Diagnosis and assessment**

    1. **History.** A detailed history must be taken from all persons involved. Quote all statements verbatim, indicating who told you what. Note the time that events occurred if possible. Suspicious findings include:

      a. Any discrepancy between the history and the physical findings.

      b. Different stories given by different people.

      c. Delay in seeking medical help.

      d. Child brought to the hospital by a parent who was not present when the trauma occurred.

      e. Repeated accidents involving the same child.

      f. Drowning or other injury in a child under 1 year of age.

    2. **Examination.** Perform a complete physical examination. Look for signs of deprivation or neglect, such as poor growth or poor hygiene. Observe the child's behavior during the examination. Excessively anxious or clinging behavior may be a clue. Proper recording is essential because the chart may be subpoenaed.

      a. **Bruises and welts.** Clearly document all injuries with drawings. Measure and date all bruises. **Accidental** bruises occur over the bony prominences—the lower legs, forearms, forehead, and chin. These bruises tend to be peripheral. **Inflicted** bruises occur on the sides of the face, behind the ears, and on the upper lip and frenulum. Elsewhere, they are seen on the buttocks and lower back, on the upper arms and legs, and on the scalp and genitalia. They are often central in distribution. Bruises in different stages of healing, linear bruises, and bruises made by belt buckles, ropes, or hand prints are particularly suggestive of child abuse. Traction alopecia may be caused by hair pulling.

b. **Burns.** Burns account for about 5% of cases of physical abuse in children. Burns should arouse suspicion if they have a circumferential pattern, or if there is an absence of splash marks. Be suspicious of burns that spare the skin folds; children who are held in hot water with their hips flexed (this often occurs during toilet training) will have buttock burns, but the skin folds will be spared. Burns may reveal the shape of the instrument used to inflict injury, such as a cigarette or curling iron. Cigarette burns are not caused by accidentally walking into a burning cigarette; it is instinctive to pull away unless force is used to hold the child there.

c. **Skeletal injuries.** Look for old and new fractures. Suspicious fractures include chip fractures of the metaphysis, spiral fractures due to twisting of the limb, epiphyseal separations, and unusual fracture sites such as ribs, vertebrae, or metacarpal bones. Radiologic evidence of subperiosteal shearing and elevation, fractures of long bones in children under the age of 3, and old fractures that have not been treated should also arouse suspicion of nonaccidental injury.

d. **Brain injury and the whiplash shaken infant syndrome.** This type of injury is the primary cause of death in most fatal cases of physical abuse. Injury to the brain can result from direct trauma such as directly inflicted subdural hemorrhage or indirect trauma due to shaking. The **whiplash shaken infant syndrome** (WSIS) should be suspected in any young infant with an unexplained decrease in level of consciousness. It is most common in infants under 2 months of age, in males, and in expremature infants. Rotational shaking leads to shearing forces on the cerebral vessels, causing scattered subdural hemorrhages. Retinal hemorrhages, dislocated lenses, and bloody CSF from an atraumatic lumbar puncture make the diagnosis a near certainty. There is usually no external sign of injury in WSIS. The **tin ear syndrome** consists of ipsilateral subdural hemorrhages and should be suspected in any child with coma and bruising of the pinna.

  e. **Abdominal and gastrointestinal injury.** Internal abdominal injuries are the second most common cause of death due to child abuse. Abdominal distention may indicate rupture of the liver or spleen or traumatic pancreatitis. Check the urine for blood if this is indicated. Renal contusions often result from direct flank trauma. Check the mouth for frenulum injury, which may result from forced feeding. See Chap. 34.

C. **Documenting evidence.** After the history and physical examination, evidence must be documented for legal purposes.

  1. **Blood.** Order a complete blood count with differential and platelet counts, a prothrombin time (PT), and a partial thromboplastin time (PTT). These results will prove that the bruised child does not suffer from a blood dyscrasia and are crucial in court.

  2. **Photographs.** Pictures are better than any description. Bruises are often more vivid at 24 hours of age.

  3. **X rays.** Consider a skeletal survey in infants and young children when there is a strong suspicion of physical abuse.

D. **Intervention.** Following treatment of the injury, the physician must act to protect the child. In doing so, a firm but nonjudgmental attitude should be maintained. Notification of local social service and law enforcement agencies is essential. If the child is brought to the hospital by the alleged abuser, it may be necessary to hospitalize the child to remove him from the abusive environment. If intervention is not carried out, the child has a 5–10% chance of returning dead the next time.

II. **Neglect.** Neglect is not so obvious as abuse. Accordingly, it is more difficult to recognize. Situations that should arouse suspicion include failure to thrive, developmental delay (if there is no obvious medical explanation), poor hygiene, and delayed immunizations.

III. **Sexual abuse.** Child sexual abuse is the involvement of developmentally immature children and adolescents in sexual activities that they do not fully comprehend and to which they cannot give informed consent. Sexual abuse is the most frequent form of abuse; an estimated one in four females and one in ten males have been sexually abused by the age of 18. Virtually all of the offenders are males, and the majority are acquaintances of the child or family members. Eighty-five percent of victims are female.

A. **The situation**

  1. **The offender.** The sexual abuse offender is rarely criminal or psychotic. He often has poor family relationships and low self-esteem, is sexually insecure, and engages in sexual activities with children to gain a feeling of power and control. One-third have been molested as children.

  2. **The mother.** The child's mother is often passive and

dependent and is unable to protect the child. She may be aware of the problem but is afraid to say anything for fear of disrupting the family.

**3. The child.** Outwardly the model child, the victim is often angry and afraid and feels trapped. In many cases the abuse continues for years.

**B. Diagnosis and assessment.** In the first place, think of the diagnosis; overcome the tendency to disbelieve.

1. **Medical indicators** of sexual abuse include recurrent vulvovaginitis and vaginal discharge, sexually transmitted disease in a prepubertal child, perineal bleeding or trauma, and pregnancy. Recurrent somatic symptoms, such as abdominal pain without a medical cause, may reflect the psychologic upheaval often present in the sexually abused child.

2. **Behavioral indicators** depend on the child's age. Examples of such signs are conversion reaction, overly mature or seductive behavior, use of sexual terminology inappropriate for age, regressive behavior, secondary enuresis or encopresis, sleeping and eating disorders, poor school performance, running away from home, and promiscuity.

3. **History.** Interview the parent, alone if possible, before dealing with the child. A minimum number of people should be present. Do not ask leading questions and quote the parent verbatim in your history.

   Determine exactly what happened and when it happened. Interview the child using simple terms that he or she can understand. If you ask the question, you will often get the answer; children rarely lie about this issue. Anatomically correct dolls may be used to reenact the event. It is important to determine if ejaculation occurred and whether the child had a bath afterward. Children may retract their statements, so record what they say carefully; they may tell their story only once.

   Other relevant data in the history include the presence of dysuria, pain on defecation, constipation, vaginal or anal bleeding, previous trauma to the perineal area, and a menstrual history.

   Record the child's emotional state. The child must be assured that the story is believed and that he or she will not be punished.

4. **Physical examination.** Positive findings are found in 35–75% of cases. In the general examination record the height, weight, general development, and any evidence of neglect or physical trauma. Note the appearance of the clothing and any staining by secretions or blood. Before beginning a genital examination, explain to the child what you are about to do and that it is not painful. Examine a young child in the mother's lap and use the frog-leg or knee-chest position. Penetration injuries to the vagina tend to occur below an imaginary line that runs from the 3 to the 9 o'clock positions (Fig. 39-1). Most injuries are external. Masturbation does not cause genital in-

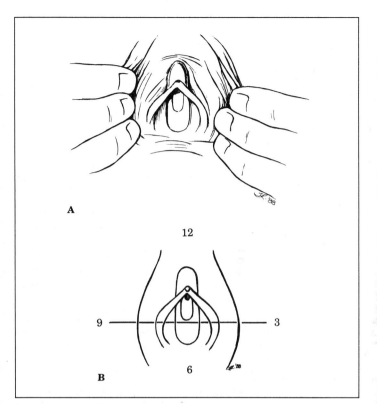

**Fig. 39-1. A. Separation technique for genital examination. B. Vaginal penetrating injuries tend to occur below the line running from the 3 o'clock to the 9 o'clock positions.**

juries (see Chap. 18 for examination technique). A knowledge of the normal anatomy is essential. There are several types of hymens such as crescentic, septate, and cribriform. A rough guide to hymenal size is given in Table 39-1.

5. **Physical evidence of abuse**
   a. **Genital fondling.** Genital fondling is more common in the younger child. There is often no physical evidence of this type of abuse. Acute signs include redness, bruising, edema, and hymenal abrasions. Chronic signs include hymenal rounding and scarring and vulval hypopigmentation or hyperpigmentation.
   b. **Vaginal sexual abuse.** Acute signs include redness, abrasions of the hymen, hymenal transection, and pubococcygeal spasm. Chronic signs include healed hymenal transections, rounded hymenal remnants, a spacious introitus, and pubococcygeal laxity.

**Table 39-1. Hymen size in children**

| Age | Hymenal size (cm) |
| --- | --- |
| Birth | 0.4 |
| 2 mo–7 yr | 0.5 |
| 7–10 yr | 0.7 |
| 10 yr | 1.0 |

      c. **Anal assault.** For acute signs of anal assault, see Chap. 40. Chronic signs of anal assault are laxity, anal tags, healed fissures, and thickened, pigmented skin.

   6. **Collection of specimens.** All samples collected become legal evidence and must be kept in a locked box. They should be delivered directly to the laboratory or handed to the police to ensure continuity of evidence.

      a. **Screening for gonorrhea and Chlamydia.** Take saline-moistened swabs from the vagina, mouth, and rectum. Repeat in 5–7 days.

      b. **Seminal fluid.** Use a moistened swab or feeding tube to obtain a vaginal sample for sperm detection. Use protein 30 if indicated; do not use saline. Note: sperm can survive for up to 3 days in the vagina.

**C. Treatment**

   1. Treat any injuries.

   2. Provide pregnancy prophylaxis if indicated (see Chap. 18).

   3. Give venereal disease prophylaxis if indicated (see Chap. 21, Sexually Transmitted Diseases).

   4. Emotional support of the parents and child is vital. Allow parents to express anger, guilt, or frustration. Explain that the child is likely to suffer behavioral disturbances that may include regressive behavior, anxiety, or conduct disturbance.

   5. Report the case to the social service and law enforcement agencies.

   6. About 50% of victims will have some emotional problems after the assault. Almost 20% will have long-term problems. Prognosis is related to the age at which the abuse occurred, the duration and frequency of the abuse, and the relationship of the abuser to the child.

**D. Legal testimony.** Physicians are often called to testify in court. Courts place great emphasis on physical evidence. Do not comment on abnormalities unless you are sure that they are significant. If there are other possible explanations for your findings, then state these in court. Answer concisely and respond only to the specific question asked.

**IV. Disposition.** All patients who are at risk for child abuse must be placed in emergency foster homes or be admitted to hospital.
**V. Key points**
  **A.** Child abuse is common. A high index of suspicion will help to identify the child at risk.
  **B.** Rarely, infants and young children seriously injure themselves.
  **C.** Careful documentation of the history and physical findings is necessary for adequate legal evidence. Use a systematic approach in the physical examination in any case of suspected child abuse.

**Bibliography**

Cowell, C. The gynecologic examination of infants, children, and young adolescents. *Pediatr. Clin. North Am.* 28:247, 1981.

Fuster, C., and Neuistein, L. Vaginal *Chlamydia trachomatis* prevalence in sexually abused prepubertal girls. *Pediatrics* 79:235, 1987.

Helfer, R. E. (ed.). *The Battered Child.* Chicago: University of Chicago Press, 1965.

Herman-Giddens, M., and Frothingham, T. Prepubertal female genitalia. *Pediatrics* 80:203, 1987.

Levin, A. Child abuse: Challenges and controversies. *Pediatr. Emerg. Care* 3:211, 1987.

# Rape

Christine A. Loock

Rape is a type of physical assault, not just a sexual act. Assault and rape are legal terms, not medical diagnoses. The incidences are estimated to be 1 in 3–4 females and 1 in 7–10 males under the age of 18 years. Most victims do not immediately report rape.

I. **Diagnosis and assessment.** Rape is a medical and psychologic emergency. The patient must be seen immediately, preferably by an organized team consisting of physicians, nurses, and legal and welfare agencies; use of a sexual assault/rape protocol ("rape kit") is recommended.

  A. **History.** In younger children, obtain information from the social worker or parents (see Chap. 39). Adolescent victims should be interviewed in a quiet, nondistracting environment. Carefully document the history and its source, quoting the victim verbatim as much as possible. Inquire about the time, place, and nature of the alleged assault and obtain a description of the assailant. Determine if there was penetration or ejaculation and ask about other injuries. Obtain a past medical history including age at menarche, last menstrual period, contraception methods used, and allergies. Inquire about postassault activities such as bathing, douching, clothing changes, and recent coitus. In writing the emergency medical report use the term "history of sexual assault."

  B. **Examination.** (For age-specific techniques see Chap. 18.) The examiner must be gentle, reassuring, empathetic, and respectful of the child's modesty—this is often the child's first gynecologic examination. Allow parents to stay if they are supportive. Never conduct the examination alone; always obtain the assistance of another physician or nurse.

    1. **General examination.** Note the general appearance, including clothing and emotional state. Examine the integument for abrasions, hematoma, and lacerations. Look at the oral cavity, breasts, genitalia, and note the Tanner stage. When possible, take a photograph of the patient prior to the detailed examination.

    2. **Genital examination.** Ask the patient to point with the finger to the area or areas of the alleged assault. Document areas of trauma on an anatomic drawing or with photographs if possible. Describe the labia and hymen and record the presence of abrasions, hematomas, and lacerations. The normal virginal hymen may have a central slitlike opening, and the labia may be hyperemic in the normal prepubertal female. Hymenal lacerations most often occur near the posterior fourchette and may extend between the 3, 5, 7, and 9 o'clock positions. Penetration can occur without rupture when there has been previous atraumatic stretching (tampons, foreplay). If there

are signs of pelvic injury, consult a gynecologist for possible examination under anesthesia (see Chap. 18).

   3. **Anal examination.** Look for and document perineal and rectal injury. Anal tears and fissures follow violent assault. Anal laxity occurs for the first few hours, followed by spasm. If there is any sign of injury, further investigation with proctoscopy or sigmoidoscopy is indicated.

**C. Investigations**

   1. **Medical investigations.** In the adolescent female, obtain a Pap smear for routine analysis and sperm identification. Samples for cultures should be taken from appropriate sites for gonorrhea and *Chlamydia,* including the mouth, perineum, rectum, vagina, and endocervix. If the history is uncertain, take cultures from all sites. Viral cultures for herpes simplex virus and human papilloma virus (condyloma accuminata) should be obtained when indicated. In the prepubertal female investigations may be limited to swabs and cultures of samples from the throat, rectum, and vaginal introitus as indicated. Refer to Chap. 18 for appropriate examination techniques. Perform a pregnancy test on patients at risk (see Chap. 18) and perform serologic tests for syphilis at the first follow-up visit and in 6–8 weeks' time.

   2. **Legal investigations.** Evidence collected for forensic purposes includes clothing, fingernail scrapings, dried secretions for acid phosphatase testing, and other articles such as tampons or kerchiefs. Obtain pubic hair by combing onto paper and sealing the paper, comb, plucked hair, and combings in a plastic bag. Sperm identification is performed by taking swabs of the mouth up to 6 hours after the assault, the rectum up to 24 hours later, and the vaginal pool or endocervix up to 24 hours after the assault. Include swabs for wet mount, *Gonococcus* culture, permanent fixation, and acid phosphatase identification (place the swabbed specimen in a plain tube). A Wood's lamp examination may show fluorescence in areas of ejaculate; these areas should be swabbed with a saline-moistened cotton swab and placed on a slide to dry. Obtain a serum specimen for a syphilis serology. All evidence should be labeled and stored in a sealed bag or locked box until it is given to authorities; do not leave medical evidence unattended until it is handed over.

**II. Management.** Management of severe injury takes precedence. Get help from a gynecologist or surgeon when there is a question of serious trauma (see Chap. 18). Collect evidence and a full history for written documentation (see sec. **I.A** above). Reporting of an alleged history of sexual assault to law enforcement agencies is mandatory. Arrangements for psychotherapeutic counseling and follow-up for the patient, parents, and the victim's partner should be initiated in the emergency department.

   **A. Antibiotics.** Antibiotic therapy for gonorrhea and *Chlamydia* infection is indicated when the victim has been assaulted by a stranger. When the assailant is known, therapy may be withheld unless there is evidence of infection in the assailant or the victim (see Chap. 21, Sexually Transmitted Diseases).

   **B. Pregnancy prevention.** Offer the morning-after pill to adolescent females at risk for pregnancy who deny consensual intercourse since their last period. Treatment must be started within 72 hours of the assault. Because of the association of this drug with fetal anomalies, follow-up after administration is mandatory. See Chap. 18.

**III. Disposition.** Admit all patients with evidence of internal or multiple trauma.

**IV. Key points**

   **A.** Physicians do not diagnose rape or sexual assault. Careful use of terminology and verbatim reports in history taking, combined with careful anatomic descriptions, drawings, and photographs, will supply evidence for the court.

   **B.** Give antibiotics when the assailant is unknown and offer contraception to females at risk for pregnancy.

### Bibliography

Anderson, S. C., and Berliner, L. *Evaluation of the Child Sexual Assault Patient in the Health Care Setting: A Medical Training Manual.* Seattle: Sexual Assault Center, University of Washington, 1983.

Aziz, A., and McIntyre, L. Sexual abuse and sexually transmitted disease in children. *Can. Med. Assoc. J.* 134, 1986.

Enos, W. F., et al. Forensic evaluation of the sexually abused child. *Pediatrics* 78(3):385, 1986.

Glaser, J. B., et al. Sexually transmitted disease in victims of sexual assault. *N. Engl. J. Med.* 315(10):625, 1986.

White, S. T., Loda, F. A., Ingram, D. L., et al. Sexually transmitted disease in sexually abused children. *Pediatrics* 72:16, 1983.

# Head Injury

## David D. Cochrane

The clinical spectrum of head injury in children varies from the common bump on the head without neurologic sequelae to severe trauma causing death. Motor vehicle accidents, falls, and nonaccidental injuries account for the majority of cases. A neurosurgeon should be consulted when there is any doubt about diagnosis or treatment.

I. **Pathology of injury.** Diffuse brain injury results in an altered level of consciousness, whereas focal injury causes a localized deficit or depressed skull fracture.

A. **Diffuse injury.** Acceleration-deceleration or rotational forces result in diffuse axonal damage. Mild injury dazes the child. Severe injury results in coma. Diffuse brain injury is followed by posttraumatic amnesia; a low Glasgow coma scale score is characteristic (see Table 41-1).

B. **Focal injury.** Focal injury is the result of impact forces applied to the brain. It is detected by noting the most abnormal motor response (see Table 41-1) and abnormalities of pupil reaction or extraocular movements. Clinical findings may be dramatic, as in the child with compound skull fracture and dense hemiplegia due to motor cortex injury.

II. **Diagnosis and assessment**

A. **History.** Determine how, when, and where the trauma occurred and whether the child uttered a recognizable word following the injury. A comatose patient who was able to speak after injury usually has a treatable complication such as an intracranial hematoma, seizure, cerebral swelling, or shock. Paramedics, family, and Medic-alert tags are important sources of information in the comatose or nonverbal child.

Ask about a past history of seizures, migraine, hydrocephalus, medications, allergies, and immunizations. In the older child and adolescent, determine if alcohol or drugs were used prior to the injury.

When the histories taken from different people are contradictory, when the history does not fit the physical findings, or when there is a skull fracture or intracranial injury in children less than 1 year of age without a history of significant trauma, suspect nonaccidental injury. Nonaccidental injury is the most common cause of traumatic coma in patients under 1 year of age (see Chap. 39).

B. **Examination**

1. Begin with an assessment of the airway, breathing, and circulation. Head injury is an unlikely cause of hypotension in older children and adults; in the absence of severe scalp bleeding, assume that hypotension is due to blood loss in the abdomen, chest, or extremities. In infants, however, shock can result from blood loss into the subgaleal space (scalp laceration) or subdural space.

**Table 41-1. Glasgow Coma Scale**

| Parameter | Score |
| --- | --- |
| Eye opening | |
|   Spontaneously | 4 |
|   To speech | 3 |
|   To pain | 2 |
|   Nil | 1 |
| Best motor response | |
|   Obeys commands | 6 |
|   Localizes stimuli | 5 |
|   Withdraws | 4 |
|   Abnormal flexion | 3 |
|   Extensor responses | 2 |
|   Nil | 1 |
| Verbal response | |
|   Oriented | 5 |
|   Confused | 4 |
|   Inappropriate | 3 |
|   Incomprehensible | 2 |
|   Nil | 1 |

Note: The Glasgow Coma Scale forms an assessment base for diffuse, not focal, brain dysfunction. Since the best motor response is recorded, hemiplegia would not be reflected in the score. Stimuli for motor testing are nail bed pressure or supraorbital stimulation (localizing requires that the hand move to the chin with supraorbital stimulation).

2. The presence of a fixed dilated pupil, or of bradycardia, arterial hypertension, and irregular or slow respirations (Cushing's triad) suggests raised intracranial pressure; these children must be attended to immediately. Conversely, these findings are not always seen in children with intracranial hypertension.

3. Perform a complete neurologic assessment in all children with head trauma. Feel the fontanel and examine the pupils, extraocular movements, and motor responses to determine whether there are focal signs. Use the Glasgow Coma Scale as a measure of the severity of diffuse injury—it should be repeated to monitor neurologic status. Complete the neurologic examination by assessing the cranial nerves. Perform funduscopy to search for hemorrhage or papilledema and examine the motor system (reflexes, coordination, and, if possible, gait). Look for any discrepancies between the right and left sides suggesting a focal lesion.

III. **Patterns of head injury in children.** Injury may be categorized according to the patient's age, mechanism of injury, and severity.

A. **Mild head injury** (pediatric concussion syndrome). Concussion is a traumatic disturbance in neurologic function followed by full recovery. Typically, it occurs following a mild injury such as a fall from a changing table or high chair, or down a flight of stairs. There may be a period of pallor and limpness, but most children cry immediately and are irritable. Persistent vomiting is characteristic. In the older child, concussion can be diagnosed by a history of loss of consciousness or the presence of posttraumatic amnesia. In the nonverbal child the diagnosis may be impossible to confirm. There is no evidence of increased intracranial pressure or focal signs of neurologic dysfunction. Subgaleal hematomas and underlying linear skull fractures are commonly associated.

    **1. Management.** In the majority of these infants and children no specific treatment is needed.

**B. Moderate head injury.** Moderate injuries are most commonly seen in the older child involved in motor vehicle trauma as a pedestrian or cyclist. Typically, an initial period of unconsciousness is followed by recovery. Subsequently, there may be variation in the level of consciousness; deterioration to a grossly abnormal level of function such as decerebrate posturing can occur. There are usually no clear localizing neurologic signs, and the intracranial pressure, if measured, is normal. Computed tomographic (CT) scans should be obtained because of the fluctuating level of consciousness; scans are usually normal or show only subarachnoid hemorrhage.

    **1. Management.** Treatment includes admission for observation and any necessary supportive therapy. Recovery may take days, during which time the child may have periods of confusion or agitation.

**C. Severe head injury.** Severe injury is usually the result of high-velocity motor vehicle accidents. It is most common in older children and adolescents. Loss of consciousness is immediate, and neurologic impairment is profound. Following impact, the patient may exhibit one of two patterns of clinical dysfunction: incomplete initial recovery of function, or no initial recovery.

    **1. Incomplete initial recovery.** Initially deeply unconscious, these children may improve to the state of obeying commands by opening the eyes or, rarely, to talking. Within minutes or hours the victim's condition deteriorates, and decerebration, pupil irregularity or dilatation, bradycardia, pallor, and an absent response to pain develop. CT scans show diffuse cerebral swelling with compression or obliteration of the subarachnoid spaces.

        **a. Management.** These children require aggressive therapy (see sec. **IV.B** below, and Chap. 22, Increased Intracranial Pressure) with intubation and hyperventilation. Mannitol should be avoided because it may worsen the clinical outcome. Recovery is usually complete within a few days.

    **2. No initial recovery.** These patients are rendered unconscious by the impact and arrive deeply unconscious with abnormal motor responses and pupillary and respiratory irregularities. They remain unchanged neurologically. CT may show brain swelling with hemorrhage into the deep white matter, dorsal midbrain, or intraventricular or subarachnoid areas. Aggressive treatment is required (see sec. **IV.B** and Chap. 22, Increased Intracranial Pressure).

**D. Head injury in the newborn.** Skull fractures can occur in utero or as a result of delivery. Injury to the craniocervical junction, facial nerve, or brachial plexus may also occur. Posterior fossa subdural hematoma may occur with a difficult vertex or breech presentation. Clinical signs of brain dysfunction are usually nonspecific and include irritability, lethargy, pallor, vomiting, and poor feeding. Characteristic features of a posterior fossa injury include vomiting, coma, and facial palsy. Depressed fractures may be difficult to diagnose when there is subgaleal edema (caput) or hematoma.

**E. Skull fracture.** A skull fracture reflects the violence to which the head has been subjected. Fractures may be compound or closed, and linear, depressed, or comminuted. They may involve the calvarium (superior portions of the frontal, occipital, parietal bones) or the skull base.

    **1. Simple closed linear fractures.** Injuries of the calvarium are common in infants and children and usually result from short distance falls. It may be difficult to differentiate fracture lines from sutures. Widely splayed fractures or sutures reflect significant injury and are often associated with intracranial hypertension and brain injury.

    **2. Depressed fractures.** Depressed fractures may be open or closed. Children with uncomplicated, closed, depressed fractures should be referred to a neurosurgeon and admitted to the hospital. Compound fractures require early meticulous surgical debridement and antibiotic coverage with intravenous anti-staphylococcal agents such as cloxacillin, oxacillin, or erythromycin. Immunize children at risk for tetanus (see Appendix I).

    **3. Basal fractures.** Temporal bone fractures are diagnosed clinically in the child with hemorrhagic otorrhea, hemotympanum, or mastoid bruising (Battle's sign). Fracture of the anterior floor of the cranial fossa is suggested by subscleral hemorrhage, periorbital ecchymosis (racoon's eyes), and hemorrhagic rhinorrhea. All basal fractures are compound and should be treated as such (see sec. **III.E.2** above).

**IV. Management principles in children with head injury**

  **A. Minor injury**

    **1. General considerations.** Children with uncomplicated minor head injury may be sent home. Parents should be instructed to wake the child every 2 hours and return immediately to the hospital if there is repeated vomiting, altered mental status, dizziness, ataxia, visual problems, or severe headache. Admit

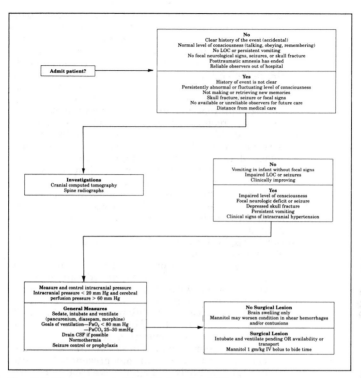

**Fig. 41-1. Management of head injury in children.**

patients with an unclear or suspicious history, an altered level of consciousness, skull fracture, seizures, neurologic signs (including posttraumatic amnesia), an inability to make or retrieve new memories, or lack of reliable follow-up (Fig. 41-1).

2. **Radiologic investigations.** Radiologic studies should be obtained when there is any suspicion of cerebral injury. In most cases a CT scan is all that is required. Skull x rays are indicated when there is suspicion of a penetrating cranial wound, depressed fracture, retained foreign body, or child abuse.

B. **Moderate or severe head injury**

1. **Resuscitation and cervical spine stabilization.** Establish an adequate airway, check breathing and circulation, and stabilize the spine with a semirigid collar or tape and sandbags (see Chap. 32). Ensuring maximum perfusion and oxygenation is vital to recovery from brain injury. In children with moderate or severe injury, start an intravenous line and draw blood for complete blood count (CBC), cross-match, and measurement of electrolytes and blood gases.

Give oxygen to all children who are not verbalizing normally. In infants, scalp bleeding may result in shock—control with point pressure.

**2. Initial neurologic assessment** (Table 41-1). Assess diffuse injury with the Glasgow Coma Scale. In the older child, verbal response to a question will often establish the adequacy of the airway, ventilation, and cognitive function. Look for focal injury by noting pupil reaction, extraocular movements, motor responses, respiratory pattern, and fontanel tension.

**3. CT scans.** CT scans should be obtained in the child with an impaired level of consciousness, focal neurologic deficit, seizures, or depressed skull fracture or in whom there is persistent vomiting or signs of increased intracranial pressure (papilledema, absent venous pulsations, full fontanel, diastasis of sutures, "setting-sun" sign). Do not wait for the results of the CT scan before resuscitating the brain-injured patient.

**4. Seizures.** Posttraumatic seizures occur in up to 10% of children with head injury.

**a. Impact seizures** occur within 1 minute of injury; they are usually generalized and do not recur. Children with single impact seizures do not require treatment.

**b. Early seizures** occur following trauma, often after a period of lucidity. The postictal state may be confused with deterioration secondary to intracranial hypertension. These seizures can be repetitive, and the patient may present with status epilepticus. Early and aggressive treatment is required (see Chap. 22, Increased Intracranial Pressure; Seizures).

**5. Increased intracranial pressure.** Head-injured children with an impaired level of consciousness, focal neurologic deficit, or recurrent seizures are included in this group. Effective treatment requires the skills of specialists in intensive care, anesthesia, neurology, and neurosurgery for management with intubation, hyperventilation, and sedation (see Chap. 22, Increased Intracranial Pressure).

**V. Disposition.** Children with penetrating skull wounds, compound or depressed fractures, or associated brain injury require CT scan and admission to hospital. Children suspected of nonaccidental injury should be admitted pending investigation by authorities.

**VI. Key points**

**A.** The comatose child who has spoken since the injury has a treatable complication of trauma.

**B.** In children, hypotension is almost never due to head injury; the exception is the infant with severe scalp or subdural bleeding.

**C.** Children with a focal abnormality or evidence of raised intracranial pressure need urgent attention, including intubation and ventilation and urgent consultation with a neurosurgeon.

## Bibliography

Bruce, D. A., and Schut, L. Concussion and contusion following pediatric head injury. In R. L. McLaurin (ed.), *Pediatric Neurosurgery of the Developing Nervous System*. New York: Grune & Stratton, 1982.

Cooper, P. R. (ed.). *Head Injury*. Baltimore: Williams & Wilkins, 1987.

Jennett, B., and Teasdale, G. *Management of Head Injuries*. Philadelphia: F. A. Davis, 1981.

Plum, F. Clinical aspects of coma. *Clin. Neurosurg.* 18:457, 1971.

Plum, F., and Posner, J. B. *The Diagnosis of Stupor and Coma* (3rd ed.). Philadelphia: F. A. Davis, 1980.

# Appendixes

# Tetanus Prophylaxis in the Wounded or Burned Child

| Immunization status (doses) | Clean minor wounds, burns | | Tetanus prone wounds, burns | |
|---|---|---|---|---|
| | TD | TIG | TD | TIG |
| **Children Age > and Over** | | | | |
| Uncertain | Yes | No | Yes | Yes |
| 0–1 | Yes | No | Yes | Yes |
| 2 | Yes | No | Yes | No[a] |
| 3 or more | No[b] | No | No[c] | No |
| **Children Under Age 7** | DTP (0.5 ml IM) | TIG (250 U IM) | DTP (0.5 ml IM) | TIG (250 U IM) |
| Unknown or less than 3 doses | Yes[d] | No | Yes[d] | Yes |
| Three or more doses | No[e] | No | No[f] | No |

Key: TD = tetanus diphtheria; TIG = tetanus immunoglobulin; DTP = diphtheria tetanus pertussis; TIG = tetanus immune globulin.

[a] Yes if wound or burn more than 24 hours old.

[b] Yes if more than 10 years since last dose.

[c] Yes if more than 5 years since last dose.

[d] The primary immunization series should be completed.

[e] Yes, if the routine immunization schedule has lapsed (i.e., to make up for missed dose).

[f] Yes, if the routine immunization schedule has lapsed, or if more than 5 years has elapsed since last dose of DPT.

Note: TD should be given if DPT is contraindicated. Acetaminophen should be given with the dose of DPT, 10 mg/kg PO.

# Vital Signs

Table II-1. Vital signs for age

| Age | Resting heart rate (per minute) | Resting blood pressure (mm Hg) Boys | Resting blood pressure (mm Hg) Girls | Resting respiratory rate (per minute) |
|---|---|---|---|---|
| Newborn | 120 (+/- 25) | 70/50 (+/- 10/10) | 70/50 (+/- 10/10) | 45 (+/- 15) |
| 1–6 months | 140 (+/- 30) | 95/50 (+/- 10/10) | 90/50 (+/- 10/10) | 40 (+/- 10) |
| 1 year | 120 (+/- 20) | 95/55 (+/- 10/10) | 95/50 (+/- 10/10) | 35 (+/- 10) |
| 2 years | 110 (+/- 30) | 95/60 (+/- 10/10) | 95/60 (+/- 10/10) | 35 (+/- 5) |
| 4 years | 100 (+/- 35) | 90/55 (+/- 10/10) | 90/55 (+/- 10/10) | 25 (+/- 8) |
| 6 years | 95 (+/- 25) | 95/60 (+/- 10/10) | 95/55 (+/- 10/10) | 22 (+/- 7) |
| 8 years | 90 (+/- 25) | 100/60 (+/- 10/10) | 100/60 (+/- 10/10) | 22 (+/- 7) |
| 10 years | 80 (+/- 20) | 100/65 (+/- 10/10) | 100/65 (+/- 10/10) | 22 (+/- 7) |
| 12 years | 75 (+/- 20) | 105/65 (+/- 10/10) | 110/70 (+/- 10/10) | 20 (+/- 5) |
| 14 years | 70 (+/- 20) | 110/65 (+/- 10/10) | 110/70 (+/- 10/10) | 20 (+/- 5) |

Source: Adapted from Report of the Second Task Force on Blood Pressure Control in Children—1987. *Pediatrics* 79:1, 1987; J. Liebman. Tables of Normal Standards. In J. Liebman, R. Plonsey, and P. C. Gillette (eds.), *Pediatric Electrocardiography*. Baltimore: Williams and Wilkins, 1982; W. W. Waring. The History and Physical Examination. In E. L. Kendig and V. Chernick, *Disorders of the Respiratory Tract* (4th ed.). Philadelphia: Saunders, 1983.

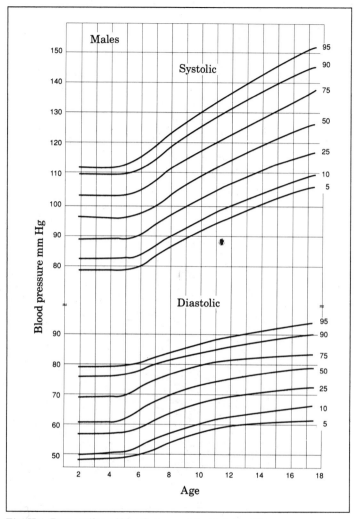

**Fig. II-1. Percentiles of blood pressure in seated males.**

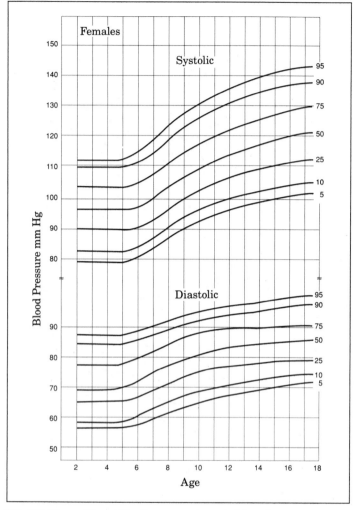

**Fig. II-2. Percentiles of blood pressure in seated females.**

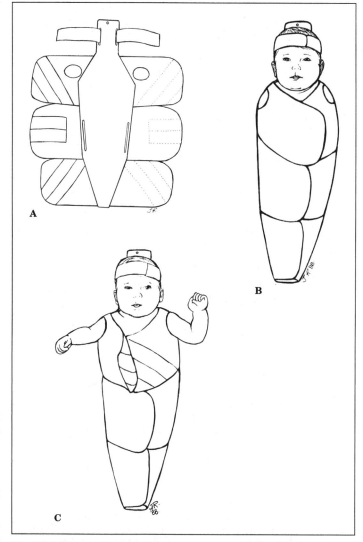

**Fig. III-1. Papoose board restraint. A. Papoose board. B. Child restrained, arms enclosed. C. Child restrained, arms free.**

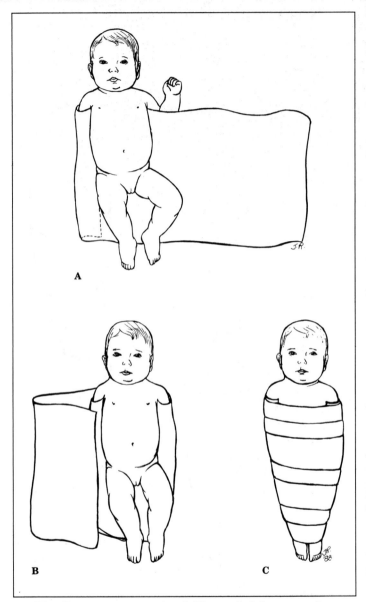

Fig. III-2. Sheet mummy restraint. A. Wrap end of sheet around arm and back. B. Wrap around other arm. C. Wrap remaining sheet around child in mummy fashion.

# Normal Laboratory Values

Anne C. Halstead, Gillian Lockitch, and
Louis D. Wadsworth

**Table IV-1. Blood gases**

| Parameter | Age | Value |
|---|---|---|
| $PO_2$ | 0–1 mo M/F | >60 mm Hg |
| | 2 mo–60 yr | >74 mm Hg |
| $PCO_2$ | 0–2 yr M/F | 26–41 mm Hg |
| | 3 yr–adult | 35–45 mm Hg |
| pH blood | | 7.35–7.45 |
| Bicarbonate | 0–2 yr M/F | 17–24 mmol/liter (mEq/liter) |
| (blood gas | 3 yr–16 yr | 18–27 mmol/liter |
| calculated) | adult | 21–29 mmol/liter |

Specimen: Heparinized whole blood, collected anaerobically, kept on ice.
Volume: 1 ml arterial blood or 250 μl arterialized capillary blood.

**Table IV-2. Urine**

| Parameter | Value |
|---|---|
| Urinalysis (routine) | |
| Specific gravity | >1.020 if no fluids taken overnight |
| Protein | Negative or trace |
| Blood | Negative |
| Glucose | Negative |
| pH | 4.5–8.0 |
| Ketones | Negative or +1 |
| Bile pigments | Negative |
| Microscopic | |
| RBC | Up to 3/hpf |
| WBC | Up to 5/hpf |
| Epithelial cells | Up to 5/hpf |
| Cellular casts | None |
| Waxy casts | None |
| Hyaline casts | Occasional/lpf |
| Granular casts | Occasional/lpf |
| Crystals | Usually not significant with notable exceptions of cystine and some amino acids. |
| Osmolality urine | 50–1200 mmol/kg (mOsm/kg) |

Specimen: Fresh random urine, no preservatives.
Volume: 10 ml is preferred, but urinalysis can be done on 1 ml.
Osmolality requires an additional 1.0 ml.

Values in Appendix IV are those used at Children's Hospital, Vancouver, British Columbia.

**Table IV-3. Chemistry**

| Test | Tube | Blood volume | Age | SI reference interval | Traditional units |
|---|---|---|---|---|---|
| Ammonia | Green | 1.0 ml on ice | higher in newborn | 5–35 µmol/L | |
| Amylase serum | Red | 0.25 ml | 0–6 mo M/F | 0–20 U/L | (IU/L) |
| | | | 6 mo–1 yr | 5–50 U/L | |
| | | | 1–adult | 30–100 U/L | |
| Aspartate aminotransferase (AST, SGOT) | Red/green | 0.25 ml | 0–5 day M/F | 35–140 U/L | (IU/L) |
| | | | 6 day–3 yr | 20–60 U/L | |
| | | | 4–6 yr | 15–50 U/L | |
| | | | 7–9 yr | 15–40 U/L | |
| | | | 10–11 yr M | 10–60 U/L | |
| | | | 12–15 yr | 15–40 U/L | |
| | | | 16–adult | 10–45 U/L | |
| | | | 10–11 yr F | 10–40 U/L | |
| | | | 12–15 yr | 10–30 U/L | |
| | | | 16–adult | 5–30 U/L | |
| Bilirubin, conjugated | Red/green | 0.25 ml | 1–19 yr M/F | <2 µmol/L | <0.1 mg/dl |
| Bilirubin, unconjugated | | | 1–19 yr M/F | 3–17 µmol/L | 0.2–1.0 mg/dl |

| Analyte | Tube color | Volume | Age | SI units | Conventional units |
|---|---|---|---|---|---|
| Calcium, serum | Red/green | 0.25 ml | 0–1 yr M/F | 1.87–2.49 mmol/L | 7.5–10.0 mg/dl |
| | | | 1–3 yr | 2.17–2.44 mmol/L | 8.7–9.8 mg/dl |
| | | | 4–9 yr | 2.19–2.51 mmol/L | 8.8–10.1 mg/dl |
| | | | 10–11 yr | 2.22–2.51 mmol/L | 8.9–10.1 mg/dl |
| | | | 12–13 yr | 2.19–2.64 mmol/L | 8.8–10.6 mg/dl |
| | | | 14–15 yr | 2.29–2.66 mmol/L | 9.2–10.7 mg/dl |
| | | | 16–adult | 2.22–2.66 mmol/L | 8.9–10.7 mg/dl |
| Calcium, ionized | Red/green | 0.25 ml on ice | 0–5 day M/F | 0.9–1.3 mmol/L | 3.6–5.4 mg/dl |
| | | | 6 day–adult | 1.1–1.3 mmol/L | 4.4–5.4 mg/dl |
| Creatinine, serum | Red/green | 0.25 ml | 0–1 yr M/F | 10–90 μmol/L | 0.1–1.0 mg/dl |
| | | | 1–3 yr | 10–50 μmol/L | 0.1–0.6 mg/dl |
| | | | 4–6 yr | 10–60 μmol/L | 0.1–0.7 mg/dl |
| | | | 7–9 yr | 20–60 μmol/L | 0.3–0.7 mg/dl |
| | | | 10–13 yr | 40–90 μmol/L | 0.4–1.0 mg/dl |
| | | | 14–adult | 50–110 μmol/L | 0.6–1.2 mg/dl |
| Sodium, serum | Red/green (lithium heparin) | 0.25 ml | | 135–145 mmol/L | (mEq/L) |
| Potassium, serum | Red/green | 0.25 ml | 0–5 yr M/F | 3.5–5.5 mmol/L | (mEq/L) |
| | | | 5–adult | 3.5–5.0 mmol/L | (mEq/L) |
| Chloride, serum | Red/green | 0.25 ml | | 95–107 mmol/L | (mEq/L) |
| Bicarbonate (total $CO_2$) | Red/green | 0.25 ml | 0–5 yr M/F | 18–26 mmol/L | (mEq/L) |
| | | | 6–adult | 23–34 mmol/L | (mEq/L) |
| Anion gap | By calculation | | | 8–14 mmol/L | (mEq/L) |

**Table IV-3.** (continued)

| Test | Tube | Blood volume | Age | SI reference interval | Traditional units |
|---|---|---|---|---|---|
| Glucose fasting serum | Red/green | 0.25 ml | 0–1 yr M/F | 3.3–5.6 mmol/L | 60–100 mg/dl |
| | | | 1–6 yr | 4.1–7.0 mmol/L | 75–125 mg/dl |
| | | | 7–adult | 3.9–5.9 mmol/L | 70–105 mg/dl |
| Lactate | Venous, no tourniquet, gray | 1.0 ml on ice | | 0.5–2.2 mmol/L | |
| Magnesium | Red/green | 0.25 ml | 0–2 mo | 0.66–0.95 mmol/L | 1.6–2.3 mg/dl |
| | | | 3 mo–12 yr | 0.78–1.03 mmol/L | 1.9–2.5 mg/dl |
| | | | 13 yr–adult | 0.74–1.00 mmol/L | 1.8–2.4 mg/dl |
| Osmolality, serum | Red | 0.5 ml | | 285–295 mmol/kg | (mOsm/kg) |
| Phosphorus, serum | Red/green | 0.25 ml | 0–5 day M/F | 1.55–2.65 mmol/L | 4.8–8.2 mg/dl |
| | | | 6 day–1 yr | 1.29–2.58 mmol/L | 4.0–8.0 mg/dl |
| | | | 1–3 yr | 1.25–2.10 mmol/L | 3.9–6.5 mg/dl |
| | | | 4–6 yr | 1.30–1.75 mmol/L | 4.0–5.4 mg/dl |
| | | | 7–11 yr | 1.20–1.80 mmol/L | 3.7–5.6 mg/dl |
| | | | 12–13 yr | 1.05–1.75 mmol/L | 3.3–5.4 mg/dl |
| | | | 14–15 yr | 0.95–1.75 mmol/L | 2.9–5.4 mg/dl |
| | | | 16–adult | 0.90–1.50 mmol/L | 2.8–4.6 mg/dl |

| Analyte | Color | Volume | Age | | |
|---|---|---|---|---|---|
| Protein, total serum | Red | 0.25 ml | 0–1 yr M/F | 5.4–7.0 gm/dl | 54–70 gm/L |
| | | | 1–3 yr | 5.9–7.0 gm/dl | 59–70 gm/L |
| | | | 4–6 yr | 5.9–7.8 gm/dl | 59–78 gm/L |
| | | | 7–9 yr | 6.2–8.1 gm/dl | 62–81 gm/L |
| | | | 10–adult | 6.3–8.6 gm/dl | 63–86 gm/L |
| Urea, serum | Red/green | 0.25 ml | 0–5 day M/F | 2–19 mg/dl | 0.7–6.7 mmol/L |
| | | | 6 day–1 yr | 5–23 mg/dl | 1.8–8.2 mmol/L |
| | | | 1–3 yr | 5–17 mg/dl | 1.8–6.0 mmol/L |
| | | | 4–13 yr | 7–18 mg/dl | 2.5–6.4 mmol/L |
| | | | 14–adult | 8–21 mg/dl | 2.9–7.5 mmol/L |
| Uric acid, serum | Red/green | 0.25 ml | 0–1 yr M/F | 1.9–7.9 mg/dl | 115–470 µmol/L |
| | | | 1–3 yr | 1.8–5.0 mg/dl | 105–300 µmol/L |
| | | | 4–6 yr | 2.2–4.7 mg/dl | 130–280 µmol/L |
| | | | 7–9 yr | 2.0–4.9 mg/dl | 120–295 µmol/L |
| | | | 10–11 yr M | 2.3–5.4 mg/dl | 135–320 µmol/L |
| | | | 12–13 yr | 2.7–6.7 mg/dl | 160–400 µmol/L |
| | | | 14–15 yr | 2.4–7.8 mg/dl | 140–465 µmol/L |
| | | | 16–adult | 4.0–8.6 mg/dl | 235–510 µmol/L |
| | | | 10–11 yr F | 3.0–4.7 mg/dl | 180–280 µmol/L |
| | | | 12–15 yr | 3.0–5.8 mg/dl | 180–345 µmol/L |
| | | | 16–adult | 3.0–5.9 mg/dl | 180–350 µmol/L |

**Table IV-4. Toxicology**

| Test | Tube | | Toxic levels | | Traditional units |
|---|---|---|---|---|---|
| Acetaminophen | Red/green | 0.5 ml | 4 hr post dose | >1300 µmol/L | >200 µg/ml |
| | | | 12 hr post dose | >300 µmol/L | >50 µg/ml |
| Ethanol | Red/green | 1.0 ml | Intoxication | 17–65 mmol/L | 80–300 mg/dl |
| | Send to laboratory immediately | | Fatal | 80–160 mmol/L | 375–750 mg/dl |
| Ethylene glycol | Red | 0.4 ml | Treat | >3.2 mmol/L | >20 mg/dl |
| | Send to laboratory immediately | | Consider dialysis | >8.1 mmol/L | >50 mg/dl |
| Iron serum | Red | 1.0 ml | (4–6 hr post dose) | >55 µmol/L | >300 µg/dl |
| | Iron | | Treat | >90 µmol/L | >500 µg/dl |
| | | | **Normal for age** | | |
| | | | 0–6 mo M/F | 4–13 µmol/L | 22–73 µg/dl |
| | | | 7 mo–1 yr | 4–18 µmol/L | 22–100 µg/dl |
| | | | 1–5 yr | 4–25 µmol/L | 22–140 µg/dl |
| | | | 6–9 yr | 7–25 µmol/L | 39–140 µg/dl |
| | | | 10–13 yr M | 5–24 µmol/L | 28–134 µg/dl |
| | | | 14–adult | 6–29 µmol/L | 33–162 µg/dl |
| | | | 10–13 yr F | 8–26 µmol/L | 45–145 µg/dl |
| | | | 14–adult | 5–33 µmol/L | 28–185 µg/dl |
| Methanol | Red | 4.0 ml | Treat | >6.2 mmol/L | >20 mg/dl |
| | Send to laboratory immediately | | Consider dialysis | >15.6 mmol/L | >50 mg/dl |
| Salicylate | Red/green | 0.5 ml | Symptoms may occur | >2.2 mmol/L | 30 mg/dl |

**Table IV-5. Therapeutic drugs**

| Drug | Tube | Therapeutic range | Sample time | Time to steady state |
|---|---|---|---|---|
| Carbamazepine | Red/green 0.5 ml | 25–50 μmol/L (6–12 μg/ml) | Pre-AM dose | Variable |
| Digoxin | Red/green 1.0 ml | 1.3–2.8 nmol/L (1.0–2.2 ng/ml) | Predose (6 h postdose) | 5–7 days |
| Phenytoin | Red/green 0.5 ml | 40–80 μmol/L (10–20 μg/ml) | Pre-AM dose | 4–7 days |
| Phenobarbital | Red/green 0.5 ml | 65–170 μmol/L (15–40 μg/ml) | At least 2 hr after IV load finished; pre-AM dose | 10–14 days |
| Theophylline | Red/green 0.5 ml | Apnea 28–55 μmol/L (5–10 μg/ml) Asthma 55–110 μmol/L (10–20 μg/ml) | Short acting: 1–2 hr post dose Long acting: 4–6 hr post dose | |
| Valproic acid | Red/green 0.5 ml | 350–700 μmol/L (50–100 μg/ml) | Pre-AM dose | 3–5 days |

**Table IV-6. Expected normal hematology values**

| Age | WBC ×10⁹/L | RBC ×10¹²/L | Hgb (gm/L) | Hct | Mean cell volume (fL) | Mean corpuscular hemoglobin (pg) | Mean corpuscular hemoglobin concentration (gm/L) | Platelets ×10⁹/L | Reticulocytes ×10⁹/L |
|---|---|---|---|---|---|---|---|---|---|
| Cord | 9.0–30.0 | 3.90–5.50 | 140–190 | | 98.0–118 | | | 120–450 | 100–300 |
| 1 day | 9.0–30.0 | 4.00–6.60 | 150–250 | | 95.0–121 | | | 120–450 | 100–300 |
| 1 wk | 5.0–20.0 | 3.90–6.30 | 149–229 | 0.420–0.600 | 88.0–126 | 31.0–37.0 | 300–366 | 140–350 | 100–300 |
| 4 wk | 5.0–19.5 | 3.30–5.30 | 102–182 | 0.390–0.630 | 86.0–124 | 29.0–36.0 | 280–360 | 140–350 | 100–300 |
| 8 wk | 5.5–18.0 | 2.70–4.90 | 91–131 | 0.280–0.420 | 77.0–105 | 26.0–34.0 | 290–370 | 140–350 | 100–300 |
| 6 mo | 6.0–18.0 | 3.10–4.50 | 101–129 | 0.290–0.410 | 74.0–108 | 25.0–35.0 | 290–360 | 140–350 | 40–120 |
| 1 yr | 6.0–18.0 | 3.70–5.30 | 107–131 | 0.330–0.390 | 70.0–86.0 | 23.0–31.0 | 300–360 | 180–440 | 40–120 |
| 5 yr | 6.0–16.0 | 3.90–5.30 | 107–147 | 0.340–0.400 | 75.0–87.0 | 24.0–30.0 | 310–370 | 180–440 | 40–120 |
| [a]6–11 yr M | 3.9–10.2 | 4.05–5.15 | 118–146 | 0.353–0.428 | 77.1–91.5 | 25.8–31.7 | 330–351 | 180–440 | 30–180 |
| [a]6–11 yr F | 3.9–10.2 | 4.05–5.15 | 118–146 | 0.353–0.428 | 77.1–91.5 | 25.0–33.8 | 330–351 | 180–440 | 30–180 |
| [a]12–15 yr M | 3.9–10.2 | 4.43–5.53 | 125–165 | 0.368–0.473 | 77.1–91.5 | 25.8–31.7 | 330–351 | 180–440 | 30–180 |
| [a]12–15 yr F | 3.9–10.2 | 4.05–4.98 | 117–149 | 0.351–0.436 | 77.1–91.5 | 25.8–31.7 | 330–351 | 180–440 | 30–180 |
| [a]16–18 yr M | 3.9–10.2 | 4.41–5.71 | 131–169 | 0.380–0.489 | 75.7–94.9 | 25.0–33.8 | 330–355 | 165–397 | 30–180 |
| [a]16–18 yr F | 3.9–10.2 | 4.00–4.87 | 117–149 | 0.351–0.436 | 80.0–94.8 | 25.0–33.8 | 330–355 | 165–397 | 30–180 |
| [b]Adult M | 4.0–11.0 | 4.50–5.90 | 140–180 | 0.400–0.520 | 82.0–98.0 | 27.0–34.0 | 320–360 | 140–350 | 40–120 |
| [b]Adult F | 4.0–11.0 | 3.80–5.20 | 120–160 | 0.350–0.470 | 82.0–98.0 | 27.0–34.0 | 320–360 | 140–350 | 40–120 |

Data adapted from M. L. Willoughby. *Pediatric Hematology.* New York: Churchill, 1977. W. Williams. *Hematology.* New York: McGraw-Hill, 1988. D. Nathan and F. Oski. *Hematology of Infancy and Childhood.* Philadelphia: Saunders, 1981.

[a]Data established by Hematology Laboratory, Children's Hospital, British Columbia

[b]Data established by Hematology Laboratory, St. Paul's Hospital, Vancouver, British Columbia

Table IV-6. (continued)

| Red cell distribution width | Mean platelet volume | Automated instrument differential | | | Neutro-phils | Band | Lympho-cytes | Mono-cytes | Eosino-phils | Baso-phils |
|---|---|---|---|---|---|---|---|---|---|---|
| | | Lympho-cytes | Mono-cytes | Gran-ulocytes | | | | | | |
| — | — | — | — | — | 1.0–2.0 | 0–1.2 | 2.0–11.0 | 0.5–1.8 | 0.2–0.60 | 0–0.6 |
| — | — | — | — | — | 2.0–20.0 | 0–1.7 | 2.0–10.0 | 0.5–1.8 | 0.2–0.60 | 0–0.6 |
| — | — | — | — | — | 2.0–8.0 | 0.4–1.4 | 2.0–17.0 | 0.5–1.8 | 0.2–0.80 | 0–0.2 |
| — | — | — | — | — | 2.0–5.5 | 0.2–1.0 | 3.6–12.0 | 0–0.9 | 0–0.50 | 0–0.2 |
| — | — | — | — | — | 2.4–7.5 | 0.2–0.8 | 2.3–8.0 | 0–0.8 | 0–0.50 | 0–0.2 |
| 0.116–0.118 | 7.4–11.1 | 1.6–4.0 | 0.2–0.6 | 2.0–4.0 | 1.8–4.2 | 0–0.2 | 1.9–4.3 | 0.1–0.7 | 0–0.70 | 0–0.1 |
| 0.116–0.118 | 7.4–11.1 | 1.6–4.0 | 0.2–0.6 | 2.0–4.0 | 1.8–4.0 | 0–0.2 | 1.9–4.3 | 0.1–0.7 | 0–0.70 | 0–0.1 |
| 0.116–0.118 | 7.4–11.1 | 1.6–4.0 | 0.2–0.6 | 1.5–6.0 | 1.4–5.2 | 0–0.2 | 1.5–4.2 | 0.1–0.7 | 0–0.70 | 0–0.1 |
| 0.116–0.118 | 7.4–11.1 | 1.6–4.0 | 0.2–0.6 | 1.5–6.0 | 1.4–5.2 | 0–0.2 | 1.5–4.2 | 0.1–0.7 | 0–0.70 | 0–0.1 |
| 0.116–0.118 | 7.4–11.1 | 1.4–3.4 | 0.2–0.6 | 1.6–7.2 | 1.5–7.4 | 0–0.2 | 1.0–3.6 | 0.1–0.7 | 0–0.70 | 0–0.1 |
| 0.116–0.118 | 7.4–11.1 | 1.4–3.4 | 0.2–0.6 | 1.6–7.2 | 1.5–7.4 | 0–0.2 | 1.0–3.6 | 0.1–0.7 | 0–0.70 | 0–0.1 |
| 0.112–0.148 | 7.4–11.1 | 1.4–3.9 | 0.2–0.6 | 2.0–7.4 | 1.8–6.8 | 0–0.2 | 1.0–3.6 | 0.1–0.7 | 0–0.50 | 0–0.1 |
| 0.112–0.148 | 7.4–11.1 | 1.3–3.0 | 0.2–0.6 | 2.0–7.4 | 1.8–6.8 | 0–0.2 | 1.0–3.6 | 0.1–0.7 | 0–0.50 | 0–0.1 |
| — | — | 1.0–4.0 | 0.1–0.8 | 2.0–6.0 | 2.0–6.0 | 0–0.7 | 1.0–4.0 | 0.1–0.8 | 0–0.45 | 0–0.1 |
| — | — | 1.0–4.0 | 0.1–0.8 | 2.0–6.0 | 2.0–6.0 | 0–0.7 | 1.0–4.0 | 0.1–0.8 | 0–0.45 | 0–0.1 |

Table IV-7. Coagulation reference ranges

### Children 6–18 yr M/F[a]

| | |
|---|---|
| Prothrombin time | 10.00–11.60 seconds |
| APTT | 29.00–40.50 seconds |
| Fibrinogen | 1.85–3.80 gm/L |
| Factor VIII | 0.75–1.50 units/dl |

### Full-term infants[b]

| | Age | | | | | |
|---|---|---|---|---|---|---|
| | Day 1 | Day 5 | Day 30 | Day 90 | Day 180 | Adult |
| Fibrinogen gm/L | 1.70–4.0 | 1.60–4.6 | 1.6–3.8 | 1.6–4.00 | 1.6–4.0 | 1.6–4.0 |
| Factor VIII (units/dl) | 0.50–1.8 | 0.50–1.5 | 0.5–1.6 | 0.5–1.25 | 0.5–1.1 | 0.5–1.5 |
| Factor IX (units/dl) | 0.15–0.9 | 0.15–0.9 | 0.2–0.8 | 0.2–1.15 | 0.4–1.4 | 0.6–1.7 |

### Adults[c]

| | |
|---|---|
| Prothrombin time | 9.5–11.5 seconds |
| APTT | 24.0–37.0 seconds |

Note: Normal ranges for prothrombin times and APTT may change slightly from year to year due to reagent changes.
[a]Values established by Children's Hospital, Vancouver, B.C., 1986.
[b]Values taken from Chedoke McMaster Hospital, Hamilton, Ontario.
[c]Values established by Children's Hospital, Vancouver, B.C., October 1987.

# V

# Drug Dosage Guidelines

John J. Macready and Albert R. McDougal

The drug dosage guidelines that appear in this section are a compilation of those appearing in standard pediatric drug reference sources, a selection of pediatric journals, and experience gathered at the British Columbia Children's Hospital. Every attempt has been made to provide the most up-to-date information in a readily usable format. Because clinical experience in pediatrics is limited, there is a paucity of definitive dosage guidelines for some drugs such as, for example, the antipsychotics. In addition, for other drugs with very special applications, such as antidotes, it is advisable to consult experts in the field or the regional poison control center prior to treating the patient.

The four-column format has been designed to enable the reader to locate and interpret the necessary information quickly. The following information is included in each drug listing.

**Column 1: Drug.** The drugs are listed in alphabetical order according to generic name. In addition, where applicable, one example brand name has been included in parentheses under the generic name. Some typical dosage forms and strengths available are also included.

**Column 2: Route of administration.** The following abbreviations are used for specifying the route of administration: IV = intravenous; IA = intraarterial; IM = intramuscular; SC = subcutaneous; PO = oral; PR = rectal; ETT = endotracheal; INH = inhalation of aerosol. The routes indicated are those that are recommended for the indications and dosage guidelines of column 3.

**Column 3: Dosage.** Drug dosages are expressed as mg/kg/day divided bid, or as mg/kg/dose bid. When available, a dosage range is provided and maximum and minimum doses are specified. Indications for use have been included in this section to facilitate selection of the appropriate drug dose.

**Column 4: Comments.** In this section information such as infusion solution compatibility, method of drug infusion, dosing modifications in patients with renal or hepatic impairment, important adverse effects, and important drug interactions and contraindications are listed for each drug.

**Table V-3.** This table provides instructions for the intravenous dilution and infusion of commonly used emergency and support drugs administered as continuous infusions. Compatibility information and short comments are included.

**Table V-1. Drug dosage guidelines in infants and children**

| Drug | Route | Dosage | Comments |
|------|-------|--------|----------|
| Acetaminophen (Tylenol)<br>Elixir: 160 mg/5 ml<br>Drops: 80 mg/ml<br>Chew tabs: 80 mg<br>Tabs: 325, 500 mg<br>Suppos: 120, 650 mg | PO, PR | 10–15 mg/kg/dose, repeated q4–6 prn<br>Max: 65 mg/kg/day | Overdose results in delayed hepatotoxicity<br>Contraindicated in patients with G6PD deficiency |
| N-Acetylcysteine (Mucomyst)<br>Soln: 20% 200 mg/ml<br>Inj: 200 mg/ml (Canada, Great Britain) | PO | For *acetaminophen overdose* give 140 mg/kg/loading dose followed by 70 mg/kg/dose repeated q4h for 17 doses | Start if 4-hour acetaminophen level exceeds 140 μg/ml (1300 μmol/liter—see Chap. 27) or ingestion is severe<br>For oral use dilute 20% solution with three parts cola, orange, or grapefruit juice<br>The dilutions should be freshly prepared and administered within 1 hour.<br>If patient vomits a dose within 1 hour, repeat dose<br>Activated charcoal will adsorb N-acetylcysteine<br>IV solutions should be freshly prepared with 5% D/W and used within time indicated for dose<br>IV therapy may be associated with skin rashes and anaphylaxis |
| | IV | The total IV dose is 300 mg/kg administered in three divided doses over 20 hours as follows:<br>First dose: 150 mg/kg over 15 minutes diluted in 50–200 ml 5% D/W<br>Second dose: 50 mg/kg over 4 hours diluted in 500 ml 5% D/W<br>Third dose: 100 mg/kg over 16 hours diluted in 1 liter of 5% D/W<br>The fluid volume may be decreased in young children | |

| | | | |
|---|---|---|---|
| Acetylsalicylic acid (aspirin, ASA)<br>Chew tab: 80 mg<br>Tab: 325 mg<br>Ent tab: 325, 650, 975 mg<br>Suppos: 150, 650 mg | PO, PR<br><br><br>PO<br><br><br>PO | *Analgesic, antipyretic*<br>10–20 mg/kg/dose repeated q4–6h prn<br>Max: 3.6 gm/day<br>*Juvenile rheumatoid arthritis,*<br>*pericarditis, rheumatic fever*<br>60–100 mg/kg/day divided qid<br>*Kawasaki syndrome*<br>100 mg/kg/day divided qid until fever resolves for 36 hours, then 5–10 mg/kg/day qam | Not recommended for use as an antipyretic in children with viral infections<br>Monitor serum drug concentrations during high-dose therapy<br>Therapeutic range is 1.1–2.2 mmole/liter (15–30 mg/dl) |
| Acyclovir (Zovirax)<br>Inj: 500 mg<br>Tab: 200 mg<br>Oint: 5% | IV<br><br><br><br>PO<br>Top<br>IV | *Genital herpes simplex virus (HSV)*<br>*first episode, HSV in*<br>*immunocompromised host*<br>*(disseminated or progressive)*<br>15 mg/kg/day divided q8h<br>200 mg 5 times daily for 5–10 days<br>5% ointment 4–6 times daily<br>*HSV encephalitis, varicella in*<br>*immunocompromised host, zoster in*<br>*immunocompetent host*<br>30 mg/kg/day divided q8h | Ensure adequate hydration of patient while using this drug<br>IV dose is diluted to 10 mg/ml and infused over 60 minutes<br>Dilute dose in 5% or 10% D/W, normal saline, lactated Ringer's, or dextrose/saline<br>Adjust dose interval in patients with renal impairment |
| Alcohol (dehydrated) 100% v/v | IV<br><br><br>PO<br><br><br>IV | *Methanol poisoning*<br>Loading dose: 7.6–10 ml/kg of 10% ethanol over 30–60 min<br>0.76–1.0 ml/kg of 100% ethanol (760–1000 mg/kg) diluted to 5–10% in orange juice<br>Maintenance dose: 1.4 ml/kg/hr by continuous infusion of 10% ethanol | For IV administration, dilute to 10% concentration in 5% D/W or normal saline<br>For oral use, ethanol must be diluted to 5–10% concentration in orange juice<br>Titrate dose to provide a therapeutic level of 100–150 mg/dl |

Table V-1. (continued)

| Drug | Route | Dosage | Comments |
|---|---|---|---|
| | PO | 0.14 ml/kg/hr of 100% ethanol (140 mg/kg/hr) diluted to 5–10% in orange juice | For infusion and compatibility information see Table V-3 |
| Aminophylline<br>Inj: 25, 50 mg/ml<br>Soln: 21 mg/ml (Palaron) | IV | *Acute asthma*<br>Loading dose: with no previous theophylline, 6.25 mg/kg IV slowly over 20–30 mins; with history of theophylline use, 3 mg/kg IV as above. | Do not use for bronchospasm in infants less than 6 months of age<br>Aminophylline contains 80% anhydrous theophylline<br>For further information see Table V-3. |
| | IV | Initial maintenance dose: continuous infusion by age as shown: | Blood level monitoring is essential to keep serum theophylline level at 55–110 μmole/liter (10–20 mg/liter) |

| Age | Infusion rate (mg/kg/hr) |
|---|---|
| 26–52 weeks | $(0.01 \times$ age in weeks) $+ 0.21$ |
| 1–9 yr | 1 |
| 9–12 yr | 0.9 |
| Adolescent smokers | 0.9 |
| Adolescent nonsmokers | 0.6 |

Concomitant use of cimetidine or erythromycin may increase serum concentrations and predispose to toxicity. Measure steady state peak or trough levels: peak with rapid-release product, 1–2 hr; peak with slow-release product, 4–6 hr; trough, predose

| | | | |
|---|---|---|---|
| | PO | *Chronic asthma*<br>Maximum maintenance doses prior to serum concentration monitoring:<br><br>**Age** — **Infusion rate (mg/kg/day)**<br>1–9 yr — 30<br>9–12 yr — 25<br>12–16 yr — 22<br>>16 yr — 18<br><br>Select dose interval according to product used—max: 900 mg/day | |
| Ammonium chloride<br>Inj: 0.4, 5mEq/ml<br>Tab: 325, 500 mg<br>ENT Tab: 500, 1000 mg | IV, PO | *Acidification of urine*<br>75 mg/kg/day divided q6h | Contraindicated in patients with severe liver or renal dysfunction |
| Amoxicillin trihydrate (Amoxil)<br>Susp: 25,50 mg/ml<br>Drops: 50 mg/ml<br>Cap: 250, 500 mg<br>Chew tab: 125, 250mg | PO | *Mild to moderate infections*<br>30–40 mg/kg/day divided q8h—max: 4 gm/day | Inappropriate for severe infections<br>Increase dosage intervals in patients with reduced renal function |

**Table V-1.** (continued)

| Drug | Route | Dosage | Comments |
|------|-------|--------|----------|
| Ampicillin sodium (Penbritin)<br>Inj: 125, 250, 500, 1000, 2000 mg | IV<br><br>IV, IM | *Meningitis*<br>200–400 mg/kg/day divided q4–6h<br>*Other*<br>100–200 kg/day divided q4–6h—max: 10 gm/day | Increase dosage interval in patients with reduced renal function |
| Ampicillin trihydrate (Penbritin)<br>Susp: 25, 50 mg/ml<br>Cap: 250, 500 mg | PO | *Mild to moderate infections*<br>50–100 mg/kg/day divided q6h | Oral route inappropriate for severe infections |
| Amyl nitrite inhaler<br>Sodium nitrite IV<br>Sodium thiosulfate (cyanide antidote kit) | Inhale<br><br><br>IV | *Cyanide poisoning*<br>Inhale amyl nitrite for 30 seconds of each minute until sodium nitrite is given<br>Children over 25 kg: give 300 mg (entire ampoule) of sodium nitrite IV. Follow immediately with 12.5 gm sodium thiosulfate<br>Children under 25 kg: Adjust the dose of sodium nitrite according to the hemoglobin level | Follow manufacturer's instructions in the kit.<br>Cyanide antidotes are toxic. Avoid unnecessary therapy.<br>Give sodium nitrite at a rate of 2.5–5 ml/min and stop if systolic blood pressure is < 80 mm Hg<br>Give sodium thiosulfate at a rate of 2.5–5 ml/min |

| Hemoglobin (gm) | Initial dose 3% sodium nitrite (ml/kg) |
| --- | --- |
| 8 | 0.22 |
| 10 | 0.27 |
| 12 | 0.33 |
| 14 | 0.39 |

Children under 25 kg: adjust the sodium thiosulfate dose according to the hemoglobin level

| Hemoglobin (gm) | Initial dose 25% sodium thiosulfate (ml/kg) |
| --- | --- |
| 8 | 1.1 |
| 10 | 1.35 |
| 12 | 1.65 |
| 14 | 1.95 |
| Max | 5 |

IV, ETT    *Cardiopulmonary resuscitation*
0.02 mg/kg/dose repeated q5min prn—maximum: 2 mg/dose; minimum: 0.1 mg/dose

*Cholinergic crisis*
IV    0.05 mg/kg/dose IV prn—maximum: 2 mg/dose

Give IV undiluted over 30 seconds
Contraindicated in patients with narrow angle glaucoma
Use with caution in patients with asthma
Incompatible with sodium bicarbonate, norepinephrine, isoproterenol

Atropine
Inj: 0.3, 0.4, 0.6 mg/ml
Prefilled syringe 0.1 mg/ml

**Table V-1.** (continued)

| Drug | Route | Dosage | Comments |
|------|-------|--------|----------|
| | PO, IM | Preoperative: 0.01–0.02 mg/kg/dose 30 min preoperatively—maximum: 0.6 mg | Safety and efficacy in children has not been established |
| Bretylium (Bretylate) Inj: 50 mg/ml | IV | *Acute ventricular fibrillation* Give 5 mg/kg/dose undiluted by rapid IV push, followed by additional doses of 10 mg/kg/dose at 15- –30-min intervals until a maximum total dose of 30 mg/kg has been given | Indicated for life-threatening ventricular dysrhythmias refractory to conventional therapy Observe for hypotension |
| Calcium chloride Inj: 100 mg/ml, 10% (0.68 mM Ca²⁺/ml) (1.36 mEq Ca²⁺/ml) (27 mg elemental Ca²⁺/ml) | IV | *Cardiopulmonary resuscitation* 15–30 mg/kg (0.15–0.3 ml/kg/dose) slow IV over 1 min, repeated q10min prn—maximum: 1 gm/dose = 10 ml of 10% solution | For cardiac resuscitation only in cases of documented or suspected hypocalcemia Give undiluted solution slowly over 1 min. via central venous catheter Not to be given SC or IM— incompatible with NaHCO₃, catecholamines For dilution instructions see Table V-3 |
| Calcium gluconate 100 mg/ml; 10% (0.23 mM Ca²⁺/ml) (0.46 mEq CaH⁺/ml) (9.4 mg elemental Ca²⁺/ml) | IV | *Hypocalcemia with seizures or tetany* 2 ml/kg/dose slow IV push over 30 min | Contraindicated in patients with digoxin toxicity or hypercalcemia Monitor closely for bradycardia and dysrhythmias Incompatible with NaHCO₃, catecholamines |

| Drug | Route | Dose | Comments |
|---|---|---|---|
| Cefaclor (Ceclor)<br>Susp: 25 mg, 50 mg/ml 250, 500 mg cap | PO | 40 mg/kg/day divided q8h<br>Maximum: 2 gm/day | Inappropriate for severe infections<br>Not recommended in newborns<br>Decrease dose in patients with reduced renal function |
| Cefazolin (Ancef)<br>Inj: 500, 1000 mg | IV, IM | 50–100 mg/kg/day divided q6–8h—maximum: 6 gm/day | Increase dose interval in patients with reduced renal function |
| Cefotaxime (Claforan)<br>Inj: 0.5, 1, 2 gm | IV, IM | *Meningitis:*<br>200 mg/kg/day divided q6h<br>*Other*<br>100–200 mg/kg/day divided q6–8h<br>Maximum: 10 gm/day | Good gram-negative coverage (except pseudomonas) and CSF penetration<br>Increase dose interval in patients with reduced renal function |
| Cefoxitin (Mefoxin)<br>Inj: 1, 2 gm | IV, IM | 80–160 mg/kg/day divided q4–6h<br>Maximum: 12 gm/day | Increase dose interval in patients with reduced renal function<br>Safe use of cefoxitin in infants <3 months old has not been established |
| Ceftazidime (Fortaz)<br>Inj: 0.5, 1, 2 gm | IV, IM | *Meningitis*<br>150 kg/day divided q8h<br>*Cystic fibrosis*<br>200 mg/kg/day divided q6h | 100–150 mg/kg/day divided q8h<br>Increase dose interval in patients with reduced renal function |
| Ceftriaxone (Rocephin)<br>Inj: 0.25, 0.5, 1, 2 gm | IV<br><br>IM | *Meningitis*<br>100 mg/kg/day divided q12h<br>Maximum: 4 gm/day<br>*Other*<br>50–100 mg/kg/day divided q12–24h<br>Maximum: 2 gm/day | |

**Table V-1.** (continued)

| Drug | Route | Dosage | Comments |
|------|-------|--------|----------|
| Cefuroxime (Zinacef) Inj: 0.25, 0.75, 1.5 gm | IV, IM | *Meningitis* 200–250 mg/kg/day divided q6H *Other* 75–150 mg/kg/day divided q8H Maximum: 9 gm/day | Increase dose interval in patients with reduced renal function |
| Cephalexin (Keflex) Susp: 25, 50 mg/ml Tab: 250, 500 mg | PO | 25–50 mg/kg/day divided q6h Maximum: 3 gm/day | Inappropriate for severe infections Increase dose interval in patients with reduced renal function Shake well before use |
| Charcoal-activated Charcodote (premixed charcoal) 25, 50 gm (200 mg/ml) in sorbitol | PO | *Single dose:* Small children, 15–30 gm Children >12 yr, 50–100 gm or 1 gm/kg *Multiple dose:* 5–10 gm q2–4h | Do not give following ingestion of strong acids or alkalies Will adsorb acetylcysteine given orally Simultaneous administration of ipecac is not recommended |
| Chloral hydrate (Noctec) Syrup: 100 mg/ml Cap: 500 mg | PO, PR | *Sedative dose:* 25–50 mg/kg/dose. Repeat prn for sedation. Maximum: 75 mg/kg/dose or 1 gm/dose | May cause excitement in patients with pain Lacks analgesic effects Dilute oral dose with water or milk |
| Chloramphenicol (Chloromycetin) Inj: 1 gm Liq: 31.25 mg/ml Cap: 250 mg | IV, PO | 50–100 mg/kg/day divided q6h Maximum: 4 gm/day | Serum level monitoring recommended to keep peaks <25 mg/liter, troughs <10 mg/liter Do not use palmitate liquid form in infants <1 yr of age or in cystic fibrosis patients |

| Drug | Route | Dose | Comments |
|---|---|---|---|
| Cimetidine (Tagamet)<br>Liq: 60 mg/ml<br>Tab: 200, 300, 400 mg, 600 mg<br>Inj: 150 mg/ml | IV, PO | 20–40 mg/kg/day divided q6h or tid before meals and at bedtime<br>Maximum: 1200 mg/day | Leukopenia has been associated with excessive doses<br>Reduces metabolism of some drugs (e.g., theophylline, anticonvulsants) |
| Clindamycin (Dalacin C)<br>Inj: 150 mg/ml<br>Susp: 15 mg/ml<br>Cap: 150 mg | IV, IM<br><br>PO | 25–40 mg/kg/day divided q6–8h<br>Maximum: 4 gm/day<br>10–30 mg/kg/day divided q6h<br>Maximum: 2 gm/day | Reduce dose in patients with marked hepatic or renal impairment<br>Not indicated in patients with meningitis |
| Cloxacillin (Orbenin)<br>Inj: 250, 500 mg, 2 gm<br>Susp: 25 mg/ml<br>Cap: 250, 500 mg | IV, IM<br><br>PO | 100–200 mg/kg/day divided q4–6h<br>Maximum: 12 gm/day<br>50–100 mg/kg/day divided q6h<br>Maximum: 4 gm/day | Oral administration of higher doses often causes gastritis |
| Codeine phosphate<br>Tab: 15, 30, 60 mg<br>Syrup: 5 mg/ml<br>Inj: 30, 60 mg/ml | IM, SC,<br>PO | *Analgesic*<br>0.5–1.0 mg/kg/dose q4–6h prn<br>Maximum: 1.5 mg/kg/dose or 5 mg/kg/day | Codeine can cause constipation, respiratory depression, and hypotension<br>Maximum dose should not be given for longer than 24 hours<br>Specific antidote for narcotic overdose is naloxone, 0.01–0.1 mg/kg IV or IM |
| Cortisone acetate (Cortone)<br>Inj: 50 mg/ml | IM | Antiinflammatory/immunosuppressive<br>1–5 mg/kg/day IM as single daily dose or divided q12h | Shake suspension well<br>Inject IM dose deep into gluteal muscle |

*Idiosyncratic or dose-related bone marrow suppression occurs*
*Reduce dose in patients with renal or hepatic dysfunction*

**Table V-1.** (continued)

| Drug | Route | Dosage | Comments |
|------|-------|--------|----------|
| Cotrimoxazole (trimethoprim-sulfamethoxazole [TMP-SMX], Bactrim, Septra) | IV, PO | *Severe infections, Pneumocystis* 20 mg (TMP)/kg/day divided q6h | IV route is used when oral form cannot be administered |
| Inj: 16 mg TMP/80 mg SMX/ml | PO | *Bacterial infections* 6–12 mg (TMP)/kg/day divided q12h or 0.31–0.63 ml/kg/day of liquid preparation divided q12h | IV dose to be diluted, 5 ml in 125 ml IV fluid, given over 30–60 min |
| Tab: 80 mg TMP/400 mg SMX | | | Dilute dose in 5% D/W 0.9% NaCl, or Ringer's solution |
| DS tab: 160 mg TMP/800 mg SMX | | *Prophylaxis for otitis media or urinary tract infections* | Adjust dosage in patients with reduced renal function |
| Ped tab: 20 mg TMP/100 mg SMX | | 5 mg (TMP)/kg/day | |
| Liq: 8 mg TMP/40 mg SMX/ml | | | |
| Deferoxamine (Desferal) | IM | *Mild intoxication* 50 mg/kg q6h | Hypotension or shock may occur if IV rate exceeds 15 mg/kg/hr |
| Inj: 500 mg | IV | *Severe intoxication* Continuous infusion: 15 mg/kg/hr for 4 hr, then 2–5 mg/kg/hr until urine color has been normal for 24 hr or serum iron is <50 μmol/liter (<300 μg/dl) | Compatible with normal saline, 5% D/W, lactated Ringer's |
| | | | Contraindicated in renal failure |
| | | Maximum dose: Do not exceed 6 gm/24 hr or 120 mg/kg, whichever is less | Consult poison control center |

| Drug | Route | Dose | Comments |
|---|---|---|---|
| Dexamethasone sodium phosphate<br>Inj: 4 mg/ml<br>Tab: 0.5, 0.75, 4 mg | IM, IV | *Increased intracranial pressure with tumor*<br>Initial dose: 1–2 mg/kg IV, then 0.25–0.50 mg/kg/day divided q6h | Give IV direct slowly over 3–5 min<br>For intermittent IV administration dilute with equal volume of fluid and infuse over 10 min |
| | IV, IM, PO | *Croup, extubation*<br>0.25–0.50 mg/kg/dose q6h prn beginning 24 hours prior to extubation and continuing for 4–6 doses afterwards | |
| | IM, IV | *Croup, acute*<br>0.6 mg/kg in a single dose | |
| | IM | *Antiinflammatory action or immunosuppression*<br>0.043–0.150 mg/kg/day IM in a single dose | |
| Dextrose (glucose)<br>Inj: 500 mg/ml | IV | 0.5–1 gm/kg/dose IV or 1–2 ml/kg/dose of 50% solution | In young children dilute 50% solution 1:1 with sterile water to make a 25% solution. |
| Diazepam (Valium)<br>Inj: 5 mg/ml | IV | *Status epilepticus*<br>0.3 mg/kg/dose q10–30 min for two doses | Give undiluted by slow IV push over 2 minutes<br>Diazepam has a short duration (20 min) of AC activity and therefore should be followed by phenytoin in children with status epilepticus<br>May cause hypotension and apnea when given IV |
| | PR | 0.5 mg/kg/dose PR for one dose<br>Maximum: 10 mg/dose<br>*Sedation*<br>0.1 mg/kg/dose | Parenteral preparation can be used PR by means of a catheter placed in the rectum |

$40 \times 3$

**Table V-1.** (continued)

| Drug | Route | Dosage | Comments |
|---|---|---|---|
| Dicloxacillin (Dynapen)<br>Cap: 250 mg<br>Susp: 12.5 mg/ml | PO | 12–25 mg/kg/day divided q6h | Rectal administration gives adequate serum levels in 4–10 min<br>Gastrointestinal disturbances such as nausea, epigastric discomfort, flatulence, and loose stools have been noted in patients treated with dicloxacillin |
| Diazoxide (Hyperstat)<br>Inj: 15 mg/ml | IV | *Hypertensive crisis*<br>1–3 mg/kg/dose rapid IV push, up to a maximum of 150 mg/dose undiluted over 10–30 sec. May repeat dose in 30 min and, if no effect, then repeat q3–24 hr | Must be infused rapidly via peripheral vein with patient in recumbent position<br>Avoid extravasation<br>Overdosage may cause Hyperglycemia, ketoacidosis, hypotension, and dysrhythmias<br>Salt and water retention occurs with multiple doses of diazoxide<br>Follow with furosemide, 1–2 mg/kg IV |
| Digoxin<br>Liq: 0.05 mg/ml<br>Tab: 0.125, 0.25, 0.0625 mg<br>Inj: 0.05, 0.25 mg/ml | IV | *Congestive heart failure*<br>Total digitalizing dose—given in three divided doses (one-half, one-fourth, one-fourth) q8h<br><br>| Age | Dose (mg/kg) |<br>|---|---|<br>| Infant <2 yr | 0.035 |<br>| Child >2 yr | 0.03 | | IV doses are given undiluted over 1–5 min<br>Doses for supraventricular tachycardia may be higher<br>Oral doses are 1.25 times larger than IV doses<br>Obtain ECG 6 hr after each dose to assess potential toxicity<br>Reduce maintenance dose during |

| Drug | Route | Dose | |
|---|---|---|---|
| | PO | Children over 10 yr old receive 0.5–1.0 mg; maximum total dose, 1.5 mg Maintenance dose is divided q12h. Start maintenance dose 12 hr after last portion of digitalizing dose. | concomitant administration of amiodarone or quinidine and in presence of reduced renal function IV dose is 0.75 times oral dose Monitoring of serum digoxin level is recommended Drug levels are monitored predose approximately 5 days after starting therapy Optimal serum digoxin level is 1–2.5 nmol/liter (0.8–2 µg/liter) For overdose management, consult a poison control center |

| Age | Dose (mg/kg/day) |
|---|---|
| Infants <2 yr | 0.01 |
| Children >2 yr | 0.008 |
| Children >10 yr | 0.125–0.25 mg/day |

Maximum: 0.25 mg/day

| Drug | Route | Dose | |
|---|---|---|---|
| Dimenhydrinate (Gravol) Tab: 15, 50 mg Liq: 3 mg/ml Inj: 10, 50 mg/ml Suppos: 50, 100 mg | IV, IM, PO, PR | 5 mg/kg/day divided q6h prn Maximum: 300 mg/day | May be given by slow IV push. Dilute 50 mg/ml concentration to a concentration not exceeding 5 mg/ml and infuse over 2 min |
| Dimercaprol (BAL in oil) Inj: 100 mg/ml (10%) | IM | *Severe arsenic or gold poisoning* 3 mg/kg q4h for 2 days, q6h for 1 day, then twice daily for 10 days to recovery *Acute mercury poisoning* 5 mg/kg once, followed by 2.5 mg/kg once or twice daily for 10 days *Severe lead poisoning* When serum lead levels are higher than 100 µg/dl with or without | Dimercaprol is administered undiluted by deep IM injection only Use separate site for EDTA when this drug is used To obtain maximum benefit, use within first 4 hr of ingestion Maintain an alkaline urine during treatment to protect the kidneys Use cautiously in patients with reduced renal function |

**Table V-1.** (continued)

| Drug | Route | Dosage | Comments |
|---|---|---|---|
| | | symptoms, give 4 mg/kg q4h for 3–7 days with EDTA | Contraindicated in patients with impaired liver function except those with postarsenic jaundice |
| Diphenhydramine (Benadryl)<br>Cap: 25, 50 mg<br>Liq: 2.5 mg/ml<br>Inj: 50 mg/ml | IV, IM, PO | *Anaphylaxis*<br>1–2 mg/kg/dose<br>*Antihistamines*<br>5 mg/kg/day divided q6–8h | Dose may be given by slow IV push undiluted over 3–5 minutes<br>Use with caution in infants and young children |
| | IV, IM | *Treatment of extrapyramidal symptoms*<br>1–2 mg/kg/dose repeated q6h prn<br>Maximum: 300 mg/day and 50 mg/dose | Contraindicated in neonates and in patients receiving MAO inhibitors<br>Incompatible with cephalothin hydrocortisone |
| Docusate (Colace)<br>Liq: 4 mg/ml<br>Drops: 10 mg/ml<br>Cap: 100 mg | PO | *Laxative*<br>5 mg/kg/day divided bid or tid or as a single daily dose | Dilute drops in milk, juice, or formula to mask bitter taste<br>Requires 1–3 days for effect |
| Dopamine (Intropin)<br>Inj: 40 mg/ml | IV | *Renal*<br>2–5 μg/kg/min<br>*Inotrope*<br>5–8 μg/kg/min<br>*Vasoconstrictor*<br>>10 μg/kg/min<br>Range: 2–20 μg/kg/min<br>Maximum: 25 μg/kg/min | When possible, give through central line by continuous infusion using infusion control device in an intensive care area<br>Monitor closely for extravasation to avoid necrosis. If extravasation occurs, manufacturer suggests infiltrating area with phentolamine, |

| Drug | Route | Dosage | Comments |
|---|---|---|---|
| EDTA (calcium disodium versenate) Inj: 200 mg/ml | IM | *Lead poisoning* When lead (blood) concentration is 25–100 µg/dl, use EDTA alone, 1 gm/m²/day for 3–5 days. When lead (blood) levels are >100 µg/dl, use EDTA in conjunction with dimercaprol: 1.5 gm/m²/day for 3–5 days two courses, with a rest period of 2–4 days between courses | 1 mg/ml in normal saline, to reverse vasoconstrictor effect. Incompatible with alkaline solutions. For further information see Table V-3. Deep IM injection is the preferred route. Use a separate site for dimercaprol when it is combined with EDTA. To minimize pain at injection site dilute each dose with an equal volume of 1% procaine. Do not give >5 ml per injection site. Monitor urinalysis daily for renal tubular damage. Consult a poison control center. |
| Epinephrine (Adrenalin) Inj: 1:10,000 (0.1 mg/ml) | IV, ETT | *Cardiopulmonary resuscitation* 0.01 mg/kg (or 0.1 ml/kg) of 1:10,000 solution. May repeat q5min as required. Minimum: 1 ml of 1:10,000 solution *Inotropic* 0.05–1.00 µg/kg/min by IV infusion | Give undiluted IV slowly over 1 min, preferably through a central line. 1:1000 solution *must be diluted* before IV or ETT use. May cause tachycardia, increased BP, ventricular fibrillation. Incompatible with alkaline solutions ($NaHCO_3$). For further information see Table V-3. |
| Epinephrine Inj: 1:1000 (1 mg/ml) | SC | *Bronchodilator; anaphylactic shock* 0.01 ml/kg/dose of 1:1000 solution SC. May repeat q15min for three to four doses or q4h prn. Maximum single dose: 0.3 ml | SC route not suitable for cardiac arrest |

**Table V-1.** (continued)

| Drug | Route | Dosage | Comments |
|------|-------|--------|----------|
| Epinephrine, racemic<br>Soln: 2.25% | | *Croup*<br>Usual doses—children <1 yr, 0.25 ml; children >1 yr, 0.5 ml or 0.05 ml/kg/ dose diluted in 2.5 ml of normal saline via nebulizer prn to maximum of q1h.<br>Maximum dose 0.5 ml | |
| Erythromycin—many preparations: (Erythrocin, Ilotycin)<br>Inj: lactobionate, 500 mg, 1 gm; glucceptate, 500 mg, 1 gm<br>Tab: base, 250 mg<br>Cap: sprinkle cap, 250 mg<br>Susp: estolate,<br>Stearate, 25, 50 mg/ml; ethyl succinate, 40, 80 mg/ml | IV<br><br>PO | *Severe infections*<br>20–50 mg/kg/day divided q6h<br>20–40 mg/kg/day divided q6–12h | Give IV by slow infusion over 60 min and dilute dose to 1–5 mg/ml<br>Gastrointestinal upset is common with oral route<br>Estolate preparation is well absorbed<br>Erythromycin increases serum levels of digoxin, theophylline and carbamazepine |
| Erythromycin ethylsuccinate/ sulfisoxazole (Pediazole)<br>Susp: 40 mg/ml erythromycin and 120 mg/ml sulfisoxazole | PO | *Acute otitis media*<br>50 mg/kg/day (erythromycin component) divided q6h for 10 days, or 0.3 ml/kg/dose repeated q6h for 10 days | |

| Drug | Route | Dose | Comments |
|---|---|---|---|
| Fenoterol (Berotec)<br>Soln: 0.1% (1 mg/ml)<br>Inhaler: 200 µg per puff<br>Tab: 2.5 mg | Inhale, soln<br><br>PO<br><br>Puffs | 0.03 ml/kg/dose diluted in 2–3 ml normal saline via nebulizer qid prn<br>Maximum: 4 mg/day<br>0.04 mg/kg/day divided tid or qid<br>Maximum: 15 mg/day<br>1–2 puffs q4–6 prn | |
| Fentanyl (Sublimaze)<br>Inj: 50 µg/ml | IV<br><br>IV<br>IV | *Anesthesia*<br>1–5 µg/kg/dose over 5 min<br>*Analgesia*<br>1–2 µg/kg/dose<br>*Continuous infusion*<br>1–2 µg/kg/hr | Potent narcotic<br>Rapid onset<br>May cause delayed respiratory depression and chest wall immobility<br>For further information, see Table V-3<br>Specific antidote for narcotic overdose is naloxone 0.01–0.10 mg/kg IV |
| Ferrous sulfate (Fer-In-Sol)<br>Drops: 125 mg/ml<br>Liq: 30 mg/ml<br>Tab: 300 mg | PO | *Iron deficiency anemia*<br>Therapeutic dose—6 mg/kg/day of elemental iron divided tid; prophylactic dose—0.5–2.0 mg/kg/day of elemental iron as a single dose or divided bid or tid | Liquid preparations stain teeth<br>If gastrointestinal irritation occurs, give with meals<br>300 mg ferrous sulfate = 60 mg elemental iron |
| Flucloxacillin (Fluclox)<br>Cap: 250, 500 mg<br>Susp: 125, 250 mg/5 ml | PO | 25–100 mg/kg/day divided q6h<br>Maximum: 4 gm/day | Gastrointestinal disturbances occur in some patients |
| Furosemide (Lasix)<br>Liq: 10 mg/ml<br>Tab: 20, 40 mg<br>Inj: 10 mg/ml | PO<br><br>IV | 0.5–2 mg/kg/dose up to 6 mg/kg/dose repeated q6–8h prn<br>Maximum: 6 mg/kg/dose<br>0.5–1.0 mg/kg/dose up to 6 mg/kg/dose q2–8h prn | May potentiate ototoxicity and nephrotoxicity of other drugs<br>May cause hypokalemia, alkalosis, dehydration, hypercalciuria |

**Table V-1.** (continued)

| Drug | Route | Dosage | Comments |
|---|---|---|---|
| | | Maximum: 6 mg/kg/dose | For IV injection give undiluted slowly over 1–2 min<br>Large dose should be infused at a rate not to exceed 4 mg/min<br>Incompatible with acidic solutions (e.g., ascorbic acid, epinephrine, norepinephrine) |
| Gentamicin (Garamycin)<br>Inj: 10, 40 mg/ml | IV, IM<br><br>IV | 3–7.5 mg/kg/day divided q8h<br>Maximum initial dose: 100 mg<br>*Cystic fibrosis*<br>12 mg/kg/day divided q8h | Serum level monitoring recommended to keep peaks 5–10 mg/liter, troughs less than 2 mg/liter<br>Peaks will be higher in patients with cystic fibrosis<br>Increase dosing interval in patients with reduced renal function |
| Glucagon<br>Inj: 1 mg glucose | IV, IM,<br>SC | *Hypoglycemia*<br>0.03 mg/kg/dose; may repeat in 20 min if necessary<br>Maximum: 1 mg/dose | 1 unit = 1 mg<br>Hyperglycemic effect is brief—follow with dextrose infusion<br>Cardiostimulatory effect is seen with high doses<br>See Dextrose |
| Haloperidol (Haldol)<br>Liq: 2 mg/ml<br>Inj: 5 mg/ml<br>Tab: 0.5, 1, 2, 5, 10, 20 mg | PO | *Agitation/psychosis/delirium*<br>Initial dose: 0.5 mg/dose, then 0.01–0.1 mg/kg/dose q2h until symptoms controlled | Dosages in young children are not well established<br>Not recommended for children <8 years old |

| Drug | Route | Dose | Comments |
|---|---|---|---|
| | IV, IM | Initial dose: 0.25–0.5 mg per dose, then 0.005–0.05 mg/kg/dose q2h until symptoms controlled. Alternatively, give q30min prn— | Use minimum effective dose in children to avoid EPS, hypotension. EPS are more common in teenage males |
| | IV | 8–12 yr, 1 mg with lorazepam 0.5 mg | Treat acute dystonias with benztropine, 0.5–2.0 mg IM or PO |
| | IM | 12–15 yr, 3 mg with lorazepam 1 mg | Give IV doses undiluted slowly over 2–5 min |
| | PO | >15 yr, 5 mg with lorazepam 2 mg | |
| Hydralazine (Apresoline) Tab: 10, 25, 50 mg Inj: 20 mg/ml | IV, IM | *Hypertension* 0.1–0.2 mg/kg/dose repeated q4–6h prn | Give by slow IV push over 3–5 min Reflex tachycardia may occur |
| | PO | Maintenance dose: 0.75–7.0 mg/kg/day divided q6h Maximum: 7 mg/kg/day or 200 mg/day, whichever is less | |
| Hydrocortisone sodium succinate (Solu-Cortef) Inj: 100, 250, 500 mg, 1 gm | IV | *Status asthmaticus* Initially, 4–8 mg/kg/dose once, then 16 mg/kg/day divided q6h for 5 days | For direct injection give slowly over 5–10 min Dilute intermittent IV injections to 1 mg/ml. Give over 30 min May be given by continuous infusion at a concentration of 1 mg/ml in 5% D/W or normal saline |
| Hydroxyzine (Atarax) Cap, 10, 25, 50 mg Liq: 2 mg/ml Inj: 50 mg/ml | PO | *Antihistamine* 2 mg/kg/day divided tid or qid | Hydroxyzine should not be given IV Dry mouth, drowsiness, convulsions may occur |
| | IM | *Antiemetic* 1.1 mg/kg/dose repeated q4–6 h prn; maximum, 400 mg/day | |

**Table V-1.** (continued)

| Drug | Route | Dosage | Comments |
|------|-------|--------|----------|
| Indomethacin (Indocid)<br>Cap: 25, 50 mg<br>Suppos: 50, 100 mg | PO | *Antiinflammatory agent*<br>In children >14 yr, 1.5–3.0 mg/kg/day divided tid with meals; maximum: 200 mg/day | |
| Insulin regular (Toronto, Iletin, Novolin, Humulin R)<br>Inj: 100 units/ml | IV | *Diabetic ketoacidosis*<br>0.1 units/kg by IV push, then 0.1 units/kg/hr by continuous infusion | Only regular insulin is given by IV route<br>Slow IV push may be given undiluted over 15–20 min<br>For continuous infusion dilute in normal saline to concentration of 0.1 unit/ml; see Table V-3<br>Preflush tubing of IV apparatus prior to use |
| Ipecac syrup (do not use fluid extract) | PO | <table><tr><td>Age</td><td>Dose</td></tr><tr><td>6–9 mo</td><td>5 ml</td></tr><tr><td>9–12 mo</td><td>10 ml</td></tr><tr><td>1–12 yr</td><td>15 ml</td></tr><tr><td>>12 yr</td><td>30 ml</td></tr></table><br>For children over 1 yr dose may be repeated in 20 min if no emesis results | Not recommended for children under 6 mo or in those who have ingested acids, alkali, tricyclics, or hydrocarbons, or in those with a decreased level of consciousness<br>Follow dose with 5 ml/kg water or fluids to maximum of 300 ml |
| Isoetharine (Bronkosol)<br>Inhaler soln: 1% 10 mg/ml; many preparations available | Inhale | 0.01 ml/kg/dose (max. 0.5 ml) of 1% solution diluted with 1.5 ml normal saline q2–6h | Tachycardia, tremor, palpitations<br>Contains bisulfite as preservative |

| Drug | Route | Dose | Comments |
|---|---|---|---|
| Isoproterenol (Isuprel)<br>Inj: 0.2 mg/ml 1:5000 | IV<br><br>IV<br>IV | *Inotrope*<br>0.05–0.5 µg/kg/min<br>*Bronchodilator*<br>0.1–0.8 µg/kg/min<br>Bradycardia: Start at 0.05–0.1 µg/kg/min, then increase dose to maximum 1 µg/kg/min | ECG monitoring is required during IV administration<br>Watch for tachycardia dysrhythmias, and signs of acute myocardial ischemia<br>Monitor fluid volume to maintain central venous pressure<br>For further information, see Appendix V, Part 3<br>Incompatible with $NaHCO_3$, lidocaine, aminophylline, epinephrine |
| Ketamine (Ketalar)<br>Inj: 10, 50 mg/ml | IV<br><br>IM | *General anesthesia*<br>1–4 mg/kg (average: 2 mg/kg); give slowly over 60 sec<br>6–13 mg/kg (average: 10 mg/kg) | 2 mg/kg will give 5–10 min of surgical anesthesia<br>10 mg/kg IM will produce 10–25 min of surgical anesthesia<br>Rapid IV administration can produce respiratory depression, laryngospasm, or airway obstruction. Give atropine predose<br>Premedication with diazepam will reduce the incidence of emergence reactions |
| Lactulose (Cephulac)<br>Liqd: 666.7 mg/ml | PO | *Acute hepatic encephalopathy*<br>1–2 ml/kg/dose by NG tube given q4–6h until watery diarrhea occurs, then reduce dose (see Chap. 16, Liver Failure) | Dose depends on indications for use—see Chap. 16, Liver Failure<br>Contraindicated in galactosemia<br>May be given as enema in patients with ileus |

**Table V-1.** (continued)

| Drug | Route | Dosage | Comments |
|------|-------|--------|----------|
| Lidocaine (Xylocaine)<br>Inj: 20 mg/ml, 200 mg/ml<br>Soln: 0.4% in 5% D/W (1 gm/250 ml) | IV, ETT | *Mild chronic encephalopathy*<br>Children <1 yr, 2.5 ml PO bid to produce daily soft stool<br>Older children and adults, 10–30 ml tid<br>*Ventricular dysrhythmias*<br>Loading dose: 0.5–1.0 mg/kg; repeat q5–10min prn to desired effect<br>Maximum: 100 mg/dose or 5 mg/kg<br>Maintenance infusion: 20–50 μg/kg/min | Administer loading doses at a rate not greater than 25–50 mg/min<br>Reduce dose in patients with hepatic or renal dysfunction<br>Therapeutic level: 6–21 μmol/liter (1.5–5.0 mg/liter) |
|  | IV | Maximum: 4 mg/min or 5 mg/kg/24 hrs<br>*Seizure control*<br>Loading dose: 3 mg/kg at rate not >25 mg/min<br>Maintenance infusion: 5–10 mg/kg/hr | Adverse effects: hypotension, bradycardia, seizures, asystole, and respiratory arrest<br>Contraindicated in patients with severe heart block. Significant widening of QRS complex or ventricular slowing suggests toxicity |
| Lorazepam (Ativan)<br>SL tab: 1, 2 mg<br>Oral tab: 0.5, 1, 2 mg<br>Inj: 4 mg/ml | SL, PO | *Preoperative sedation*<br>0.05 mg/kg/dose | Pediatric use not FDA approved<br>May cause apnea and hypotension when given IV |
|  | IV | *Status epilepticus*<br>0.05 mg/kg/dose; may repeat q15min prn for two doses<br>Maximum: 2 mg/dose, 8 mg q12h | Dilute injection with equal volume of normal saline or 5% D/W and administer at a rate not to exceed 2 mg/min |

| Drug | Route | Dose | Comments |
|---|---|---|---|
| Magnesium citrate 5% (Citromag) | PO | *Cathartic* 4 ml/kg/dose Maximum: 200 ml/dose | Use caution in patients with reduced renal function |
| Maalox Susp: aluminum hydroxide 200 mg, magnesium hydroxide 200 mg/5 ml Tab: equivalent to 10 ml of suspension | PO | *Antacid* 0.5 ml/kg/dose after feeds or Infants, 2–5 ml after feeds, Children, 5–15 ml PO after meals and at bedtime | Aluminum and magnesium toxicity may occur in patients with renal failure |
| Magnesium sulfate Inj: 500 mg/ml = 2 mM/ml or 4 mEq/ml magnesium | IM, IV | *Hypomagnesemia* Initial dose: 25–50 mg/kg/dose (0.1–0.2 mmol/kg/dose) q4–6h for three to four doses; may repeat if necessary | For IV use, dilute to 10 mg/ml and infuse over 60 min Give IM doses as a 20% solution in children |
| | IV | Maintenance dose: 0.1–0.2 mmol/kg/day or 25–50 mg/kg/day Maximum: 1000 mg/day | Monitor blood pressure during infusion Caution needed in patients receiving digitalis preparations or those with impaired renal function |
| | PO | Cathartic: 250 mg/kg/dose q4–6h | Overdose results in CNS and respiratory depression, dysrhythmias, hypotension. Monitor for diminished deep tendon reflex Monitor magnesium levels Antidote: Calcium |
| Mannitol (Osmitrol) Soln: 5, 10, 15, 20% | IV | *Acutely increased intracranial pressure with decompensation* 0.25–1.0 gm/kg/dose over 10–30 min. May repeat q2h prn | Adjust rate to produce urine output of 5–10 ml/kg/hr Solutions of more than 20% should be administered with an inline filter |

**Table V-1.** (continued)

| Drug | Route | Dosage | Comments |
|------|-------|--------|----------|
| | | Maximum: 2 gm/kg/dose | Use only solutions that are clear and crystal free<br>May cause circulatory overload and electrolyte imbalances<br>Place Foley catheter prior to administration |
| Meperidine (Demerol)<br>Inj: 50, 75, 100 mg<br>Tab: 50 mg | IV<br>IM<br>SC<br>PO | *Analgesia*<br>1.0–1.5 mg/kg/dose. May repeat q3–4h prn<br>Maximum: 2 mg/kg/dose or 100 mg/dose, whichever is less | Dilute IV dose in small volume of IV fluid and give over 2–3 min<br>May cause respiratory depression, hypotension<br>Specific antidote for narcotic overdose: naloxone 0.01–0.10 mg/kg<br>Use with caution in patients with asthma, increased intracranial pressure, or cardiac dysrhythmias |
| Methylene blue<br>Inj: 1% (10 mg/ml) | IV | *Methemoglobinemia*<br>1–2 mg/kg/dose (0.1–0.2 ml/kg/dose) over 5 min. May repeat after 1 hour if cyanosis persists.<br>Maximum: 7 mg (0.7 ml)/kg | |
| Metronidazole (Flagyl)<br>Tab: 250 mg<br>Cap: 500 mg<br>Inj: 5 mg/ml<br>Premixed: 100 ml | PO<br><br><br>IV | *Anaerobic infections*<br>15–35 mg/kg/day divided q8h<br>Maximum: 2 gm/day<br>30 mg/kg/day divided q6h<br>Maximum: 4 gm/day IV | Avoid alcohol or alcohol-containing products with this drug.<br>Combination may cause disulfuram reaction<br>Dose reduction is recommended in |

| | | | |
|---|---|---|---|
| Inj: 500 mg lyophilized powder for reconstitution | PO | *Giardiasis*<br>15 mg/kg/day divided tid for 7 days<br>Maximum: 750 mg/day | patients with liver impairment<br>Administer IV not faster than 5 ml/min |
| | PO | *Amoebiasis*<br>35–50 mg/kg/day divided tid for 7–10 days<br>Maximum: 2.25 gm/day | |
| | PO | *Trichomonas vaginalis*<br>Children >13 yr, 2 gm one dose only | |
| Methylprednisolone sodium succinate (Solu-Medrol)<br>Inj: 40, 125, 500 mg, 1 g | IV | *Status asthmaticus*<br>Initial dose: 1–2 mg/kg<br>Subsequent dose: 2–8 mg/kg/day divided q6h for 1–5 days | Use diluent provided for reconstitution<br>In emergencies give IV undiluted over 5 min<br>For intermittent infusions, dilute to maximum concentration of 60 mg/ml in 5% D/W<br>Give over 20–30 min |
| Morphine<br>Inj: 2, 10, 15 mg/ml | IV, IM, SC | *Analgesia*<br>0.1–0.2 mg/kg/dose q4h prn<br>Maximum: 15 mg/dose | Give IV diluted 1 mg/ml slowly<br>For intermittent IV use, give IV undiluted slowly over 3–5 min<br>Give IM undiluted |
| | IV, SC | Continuous infusion—average: 0.01–0.04 mg/kg/hr | Begin with lowest dose and titrate as required to achieve adequate pain control<br>May cause hypotension and respiratory depression especially in infants less than 1 year old |

**Table V-1.** (continued)

| Drug | Route | Dosage | Comments |
|------|-------|--------|----------|
| Naloxone (Narcan)<br>Inj: 0.02, 0.40 mg/ml | IV | *Narcotic antagonist*<br>0.01 mg/kg/dose. If ineffective, give 0.1 mg/kg/dose. If ineffective, give 0.2 mg/kg/dose | Specific antidote for narcotic overdose is naloxone, 0.01–0.10 mg/kg/dose IV<br>For infusion information see Table V-3<br>Effect is short lived<br>Duration of action is less than that of morphine, so patients should be monitored closely<br>Must repeat dose q5–10min prn |
| Neostigmine<br>Inj: 0.5, 1.0, 2.5 mg/ml | IV | *Reversal of neuromuscular block*<br>0.04–0.06/kg/dose<br>Maximum: 2.5 mg/dose | Give together with or following atropine 0.02 mg/kg to prevent severe vagal reaction<br>Contraindicated in patients with gut, urinary obstruction, or sick sinus syndrome |
| Nitroprusside sodium (Nipride)<br>Inj: 50 mg | IV | 0.5 up to 8 µg/kg/min<br>Start with low dose (0.5–1.0 µg/kg/min) and titrate upwards to desired effect<br>Maximum cumulative dose: 2.5 mg/day | Give by continuous infusion only with an infusion control device in an intensive care area<br>Dilute in 5% D/W only and protect infusion from light<br>Monitor thiocyanate levels when treatment is longer than 48 hours and in patients with renal failure, and when dose is more than 3 µg/kg/min |

| Drug | Route | Dose | Comments |
|---|---|---|---|
| Nystatin (Nilstat)<br>Susp: 100,000 units/ml<br>Tab: 500,000 units | PO | *Oral candidiasis*<br>400,000–2,400,000 units/day divided q4–6h | Retain in mouth as long as possible before swallowing |
| Orciprenaline (Alupent)<br>Syrup: 2 mg/ml<br>Tab: 20 mg<br>Inh: 50 mg/ml<br>Aerosol: 750 µg/puff | PO<br><br><br>Inhale | 2.0 mg/kg/day divided tid or qid<br>Maximum: 20 mg/dose<br>Nebulizer: 0.01–0.03 ml/kg/dose in 3 ml normal saline q4–6h | |
| Oxacillin (Prostaphlin)<br>Inj: 250, 500, 1000, 2000, 4000 mg<br>Cap: 250, 500 mg<br>Soln: 50 mg/ml | IV, IM<br>PO | 150–200 mg/kg/day divided q6h<br>50–100 mg/kg/day divided q6H | Keep thiocyanate blood levels under 100 µg/ml (0.8 mmol/liter)<br>Prepare fresh solution q12h<br>For infusion information, see Table V-3<br>Do not administer with other drugs |
| Pancuronium (Pavulon)<br>Inj: 1, 2 mg/ml | IV | *Muscle paralysis*<br>0.05–0.10 mg/kg/dose, repeat q30min prn | To reverse effects of this drug give atropine, 0.02 mg/kg/dose or neostigmine, 0.04–0.06 kg/dose IV divided into three doses given 1–2 min apart |

**Table V-1.** (continued)

| Drug | Route | Dosage | Comments |
|---|---|---|---|
| Paraldehyde<br>Inj: 1 gm/ml | PR | *Anticonvulsant*<br>300 mg/kg/dose (0.3 ml/kg/dose) of paraldehyde diluted to a 50% solution with mineral oil or normal saline q4–6h | Give PR as a 50% solution diluted in mineral oil or normal saline<br>To make a 4% solution, mix 20 ml (20 gm) of paraldehyde with 480 ml of normal saline to make 500 ml of 4% paraldehyde |
| | IV | Loading dose: 200 mg/kg/dose (2 ml/kg/dose of 10% solution)—i.e., 1 ml of paraldehyde and 9 ml of normal saline—are given slowly over 15–20 min<br>Followed by a continuous infusion of 20 mg/kg/hr<br>(0.5 ml/kg/hr of a 4% solution) | Replace plastic tubing and syringes q4h<br>Protect solution from light<br>Adverse effects: pulmonary edema, hemorrhage, hypotension, local irritation, displacement of bilirubin from binding site<br>Reduce dose in patients with hepatic and renal impairment<br>Use with caution in patients with pulmonary disease<br>Routine use is discouraged in children except in the treatment of status resistant to initial therapy with first-line anticonvulsants |
| Penicillamine (Cuprimine)<br>Cap: 125, 250 mg | PO | *Heavy metal poisoning*<br>20–40 mg/kg/day divided qid<br>Maximum: 1.5 gm/day; for prolonged use, maximum dose is 40 mg/kg/day | Give between meals and at bedtime on empty stomach<br>For children, empty capsule into small amount of fruit juice before giving |

| Drug | Route | Dosage | Notes |
|---|---|---|---|
| Penicillin G sodium; potassium<br>Inj: 1, 5, 10 mu | IV, IM | 100,000–250,000 units/kg/day divided q4–6h<br>Maximum: 20 mu/day | Monitor urinalysis, complete blood count, differential count, platelets, renal function and liver function tests<br>600 mg = approximately 1 mu<br>Use sodium salt for large IV doses<br>1 mu = 1.7 mM sodium or potassium |
| Penicillin G benzathine (Bicillin-1200 LA)<br>Inj: 1.2 mu | IM | *Streptococcal pharyngitis*<br>Children under 27.3 kg (60 lb): 600,000 units for one dose<br>Children over 27.3 kg (60 lb): 1.2 mu for one dose | Administer by deep IM route only |
| | IM | *Rheumatic heart disease*<br>Prophylaxis: 1.2 mu once a month | |
| | IM | *Syphilis* (primary or secondary)<br>Under 1 yr duration: 50,000 units/kg once | |
| | | Maximum: 2.4 mu/dose | |
| Penicillin G procaine (Wycillin)<br>Inj: 500,000 units/ml | IM | 25,000–50,000 units/kg/day once daily or divided q12h<br>Maximum: 4.8 mu/day | Administer by deep IM route only<br>Multidose vials should be shaken thoroughly before withdrawing medication |
| Penicillin V potassium (phenoxymethyl penicillin)<br>Tab: 125, 250, 300 mg | PO | 25–50 mg/kg/day divided q6–8h<br>Maximum: 3 gm/day | 250 mg = approximately 400,000 units<br>Better absorbed than penicillin G |
| Susp: 25, 50 mg/ml | PO | *Prophylaxis in asplenics*<br>Under 5 yr, 125–250 mg bid | |
| | PO | *Prophylaxis in rheumatic fever*<br>Under 5 yr, 125–250 mg bid | |

**Table V-1.** (continued)

| Drug | Route | Dosage | Comments |
|---|---|---|---|
| Phenobarbital<br>Inj: 30, 120 mg/ml<br>Tab: 15, 30, 60, 100 mg<br>Liq: 5 mg/ml | IV<br><br>IV, IM, PO | *Status epilepticus*<br>Loading dose: 10–15 mg/kg<br>Maximum loading dose, 30–40 mg/kg<br>Maintenance dose: Start 12–24 hr after loading dose—3–5 mg/kg/day divided bid | Administer loading dose at a rate not >1 mg/kg/min or 60 mg/min, whichever is less<br>Monitoring serum drug concentrations is recommended<br>Therapeutic range is 65–170 μmol/liter (15–40 μg/ml)<br>May be given direct IV or diluted 1:1 volume/volume in IV fluids<br>Large IV doses may cause respiratory arrest or hypotension, especially when given with diazepam<br>$T_{1/2}$ = 96 hr in children |
| Phenytoin sodium (Dilantin)<br>Inj: 50 mg/ml<br>Susp: 6, 25 mg/ml<br>Chew tab: 50 mg<br>Cap: 30, 100 mg | IV<br><br>IV, PO | *Status epilepticus*<br>Loading dose: 15–20 mg/kg<br>Maximum: 1 gm/dose or 25 mg/kg<br>*Maintenance dose in epilepsy*<br>Children 5–10 mg/kg/day divided q8h | Administer at a rate not > 0.5 mg/kg/min or 50 mg/min, whichever is less, undiluted or diluted in normal saline to 5 mg/ml just prior to administration<br>Do not give in dextrose solutions<br>Maintenance dose requirements are variable in pediatric population.<br>Adjust dose to keep serum phenytoin within range of 40–80 μmol/liter (10–20 μg/ml)<br>Measure serum phenytoin level 1 hr after loading dose or before |

| Drug | Route | Dosage | Comments |
|---|---|---|---|
| | | | maintenance doses. Commence maintenance dose 6 hr after loading dose or when serum phenytoin level is less than 60 mmol/liter (15 µg/ml). If hypotension develops, slow infusion rate |
| Potassium chloride solution (Kaochlor) 20 mmol/15 ml (20 mEq/15 ml) Inj: 2mmol/ml (2 mEq/ml; 1 mmol = 1 meq) | IV, PO | 2–3 mmol/kg/day continuous IV infusion or PO in two or three divided doses | IV doses must be diluted to maximum concentration of 60 mmol/liter via peripheral line. Use infusion control device. Maximum rate, 0.5 mmol/kg/hr. Caution in patients with renal impairment or those taking potassium sparing diuretics |
| Potassium phosphate Inj: 4.4 mmol K/ml, 3.0 mmol P/ml | IV | *Uncomplicated hypophosphatemia* 0.15–0.33 mM/kg/dose; repeat as required to maintain serum phosphorus levels > 2 mg/dl (0.65 mmol/liter) | Dosage must be expressed in terms of mM $PO_4$. Dilute in normal saline and infuse over 6 hr. Use caution with added $K^+$ content. Phosphate may also be given as sodium salt. Serum potassium, phosphorus, and calcium should be monitored as a guide to dosage |
| | IV | Maintenance dose: 0.5–1.5 mM/kg/24 hr | |
| Pralidoxime (Protopam) Inj: 1 gm | | 25–50 mg/kg/dose slowly; repeat after 1 hr if weakness and fasciculations persist. Then give q8–12h prn | Use with 0.05 mg/kg atropine repeated q30–60min to maintain atropinization |

**Table V-1.** (continued)

| Drug | Route | Dosage | Comments |
|------|-------|--------|----------|
| | | Maximum: 1 gm | Administer IV infusions over 15–30 min at a rate not exceeding 200 mg/min<br>For more rapid effect, 50 mg/ml solution can be administered over 5–10 min |
| Prednisone (Deltasone)<br>Tab: 1, 5, 50 mg | PO | *Antiinflammatory/Asthma*<br>0.5–2.0 mg/kg/day in single or two divided doses. Adjust to response | Give with food or milk to avoid gastric irritation<br>Alternate day dosing recommended |
| Prochlorperazine (Stemetil)<br>Tab: 5, 10 mg<br>Liq: 1 mg/ml<br>Inj: 5 mg/ml<br>Suppos: 10 mg | IM<br><br><br><br>PO, PR | *Antiemetic or sedative*<br>In children >10 kg or >2 yr, give 0.14 mg/kg/day once only or divided q6–8h by deep IM injection<br>Maximum: 40 mg/day<br>0.4 mg/kg/day divided q6–8h | May cause extrapyramidal effects, restlessness, and excitement<br>Do not administer to children <2 years old or <10 kg<br>IV route is not recommended for use in children |
| Promethazine (Phenergan)<br>Tab: 10, 25, 50 mg<br>Liq: 2 mg/ml<br>Inj: 25 mg/ml | PO<br><br>IM, PO, PR<br><br>PO<br><br>PO | *Antihistamine*<br>0.1 mg/kg/dose repeated q6h and 0.5 mg/kg/dose qhs prn<br>*Antiemetic*<br>0.25–0.5 mg/kg/dose repeated q4–6h prn<br>*Motion sickness*<br>0.5 mg/kg/dose repeated q12h prn<br>*Sedative and preoperative*<br>0.5–1.0 mg/kg/dose q6h prn | Give IM deep in large muscle mass<br>Not recommended in children <2 years of age<br>May cause drowsiness, dystonic reactions, or paradoxical excitement in children<br>Use with caution in children with a history of sleep apnea, or in those with a family history of sudden infant death syndrome |

| Drug | Route | Dose | Comments |
|---|---|---|---|
| Propranolol (Inderal)<br>Tab: 10, 20, 40, 80 mg<br>Inj: 1 mg/ml | IV | *Antidysrhythmic*<br>0.01–0.15 mg/kg/dose q6–8h prn<br>Maximum: 3 mg/dose | Give by slow IV push at a rate not >1 mg/min and monitor ECG continuously |
| | IV | *Tetralogy spells*<br>0.05–0.10 mg/kg/dose given over 10 min | Contraindicated in second- and third-degree heart block, bronchial asthma, congestive heart failure, and sinus bradycardia |
| | PO | Maintenance dose: 0.5–4.0 mg/kg/day divided tid or qid<br>Maximum: 10 mg/kg/day | Use caution in patients with renal and hepatic disease<br>Cimetidine will reduce clearance of propranolol<br>Weight-adjusted dose is an approximation for initial therapy. Dose must be adjusted according to the therapeutic response of the patient |
| Pyrvinium pamoate (Vanquin)<br>Susp: 10 mg/ml<br>Tab: 50 mg | PO | 11 mg/kg/dose once<br>Maximum dose 1 gm | Take immediately after a meal<br>Stains clothing and teeth<br>Repeat dose after 2 weeks |
| Ranitidine (Zantac)<br>Tab: 150, 300 mg<br>Inj: 25 mg/ml | PO<br>IM<br>IV | 2.5–3.8 mg/kg/day divided q12h<br>1.25–1.9 mg/kg/day divided q6–12h<br>Maximum: 300 mg/day | Dilute IV dose in normal saline or 5% D/W to a concentration of 0.5–2.5 mg/ml and infuse over 20 min<br>Decrease dose to 25–50% in patients with severe renal impairment<br>Give IM doses undiluted |

**Table V-1.** (continued)

| Drug | Route | Dosage | Comments |
|---|---|---|---|
| Ribavirin (Virazole)<br>Vial: 6 gm | Inhale | 1 vial (6 gm)/day via SPAG-2 (small particle aerosol generator) for 3–7 days | Reconstitute vial with 60 ml sterile water for injection. Transfer contents to flask and dilute to 300 ml (20 mg/ml) with sterile water for inhalation |
| Rifampin (Rimactane)<br>Cap: 150, 300 mg | PO<br><br>PO | *Haemophilus influenza prophylaxis*<br>20 mg/kg/day once a day for 4 days<br>Maximum: 600 mg/day<br>*Meningococcal prophylaxis*<br>20 mg/kg/day divided q12h for 2 days<br>Maximum: 1200 mg/day | May discolor urine, sweat, saliva, and tears<br>A suspension of 20 mg/ml in simple syrup can be compounded for children<br>See p. 250 |
| Salbutamol, albuterol (Ventolin)<br>Liq: 0.4 mg/ml<br>Inh: 5 mg/ml<br>Metered aerosol: 100 μg/puff<br>Rotacaps: 200, 400 μg<br><br>Inj: 0.5 mg/ml | Inhale<br><br><br>Puff<br><br><br>IV | 0.01–0.03 ml/kg/dose of 0.5% inhalation solution in 3 ml of normal saline via nebulizer q20 min–4h<br>Maximum: 1 ml<br>1–2 puffs q4–6h prn<br>Maximum: 8 puffs/day<br>0.5–1.0 μg/kg/min. Increase dose as required q15min to a maximum of 10 μg/kg/min | Tachycardia, hypoglycemia<br>For infusion information see Table V-3<br>See Table V-3 for infusion |
| Sodium bicarbonate<br>Tab: 2, 4 mg<br>Inj: 8.4% (1 mmol/ml); 4.2% (0.5 mmol/ml)<br>Note: 1 mmol = 1 mEq | PO<br>IV | 0.3–0.6 mg/kg/day divided tid or qid<br>*Cardiac arrest*<br>0.5–1.0 mmol/kg/dose q10min as required for prolonged arrest or documented metabolic acidosis | Indicated in patients with metabolic acidosis with adequate ventilation<br>Use only after adequate alveolar ventilation is established |

| | | | |
|---|---|---|---|
| Sodium chloride: Available as the following solutions:<br>0.2% = 0.34 mmol/10 ml<br>0.3% = 0.56 mmol/10 ml<br>0.45% = 0.77 mmol/10 ml<br>0.9% = 1.54 mmol/10 ml<br>3.0% = 5.16 mmol/10 ml<br>5.0% = 8.6 mmol/10 ml<br>Note: 1 mmol = 1 mEq | IV | *Hyponatremia*<br>Calculate sodium deficit in mM = desired plasma sodium (mmol/liter) − current plasma sodium (mmol/liter) × 0.6 × body weight (kg) | Molecular weight of NaCl = 58.5 |
| Sodium polystyrene sulfonate (Kayexalate) | PO | *Hyperkalemia*<br>1 gm/kg/dose q6h prn | Exchanges approximately 1 mmol potassium per gram of resin (1 mEq/gram of resin) |
| | PR | 1 gm/kg/dose q2–6h prn. For rectal use, use a cleansing enema. Place resin high in the sigmoid colon. Resin should be retained for 30–45 min. Remove with saline enema. | Suspend 1 gm of resin in 4 ml of 25% sorbitol<br>Monitor serum K⁺ q12h or daily |
| Sodium thiopental (Pentothal) 1, 5 gm containers for preparation of 2.5% solutions | IV | *General anesthetic*<br>4–6 mg/kg IV push over 30 sec–1 min | Avoid extravasation<br>Monitor for respiratory depression, hypotension |
| | IV | *Seizures*<br>Loading dose: 3–5 mg/kg IV followed by 2–4 mg/kg/hr by continuous infusion | Monitoring serum drug concentrations recommended when used for seizure control |
| Succinylcholine (Suxamethonium, Quelicin) Inj: 20 mg/ml | IV | *Endotracheal intubation*<br>Infants and children: 1–2 mg/kg<br>Administer by rapid IV push over 10–30 sec. Flush with normal saline or 5% D/W | Ultra short-acting depolarizing muscle relaxant. Onset 1 min, duration 2–5 min, recovery 4–10 min<br>Monitor for bradycardia, hyperkalemia |

**Table V-1.** (continued)

| Drug | Route | Dosage | Comments |
|------|-------|--------|----------|
| Spironolactone (Aldactone)<br>Tab: 25, 100 mg<br>2 mg/ml oral suspension can be prepared | PO | 1–4 mg/kg/day as single daily dose or divided bid–qid | Contraindicated in patients with airway abnormalities, burns, hyperkalemia, demyelinating disease, open eye injury and malignant hyperthermia |
| Terbutaline (Bricanyl)<br>Tab: 2.5, 5 mg<br>Spacer: 200 doses 0.25 mg/dose<br>Inj: 1 mg/ml (USA) | PO<br>Puff<br>Inhale<br><br>SC | 0.1–0.3 mg/kg/day divided tid–qid<br>1–2 puffs qid<br>0.03 ml/kg diluted with 1.5 ml normal saline and repeated q4–6h.<br>Maximum dose 1 ml<br>0.005–0.01 kg/dose<br>May repeat in 15–30 min for 3 doses<br>Maximum dose 0.4 mg | Often combined with other diuretics for its potassium-sparing effect<br>Use KCl supplements with caution in children taking this drug<br>Manufacturer does not recommend use in children <12 years of age |
| Theophylline<br>Controlled release capsule: 50, 75, 100, 250 mg (Somophyllin 12)<br>Sustained release tablet: 100, 200, 300 mg (Theo-Dur)<br>Soln: 80 mg/15 ml (Theolair) | PO | *Asthma*<br>Maximum maintenance doses prior to serum concentration monitoring<br>Infants<br>26–52 wk − (0.2 × [age in weeks] + 5) mg/kg/day<br>Children<br>1–9 yr, 24 mg/kg/day | Measure serum theophylline levels at steady state (55–110 µmol/liter) (10–20 mg/liter)<br>Do not use as a bronchodilator in children <6 months of age<br>Select dosing interval appropriate for product selected |

| Drug | Route | Dosing | Comments |
|---|---|---|---|
| | | 9–12 yr, 20 mg/kg/day<br>Adolescents<br>18 mg/kg/day<br>Over 16 yr, 14 mg/kg/day<br>Maximum dose is 900 mg/day | |
| Ticarcillin (Ticar)<br>Inj: 1, 3, 6, 20 gm | IV, IM | *Severe infections*<br>200–300 mg/kg/day divided q4–6h<br>Maximum: 24 gm/day<br>*Cystic fibrosis*<br>600 mg/kg/day divided q6h | Each gram contains approximately 5.0 mmol (120 mg) of $Na^+$<br>Activity similar to carbenicillin<br>Increase dosing interval in patients with reduced renal function |
| Thioridazine (Mellaril)<br>Liq: 30 mg/ml, 2 mg/ml<br>Tab: 10, 25, 50, 100, 200 mg | PO | *Antipsychotic, agitation*<br>Young children: up to 3 mg/kg/day | Clinical experience is limited<br>Psychiatrist should be consulted |
| Tobramycin (Nebcin)<br>Inj: 10, 40 mg/ml | IV, IM | 3.0–7.5 mg/kg/day divided q8h<br>Maximum: 100 mg/initial dose<br>*Cystic fibrosis*<br>12 mg/kg/day divided q8h | Serum level monitoring is recommended (peaks, 5–10 mg/liter, troughs, less than 2 mg/liter)<br>Increase dosing interval in patients with reduced renal function |
| Vancomycin (Vancocin)<br>Inj: 500 mg | IV<br><br>IV<br><br>PO | *Bacterial infections*<br>40 mg/kg/day divided q6h<br>Maximum: 2 gm/day<br>*Meningitis*<br>60 mg/kg/day divided q6h<br>Maximum: 4 gm/day<br>*Pseudomembranous colitis*<br>50 mg/kg/day divided q6h<br>Maximum: 500 mg/day | Serum level monitoring is recommended. Peak is 1 hr after 1-hr infusion (25–40 mg/liter); trough is 0.5 hr before infusion (5–10 mg/liter)<br>Minimum dilution for IV use is 5 mg/ml<br>For pseudomembranous colitis use injectable product orally<br>Increase dosing interval in patients with renal impairment |

**Table V-1.** (continued)

| Drug | Route | Dosage | Comments |
|------|-------|--------|----------|
| Verapamil (Isoptin)<br>Inj: 2.5 mg/ml | IV | *Supraventricular tachycardia*<br>0.075–0.300 mg/kg/dose over 30–60 sec; may repeat once in 30 min if necessary<br>Maximum: 5 mg first dose; 10 mg repeat dose | Give IV undiluted over 2 min<br>Contraindicated in infants, in patients receiving beta blockers, in those with severe low cardiac output or significant intracardiac R-L shunts unless related to tachycardia<br>Can cause hypotension with rapid administration of large doses<br>Have calcium chloride available |
| | PO | 4–10 mg/kg/day PO divided tid or qid | |

**Table V-2. Drug dosage guidelines in neonates**

| Drug | Route | Dosage | Comments |
|---|---|---|---|
| Acetaminophen (Tylenol; Tempra) Liq: 32 mg/ml; 80 mg/ml | PO, PR | 5 mg/kg/dose q4–6h prn Maximum: 25 mg/kg/day | Overdose results in delayed hepatotoxicity Contraindicated in patients with G6PD deficiency |
| Acyclovir (Zovirax) Inj: 500 mg | IV | *Herpes simplex infections* 30 mg/kg/day divided q8h for 10–14 days | Infuse over 60 min Adverse reactions noted include transient renal dysfunction, thrombophlebitis Increase dosing interval in patients with reduced renal function |
| Albumin Inj: 25% | IV | 0.5–1.0 gm/kg/dose | 25% albumin to be diluted to 5% with normal saline |
| Amikacin (Amikin) Inj: 250 mg/ml | IM, IV | Weight >2 kg: 0–7 days old: 20 mg/kg/day divided q12h 7–28 days old: 30 mg/kg/day divided q8h | Increase dosing interval in patients with reduced renal function Monitoring of serum drug concentrations recommended |
| Aminophylline Inj: 25 mg/ml Liq: 5 mg/ml (compounded) | IV, IM | *Apnea* Loading dose: 5–6 mg/kg/dose Maintenance dose: 2–3 mg/kg/dose q12h | In older infants the dosage requirements may increase to 20–25 mg/kg/day, and the interval of administration may need to be shortened to q4–8h Adverse effects: tachycardia, hyperglycemia, and jitteriness |

**Table V-2.** (continued)

| Drug | Route | Dosage | Comments |
|------|-------|--------|----------|
| Ampicillin (Penbritin)<br>Inj: 250, 500, 1000, 2000 mg | IV | *Meningitis*<br>Weight >2 kg:<br>0–7 days: 150 mg/kg/day divided q8h<br>7 days–28 days: 200 mg/kg/day divided q6h<br>*Other*<br>Weight >2 kg:<br>0–7 days: 75 mg/kg/day divided q8h<br>7–28 days: 100 mg/kg/day divided q6h | Increase dosing interval in patients with reduced renal function |
| Atropine<br>Inj: 0.4, 0.6 mg/ml | IV, ETT | 0.01 mg/kg/dose. May repeat q10–15min prn<br>Minimum dose: 0.1 mg<br>Maximum dose: 0.04 mg/kg | Indicated for bradycardia, presumed to be vagal in origin. Premedication for intubation, not required for resuscitation |
| Calcium gluconate<br>Inj: 10% | IV | *Symptomatic hypocalcemia*<br>2 ml/kg/dose slow IV over 30 min<br>Maintenance infusion: 2–4 ml/kg/day over 24h | Contains elemental $Ca^{2+}$ 0.46 mEq/ml (9 mg/ml)<br>Monitor closely for bradycardia and extravasation |
| Cefotaxime (Claforan)<br>Inj: 500, 1000, 2000 mg | IV, IM | Weight >2 kg:<br>0–7 days: 100 mg/kg/day divided q12h<br>7–28 days: 150 mg/kg/day divided q8h | Increase dosing interval in patients with reduced renal function |
| Chloramphenicol (Pentamycetin)<br>Inj: 1000 mg | IV | Weight >2 kg:<br>0–7 days: 25 mg/kg/day once a day<br>7–28 days: 50 mg/kg/day divided q12h | Reduce dose in patients with hepatic dysfunction<br>Monitor serum drug concentrations |

| Drug | Route | Dose | Comments |
|------|-------|------|----------|
| Cimetidine (Tagamet)<br>Inj: 150 mg/ml<br>Liq: 60 mg/ml | IV, PO | Term: 15 mg/kg/day divided q4–6h | Reduce dose in patients with reduced renal function |
| Clindamycin (Dalacin C)<br>Inj: 150 mg/ml | IV | Weight >2 kg:<br>0–7 days: 15 mg/kg/day divided q8h<br>7–28 days: 20 mg/kg/day divided q6h | Reduce dose in patients with hepatic dysfunction<br>Inadequate pharmacokinetic studies in neonates |
| Cloxacillin (Orbenin)<br>Inj: 250, 500, 2000 mg<br>Susp: 25 mg/ml | PO | Weight >2 kg:<br>0–7 days: 75 mg/kg/day divided q8h<br>7–28 days: 100 mg/kg/day divided q6h | Double dose for meningitis |
| Diazepam (Valium)<br>Inj: 5 mg/ml | IV | *Seizures*<br>0.1–0.2 mg/kg/dose by slow IV push over 2 min. Repeat q5–10min prn up to total dose of 1 mg/kg | Indication: not used as a first-line anticonvulsant<br>Short-term adjunctive therapy in status epilepticus<br>Risk of CNS and respiratory depression, hypotension, and phlebitis. Contraindicated in hyperbilirubinemic neonates |
| | PR | 0.5 mg/kg/dose; parenteral preparation to be used in conjunction with a syringe and catheter inserted into rectum | |
| Digoxin (Lanoxin)<br>Inj: 0.05 mg/ml<br>Liq: 0.05 mg/ml | IV | Loading dose: Given in three divided doses (one-half, one-fourth, one-fourth) q8h<br>Preterm: 20–30 µg/kg IV<br>Full term: 40 µg/kg IV | The oral dose is 25% more than the IV dose<br>Increase dosing interval in patients with reduced renal function.<br>Monitor serum drug concentrations |

**Table V-2.** (continued)

| Drug | Route | Dosage | Comments |
|---|---|---|---|
| | | Maintenance dose: Start maintenance dose 24 hours after last loading dose in preterm neonates and 12 hours after in full-term neonates. Preterm: 6–8 µg/kg/day IV divided q12h<br>Full-term: 10–12 µg/kg/day IV divided q12h | Doses are for congestive heart failure. Higher doses may be required for the treatment of dysrhythmias. Therapeutic serum levels are 1.3–2.6 nmol/liter |
| Dopamine (Inotropin)<br>Inj: 40 mg/ml | IV | Continuous IV infusion: Initial dose: 2–5 µg/kg/min increasing gradually up to 20 µg/kg/min for desired cardiac/vascular effects | Dose depends on pharmacologic effects: Renal: 2–5 µg/kg/min<br>Inotropic: 5–10 µg/kg/min<br>Vasoconstrictive: >10 µg/kg/min |
| Epinephrine (Adrenalin)<br>Inj: 1:10,000 (0.1 mg/ml) | IV, ETT | *Asystole or severe bradycardia*<br>0.1 ml/kg/dose | |
| Erythromycin (Ilosone)<br>Susp: 50 mg/ml | PO | Weight >2 kg:<br>0–7 days: 20 mg/kg/day divided q12h<br>7–28 days: 30–40 mg/kg/day divided q8h | Reduce dose in patients with reduced liver function or markedly reduced renal function<br>Monitor serum bilirubin, alkaline phosphatase, serum transaminases<br>Adverse effects: intrahepatic cholestasis |
| Furosemide (Lasix)<br>Inj: 10 mg/ml<br>Liq: 10 mg/ml | IV, IM, PO | Term: 1 mg/kg/dose q12h<br>Maximum dose: 2 mg/kg/dose | For IV administration give slow IV push over 2–3 min<br>Adverse effects: ototoxicity, hypokalemia, hypochloremia, |

| Drug | Route | Dose | Comments |
|---|---|---|---|
| | | | hyponatremia, hypercalciuria, nephrocalcinosis, metabolic alkalosis |
| Gentamicin (Garamycin)<br>Inj: 10 mg/ml | IV | 0–7 days:<br>>35 wk GA: 2.5 mg/kg/dose q12h<br>7–28 days:<br>>35 wk PCA: 2.5 mg/kg/dose q8h | Reduce dose in patients with reduced renal function<br>Monitor serum levels |
| Glucagon<br>Inj: 1 mg | IM | *Hypoglycemia*<br>30 µg/kg/dose. Dose may be repeated after 6–12 hr | Limited use.<br>Transient effect, must be followed by IV dextrose infusion (see below) |
| | IV | 1.0–1.5 mg/day via continuous infusion over 24 hr. Infuse in dextrose solutions only; incompatible with electrolyte solutions | |
| Glucose (Dextrose)<br>Inj: 10% | IV | *Hypoglycemia*<br>0.25 gm/kg/dose (2.5 ml) followed by a continuous infusion of 5–8 mg/kg/min (3.0–4.8 ml/kg/hr) | Hyperglycemia |
| Hydralazine (Apresoline)<br>Inj: 20 mg/ml | IV, IM | *Hypertension*<br>0.1–0.5 mg/kg/dose q6h prn. Increase dose gradually in increments of 0.1 mg/kg/dose every 6 hr prn.<br>Maximum dose: 4 mg/kg/day | Dose requirements may be decreased to less than 0.15 mg/kg/dose when used in conjunction with other antihypertensives<br>Rebound tachycardia may occur. |
| Isoproterenol (Isuprel)<br>Inj: 1:5000 (0.2 mg/ml) | IV | 0.1–1.0 µg/kg/min by continuous IV infusion | Adjust rate of infusion to keep heart rate <200 bpm |
| Morphine<br>Inj: 2, 10, 15 mg/ml | IV, IM, SC | 0.025 mg/kg/dose q4h prn<br>Continuous infusion: 0.01–0.04 mg/kg/hr | Give slow IV push over 3–5 min<br>Adverse effects: respiratory depression, hypotension |

**Table V-2.** (continued)

| Drug | Route | Dosage | Comments |
|------|-------|--------|----------|
| Naloxone (neonatal Narcan)<br>Inj: 0.02 mg/ml | IV, IM, SC | 0.01–0.02 mg/kg/dose q5–10min prn | Naloxone is specific antidote<br>Duration of effect approximately 35–45 min<br>Can cause acute withdrawal in infants born to narcotic-addicted mothers |
| Oxacillin (Bactocill)<br>Inj: 250, 500 mg | IV, IM | Weight >2 kg:<br>0–7 days: 75 mg/kg/day divided q8h<br>7–28 days: 150 mg/kg/day divided q6h | |
| Pancuronium (Pavulon)<br>Inj: 2 mg/ml | IV | 0–1 wk: 0.03 mg/kg/dose<br>1–2 wk: 0.06 mg/kg/dose<br>2–4 wk: 0.09 mg/kg/dose<br>>4 wk: 0.1 mg/kg/dose<br>Administer q2–4h prn | Infuse by slow IV push over 3–5 min<br>Must be able to support ventilation<br>Effects potentiated in hypothermia, acidosis, renal impairment, hypokalemia, hypermagnesemia, and by aminoglycosides |
| Paraldehyde<br>Inj: 1 gm/ml | IV | Loading dose: 150 mg/kg/hr of a 5% solution for 3 hr<br>Maintenance dose: 20 mg/kg/hr by continuous infusion using a 5% solution | Undiluted paraldehyde contains 1 gm/ml<br>For IV administration, add 5 ml (5 gm) to 100 ml normal saline or 5% D/W to make a 5% solution.<br>Administer via an autosyringe pump with a glass syringe. IV tubing and syringe must be protected from light by wrapping. |
| | PR | 300 mg/kg/dose q4–6h prn. Dissolve dose in equal volume of mineral oil prior to administration | |

| | | | |
|---|---|---|---|
| **Phenobarbital**<br>Inj: 30, 60 mg/ml<br>Liq: 5 mg/ml | IV<br><br>IV, IM, PO | *Seizures*<br>Loading dose: 15–20 mg/kg/dose over 10 min (not > than 1 mg/kg/min)<br>Maintenance dose: 3–5 mg/kg/day divided q12–24h. First dose 24 hr after loading dose | IV tubing and syringe (if plastic) must be replaced every 4 hr<br>If seizures continue after initial loading dose, additional doses of 5 mg/kg/dose spaced at 20–30 min intervals can be given up to a total dose of 40 mg/kg to achieve plasma concentrations of up to 40 µg/ml (170 µmol/liter). Ensure adequate respiratory control if using high doses |
| **Phenytoin (Dilantin)**<br>Inj: 50 mg/ml | IV<br><br>IV | *Neonatal seizures*<br>Loading dose: 18 mg/kg slow IV (not >0.5 mg/kg/min)<br>Maintenance dose: 5–10 mg/kg/day q12–24h (first dose given when it is estimated that serum level will fall to 60 µmol/liter (15 mg/liter). | Infuse in normal saline only.<br>Rapid IV administration may cause hypotension and bradycardia<br>Indicated in neonatal seizures refractory to phenobarbital alone<br>Frequent serum level monitoring essential in first 3 weeks of life due to rapid changes in elimination rate |
| **Propranolol (Inderal)**<br>Inj: 1 mg<br>Susp: 1 mg/ml (compounded) | IV | *Dysrhythmia*<br>0.01–0.15 mg/kg/dose slow IV over 10 min. May be repeated in 10 min | Contraindicated in congestive heart failure |

**Table V-2.** (continued)

| Drug | Route | Dosage | Comments |
|------|-------|--------|----------|
| | | *Tetralogy spells* 0.1 mg/kg slow IV. May be repeated once in 15 min | |
| | PO | *Other* 0.25–1.00 mg/kg/day divided q6–8h | |
| Prostaglandin E₁ (Prostin VR) Inj: 500 μg | IV, IA | Initial dose: 0.05–0.10 μg/kg/min Maintenance dose: Once stable, may decrease initial dose by one-half or less | May cause apnea, fever, jitteriness, cutaneous flush along course of vein |
| Pyridoxine Inj: 100 mg/ml | IV IV, PO | Initial dose: 50–100 mg/dose over 1–2 min Maintenance dose: 50–100 mg/dose divided q24h | Indicated for diagnosis and treatment of pyridoxine-dependent seizures Initial dosing should be accompanied by EEG monitoring No toxicity reported with therapeutic doses |
| Sodium bicarbonate Inj: 4.2% | IV | *Documented metabolic acidosis* 0.5 mEq/kg/dose slow IV over 5 min | Ensure adequate ventilation to have an effect Hypernatremia |
| Sodium polystyrene sulfonate (Kayexalate) Susp: 0.25 gm/ml in 25% sorbitol | PR, PO | *Hyperkalemia* 1 gm/kg/dose q6h (make suspension containing 0.25 gm/ml in sorbitol 25%) | Exchanges approximately 0.5–2.0 mEq of potassium/gm of resin Monitor serum electrolytes |
| Spironolactone (Aldactone) Susp: 2 mg/ml (compounded) | PO | 1–3 mg/kg/day divided q12–24h | Monitor serum potassium |

| Drug | Route | Dose | Comments |
|---|---|---|---|
| Tobramycin (Nebecin)<br>Inj: 10 mg/ml | IV, IM | Same dose as for gentamicin. | |
| Tolazoline (Priscoline)<br>Inj: 25 mg/ml | IV | Loading dose: 1–2 mg/kg/dose IV bolus<br>Maintenance dose: 1–2 mg/kg/hr continuous infusion | Emergency release—investigational agent (Canada)<br>Monitor for hypotension |
| Vancomycin (Vancocin)<br>Inj: 500 mg vial | IV | Infants >37 wk PCA: 22.5 mg/kg/dose q12h | Monitor serum drug concentrations<br>Increase dosing interval in patients with reduced renal function |
| Vitamin K (phytonadione)<br>Inj: 1 mg/0.5 ml, 10 mg/ml | IM, SC<br><br>IM, IV | *Hemorrhagic disease of newborn*<br>Prophylaxis: 0.5–1.0 mg at birth<br>Treatment: 1 mg/kg/dose (if given IV, administer at a rate not to exceed 1 mg/min) | |

Key: GA = gestational age; PCA = postconceptional age.

## Table V-3. Infusion guidelines

| Drug | Dilution (mg or ml/50 ml IV fluid) | Infusion rate | Dose delivered | Dose range | Compatibilities and compatible solutions | Incompatibilities | Comments |
|---|---|---|---|---|---|---|---|
| Alcohol, ethyl 99% | 5 ml to make (10%) | 1.4 ml/kg/hr | 140 mg/kg/hr | Titrate to keep in therapeutic range | 5% D/W, NS | Lactated Ringer's, Ringer's soln. | Range 100–150 mg/dl |
| Alprostadil (prostaglandin E1) | $0.3 \times$ wt (kg) | 1 ml/hr | 0.1 µg/kg/min | 0.05–0.1 µg/kg/min | 5% D/W, 10% D/W, KCl, NS, epinephrine, isoproterenol | NaHCO$_3$, calcium, MgSO$_4$, aminophylline | Can cause apnea, fever, flushing |
| Aminophylline | 50 mg | 1 ml/kg/hr | 1 mg/kg/hr | Titrate to keep in therapeutic range | 5% D/W, 10% D/W, NS, D5NS, LR, calcium | Epinephrine, insulin, MVI, heparin, ascorbic acid, morphine | Therapeutic range is 10–20 mg/L (55–110 µmol/L) |
| Calcium chloride | $130 \times$ wt (kg) | 1 ml/hr | 0.5 mM/kg/day (1 mEq/kg/day) | 1–3 mEq/kg/day | Most common IV solutions, dopamine, isoproterenol, lidocaine, heparin | Epinephrine, NaHCO$_3$, phosphate, tetracycline, chloramphenicol, cefazolin | Can cause hypercalcemia Give via central line |
| Dopamine | $15 \times$ wt (kg) | 1 ml/hr | 5 µg/kg/min | 2–20 µg/kg/min | 5% D/W, 10% D/W, NS, LR, heparin, KCl, lidocaine, CaCl$_2$ | Alkaline solutions, (e.g., NaHCO$_3$), phenytoin, aminophylline | Give via central line if possible |
| Epinephrine | $0.3 \times$ wt (kg) | 1 ml/hr | 0.1 µg/kg/min | 0.05–1.00 µg/kg/min | 5% D/W, NS, heparin, dopamine, KCl vitamin B and C, | Alkaline solutions (e.g., NaHCO$_3$) | Do not mix with other drugs |

| Drug | Preparation | Rate | Concentration | Dose range | Compatible solutions | Incompatible | Comments |
|---|---|---|---|---|---|---|---|
| | | | | | calcium $Cl_2$, lidocaine | | |
| Fentanyl | 0.05 × wt (kg) | 1 ml/hr | 1 µg/kg/hr | 1–2 µg/kg/hr | 5% D/W, NS, 5% D/RL, heparin, hydrocortisone KCl, vit B and C complex | Pentobarbital, acidic solutions | Narcotic Can cause respiratory depression and chest wall immobility Antidote is naloxone |
| Insulin (CZI regular) | 5 units | 1 ml/kg/hr | 0.1 unit/kg/hr | 0.05–0.2 unit/kg/hr | NS, cimetidine, lidocaine, KCl | Aminophylline, phenytoin, phenobarbital, $NaHCO_3$ | Preflush tubing with insulin solution |
| Isoproterenol | inotrope: 0.075 × wt  bronchodilator: 0.3 × wt | 1 ml/hr  1 ml/hr | 0.025 µg/kg/min  0.1 µg/kg/min | 0.05–0.50 µg/kg/min  0.1–0.8 µg/kg/min. | NS, 5% D/W, calcium salts, heparin, KCl, MVI | Aminophylline, epinephrine, $NaHCO_3$, lidocaine, barbiturates | Discard solution after 12 hr |
| Lidocaine | 30 × wt | 2 ml/hr | 20 µg/kg/min | 20–50 µg/kg/min | Most common IV solutions, aminophylline, calcium, KCl, dopamine, heparin, insulin | $NaHCO_3$ | |
| Morphine | 0.5 × wt | 1 ml/hr | 10 µg/kg/hr | 10–60 µg/kg/hr | Most common IV solutions | Heparin | Titrate to achieve desired analgesic effect Can cause hypotension and respiratory depression Antidote is naloxone |

**Table V-3.** (continued)

| Drug | Dilution (mg or ml/50 ml IV fluid) | Infusion rate | Dose delivered | Dose range | Compatibilities and compatible solutions | Incompatibilities | Comments |
|---|---|---|---|---|---|---|---|
| Nitroprusside | 3 × wt | 1 ml/hr | 1 µg/kg/min | 0.5–8.0 µg/kg/min | Prepare solution in 5% D/W only. Discard after 12 hr | Do not mix with other drugs | Protect infusion from light |
| Nitroglycerin | 3 × wt | 1 ml/hr | 1 µg/kg/min | 1–5 µg/kg/min | 5% D/W, NS, KCl, dopamine, dobutamine, epinephrine, isoproterenol | NaHCO₃, calcium, heparin, aminophylline | Give via syringe pump with non-PVC tubing |
| Paraldehyde 1 gm/ml | 2 ml | 0.5 ml/kg/hr | 20 mg/kg/hr | Same | NS | Do not mix with other drugs | Administer in glass container. Protect from light |
| Salbutamol | 3 × wt | 1 ml/hr | 1 µg/kg/min | 1–5 µg/kg/min | 5% D/W, NS, D/S, KCl | NaHCO₃, calcium, magnesium, aminophylline | |
| Tolazoline | 25 × wt | 1 ml/hr | 0.5/mg/kg/hr | 1–2 mg/kg/hr | 5% D/W, 10% D/W, NS | | Monitor for hypotension |

Key: NS = normal saline; D5NS = 5% dextrose in normal saline; LR = lactated Ringer's solution; MVI = multiple vitamin infusion; D/S = dextrose in saline; PVC = polyvinyl chloride.

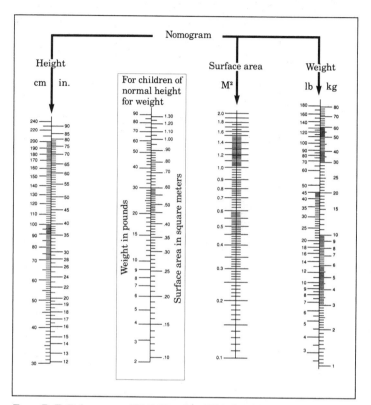

From R. E. Behrman and V. C. Vaughan III (eds.), *Nelson Textbook of Pediatrics* (13th ed.). Philadelphia: Saunders, 1987.

# Index

# Index

An italicized page number denotes a figure;
the abbreviation *t* denotes a table.